NOVEL ASPECTS OF PTHrP PHYSIOPATHOLOGY

NOVEL ASPECTS OF PTHrP PHYSIOPATHOLOGY

CLAUDIO LUPARELLO
EDITOR

Nova Biomedical Books
New York

For permission to use material from this book please contact us:
Telephone 631-231-7269; Fax 631-231-8175
Web Site: http://www.novapublishers.com

LIBRARY OF CONGRESS CATALOGING-IN-PUBLICATION DATA

Available upon request.

ISBN: 978-1-60021-857-6

Published by Nova Science Publishers, Inc. ✣ New York

CONTENTS

PREFACE

More than fifty years ago Albright hypothesized the existence of a parathyroid hormone-like factor responsible for the hypercalcemic syndrome commonly linked to malignant tumor progression. It was only in the 1980s that evidence was first produced on the isolation and characterization of the agent of such a paraneoplastic syndrome, and, differing from genuine PTH, it was denominated parathyroid hormone-related protein (PTHrP). Since then, a plethora of data on the structural and functional characterization of this protein in human and animal model systems has appeared, unveiling the participation of PTHrP in complex networks of interactions governing the differentiation and homeostasis of virtually every tissue of the body, as well as its involvement in the onset of different common pathologies. In light of its ubiquitousness and multifarious activities, and despite extensive experimentation by laboratories worldwide, a comprehensive panel of the various aspects of PTHrP physiopathology is still far from being completed. The idea of this book is to attempt to provide an appropriate ground for the discussion of modern PTHrP-related issues, and for the consideration of attentive speculation and comments on current work. It is designed to intersect all the usual lines of disciplines providing a site for presenting pertinent investigations and for discussing critical questions relevant to the entire field. Thus, this book hopes to develop a new focus and new perspectives for all those concerned with PTHrP and its pathobiology. The authors are active and busy investigators, recognized experts in their fields, but the all readily agreed to write a chapter for this audience. Contributions were prepared on the basis of scientists' own expertise and therefore, while some themes are presented in more than one chapter, every contributor has clearly added his/her own point of view and framed the topic within a specific context. This volume contains review articles that include critical discussions of controversial subjects with ample references to recent literature, and also articles incorporating original laboratory investigations and articles dealing with clinical studies. The volume opens with James F. Whitfield's plenary contribution discussing the multiple roles of the different PTHrP domains, which is followed by chapters reporting data on a variety of different model systems ranging from animal and human physiology to human pathology and cancer. In particular, Adelino Canario and coworkers begin examining structural and functional features of PTHrP in teleost fishes. PTHrP biology within the context of specific organs and tissues in mammalians and humans is reviewed by John Foley and coworkers (PTHrP and skin), John S. Torday and Virender K.

Rehan (PTHrP and lung), Pedro Esbrit and coworkers (PTHrP and kidney) and C.C. van Donkelaar (PTHrP and bone growth). The following chapter by Emanuela Maioli and coworkers is aimed at elucidating the involvement of N-terminal PTHrP in various intracellular signalling pathways, both normal and abnormal. Getting into human pathology, the opening contribution is provided by Janet Funk discussing the potential role for PTHrP in the different aspects of inflammatory responses. The final chapter, which focuses on cancer, was written by Majed S. Alokall and analyzes the general aspects of molecular targeting of PTHrP in tumors, then regulation of *PTHrP* gene expression in normal and tumor cells is reviewed by Jürgen Dittmer, and John J. Grzesiak and collaborators provide an overview of PTHrP pathobiology in various types of cancers. The last two chapters are by Fabio Caradonna and coworkers reporting on interplays between PTHrP hypermethylation and both rheumatoid arthritis and carcinogenesis, and by myself and collaborators discussing some cellular and molecular aspects of the cytotoxic effect of mid-region PTHrP on breast cancer cells. In conclusion, PTHrP has become an important area of research for almost every aspect of cell and molecular biology, so I think you will enjoy this book.

Claudio Luparello

In: Novel Aspects of PTHrP Physiopathology
Editor: Claudio Luparello, pp. 1-25
ISBN: 978-1-60021-857-6

Chapter I

PARATHYROID HORMONE-RELATED PROTEIN (PTHRP): AN ANCIENT STRING OF CYTOKINES WITH MANY KNOWN AND STILL UNKNOWN FUNCTIONS

James F. Whitfield[*]
Institute for Biological Sciences, National Research Council of Canada.

ABSTRACT

The founder of the parathyroid hormone-related protein, PTHrP, which is widely expressed throughout a mammalian body, might have appeared more than 450-500 million years ago. Unlike its 84-aminoacid cousin, PTH, it may contain 139, 141 or 173 amino acids depending on the alternative splicing of *pthrp* gene transcripts. It is neither a hormone (i.e., it is not blood borne unless the person has cancer) nor a simple autocrine or paracrine cytokine. It is a string of different cytokines each of which belongs to one of three distinct domains. It owes its name to the structural and functional resemblance of its 1-34 N-terminus in domain-1 to the endocrine parathyroid hormone's (PTH's) 1-34 N-terminus and their sharing PTHR1, the type 1 PTH receptor. But unlike PTH there are alternatively spliced *pthrp* gene transcripts for a PTHrP peptide with a NLS (nucleus-localizing sequence) between aminoacids 85 and 107 by which it can be shipped into the nucleus. Because of its NLS this PTHrP peptide is an "intracrine" instead of an autocrine / paracrine factor, which, operating independently from the PTHR1 receptor or other cell surface receptors, can bring its cytokine components to bear on gene expressions and other nuclear functions.

PTHrP components are major drivers of many different functions. For example, they are induced by mechanical stress and relax the smooth muscle cells in distended organs

[*] Correspondence concerning this article should be addressed to: James F. Whitfield, Institute for Biological Sciences, National Research Council of Canada, Building M-54, Montreal Road Campus, Ottawa, ON, Canada, K1A 0R6. E-mail: pthosteo@rogers.com; Tel: 01.613.722-2209.

such as bladder and uterus. They control endochondral bone development. The appearance of autocrine and paracrine PTHrP and the PTHR1receptor drives the proliferative shutdown that marks the start of osteoblast terminal maturation. The similarity between PTHrP's 8-11 region and endothelin-1's 6-9 region enables the PTHrP secreted by maturing osteoblasts to drive the proliferation and development of immature PTHR1-lacking osteoprogenitor cells by activating their endothelin-A receptors. Also NLS-bearing PTHrP can drive the proliferation of vascular smooth muscle cells leading to endochondral ossification of vascular atheromas They also mediate keratinocyte terminal differentiation.

But what do we know about the cytokines beyond the N-terminus of the PTHrP string? One of them is in the 67-68 region of domain-2. It drives Ca^{2+} transport from the maternal circulation through the placenta into the fetus. And it does this through yet another receptor, the putative "mid-region" receptor. Another is "osteostatin", which is in the 107-139 domain-3. This is, or contains, the highly conserved 107-111 (TRSAW) sequence. It stimulates the proliferation and maturation of osteoblastic cells; it inhibits osteoclast generation; it stimulates osteoblasts to make the angiogenic VEGF; it drives the osteogenic vascular invasion into ossifying cartilage during endochondral bone formation; and it modulates the proliferation of human and murine skin keratinocytes. And it does these at concentrations as low as 10^{-15} M via a very high-affinity receptor, the TRSAW receptor.. So there are at least three receptors for PTHrP cytokines: the thoroughly characterized PTHR1 for the N-terminal region and the "mid-region" and the TRSAW (osteostatin) receptors for the C-terminal region. Both of the latter receptors trigger Ca^{2+}surges and stimulate protein kinase C activity.. Everyone has been focusing almost exclusively on the structure and mechanism of activation of the PTHR1receptor simply because its signaling is responsible for the abilities of Lilly's USFDA-approved rhPTH-(1-34) (Forteo™) and other commercially and therapeutically promising PTHs to strongly stimulate bone growth in osteoporotic women and men. Therefore there is a lot of excitingly original work yet to be done to be done to characterize the PTHrP components and their receptors.

INTRODUCTION

"The similarities in amino acid sequences between the several mammalian parathyroid hormone-related proteins already analysed, and that of the chicken, together with the functional analysis of specific sequences have indicated that PTHrP is highly conserved and thus is likely to have a long evolutionary history."— P.M. Ingleton [2002]

The first parts of PTHrP probably appeared 450-500 million or more years ago in the emerging invertebrates and proto-vertebrates of pre-Cambrian or Cambrian oceans perhaps as Ca^{2+}-regulating neuropeptides [Hull et al., 1998, 2006]. With time, gene duplication, translocation and fusion(s) the first of the poly-functional cytokine chains appeared in the vertebrates. The nearest we can get to the earliest vertebrate PTHrP is that of saltwater fishes such as the sea bream (*Sparus aurata*) and puffer fish (*Fugu rubripes*) [reviewed by Ingleton, 2002)] The ancestor of PTHrP was probably a chain of 125 amino acids. Like the 131-173-amino acid mammalian PTHrPs, it probably had in its N-terminal "nose" a 1-34 domain which activated the ancestor of the current PTHR1 receptor that is linked to the cyclic AMP-making adenylyl cyclase. This N-terminal domain was followed by a still-functionally mysterious 38-54 domain, a nuclear transporter domain and finally a C-terminal RNA-binding domain. [Ingleton, 2002]. So early in its history PTHrP was already a collection of different functional domains separated by six dibasic-tetrabasic arginine and lysine elements five of which are "cut-here"sites tagged for endopeptidases and one of which is a "carry-me-into-the-nucleus" (NLS) tag [Ingleton, 2002; Orloff et al., 1994].

This basic structure lasted up to frogs (amphibians), but then something happened. The 38-54 domain was lost and replaced by a large and, as we shall see, functionally intriguing piece which is the ligand for a very high affinity receptor and was attached to the C-tail. This resulted in a net increase of the size of the molecule from the ancestral 125-126 amino acids to the human 139, 141 or 173 amino acids with seven instead of six multi-basic "cut-here" tags but still only one nuclear transport tag. In other words the mammalian PTHrP is a string of cytokines which could be cut out by processing proteases and then operate through their own receptors to carry out widesprerad autocrine, paracrine and intracrine functions from brain, to lungs, skin, heart, kidney, smooth muscles, placenta, bone and intestine [Clemens et al., 2001; Orloff et al., 1994; Whitfield, 2007].

As we shall see, the 1-13 part of PTHrP's N-terminal 1-34 domain is structurally and functionally homologous to PTH's 1-34 N-terminal domain. Both N-terminal peptides bind and activate the widely distributed PTHR1 receptor (i.e., the type 1 PTH/PTHrP receptor) [reviewed by Whitfield, 2007]. But they function very differently in the mammalian body. PTH is produced by parathyroid gland "chief" cells which release it in response to a falling blood Ca^{2+} concentration which causes the PTH secretion-restraining signaling from the parathyroid cell's CaSRs (Ca^{2+}-sensing receptors) to fade thereby sounding a "low-Ca^{2+}" warning. The PTH dumped into the blood in response to this warning induces kidney distal convoluted tubule cells to pick up more Ca^{2+} from the passing urine stream and reduce phosphate uptake by the proximal convoluted kidney tubule cells. And if these first-level measures don't raise the blood Ca^{2+} concentration high enough to stimulate the parathyroid cells' CaSRs, the hormone can shift to mobilizing Ca^{2+} from the huge bone stores. By contrast, a burst of expression of the PTHrP chain is part of various cell differentiation programs in virtually every organ of the body and it does not spill over into the circulation unless the person has a cancer that is continuously making and secreting large amounts of it that activate bone-resorbing osteoclasts to cause "humoral hypercalcemia of malignancy". In other words, its components normally stay where, or close to where, they are made and secreted.

Now we must stroll along the PTHrP chain that is encoded by the *pthrp* gene on human chromosome 12 and see what is known about the signaling from, and functions of, the components of the three domains (Figure 1). But before we do this it is essential to know that while the components of the PTHrP chain are variously processed and appear to be secreted there has been little interest in them following a burst of experimentation in the 1990s and the receptors that recognize them remain uncharacterized. Of course because of the current excitement over the potent bone-building 31-34-amino acid, N-terminal PTH fragments for treating osteoporosis, mending fractures and repopulating bone marrow depleted by chemotherapeutic agents, attention has been focused mainly on the PTHR1 receptor-activating domain 1 [Whitfield, 2006a,b; 2007].

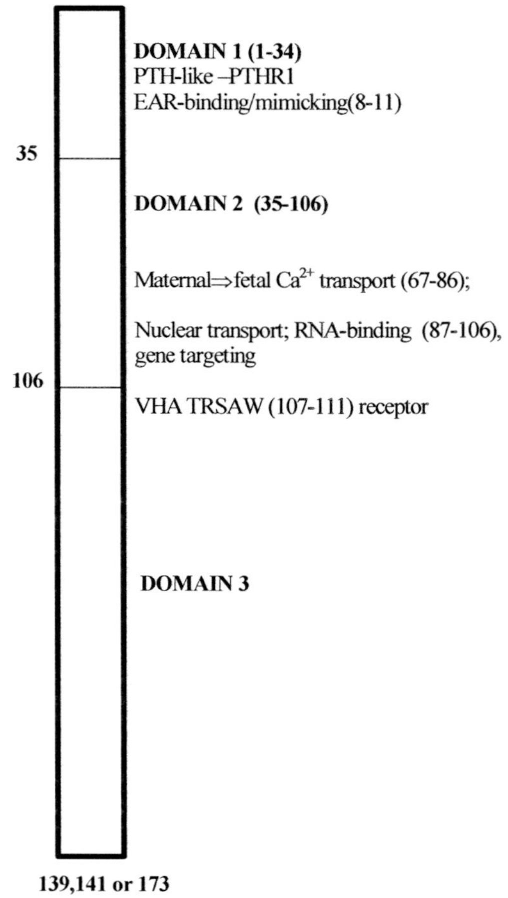

Figure 1. The three domains of PTHrP. VHA refers to the seemingly very high-affinity of the putative TRSAW receptor for the leading region of domain 3.

DOMAIN-1

A. Signals

When PTHrP's mRNA is translated into one of its constituent peptides with a so-called secretory signal sequence the peptide is directed to the Golgi apparatus where it is consigned to the secretory machinery and dumped into the medium [de Miguel et al, 2001]. But before this, the primary string of peptide "pearls" is chopped by various prohormone convertases into the individual secretory cytokine/ peptides, each with its "personal" receptor and function. One of these peptides is the N-terminal hPTHrP-(1-36) [de Miguel et al, 2001; Orloff et al., 1994; Philbrick et al., 1996; Stewart, 1996; Whitfield, 2007]. As said above, the first 13 amino acids of this peptide are 70% homologous to those of hPTH-(1-36), but the 14-36 amino acids are not although they are sterically, and therefore functionally, similar and target the same PTHR1 receptor.

Thus N-terminal 31-36- aminoacid peptides should be functionally equivalent with respect to the ability to stimulate adenylyl cyclase activity. Indeed, for example, the novel hPTHrP-(1-31)NH_2 is just as powerful a stimulator of adenylyl cyclase in ROS 17/2 rat osteoblasts as hPTH-(1-34)NH_2 [Whitfield et al.,1997].

Both N-terminal PTH and PTHrP stimulate membrane-associated PKCs (protein kinase Cs) activity [Gagnon et al., 1993; Whitfield, 2007]. D. Yang et al (2006) have found that hPTH-(1-34) has two different sites for stimulating PKCs which correspond to Janulis et al.[1993] and Jouishomme et al. [1992] 's membrane-associated PKC-only responses to picomolar PTH concentrations and both adenylyl cyclase and PKCs responses to nanonmolar PTH concentrations. Actually this two-site story began emerging when Whitfield, Isaacs et al. (2000) showed that N-terminally truncated PTH peptides, which according to Takasu et al. [1999], do *not* stimulate the PKCs-activating PLC-β1 (phospholipase β1) in HKRKB7 pig kidney cells actually stimulated membrane-associated PKC activity in these cells as well as rat kidney and bone cells provided the peptides have the 28-32 region [reviewed by Whitfield, 2007]. The story crystallized when D.Yang et al [2000] reported that when ω*t*9 murine osteoblasts were exposed to hPTH-(1-34) they of course activated adenylyl cyclase and phosphorylated and activated PKC-δ. On the other hand, [G1, R19]hPTH-(1-28) with its altered N-terminus and without the 29-34 PKC activating domain stimulated adenylyl cyclase, but not PLC or PKC-δ. However, when a 29-34 domain was attached to [G1,R19]hPTH-(1-28)'s C-tail to make [G1,R19]hPTH-(1-34), the peptide then stimulated adenylyl cyclase and PKC-δ, but it still could not stimulate PLC activity. Thus, there is a PLC-activating site (PKCs1) in the 1-20 region and a PLC-independent PKCs-activating site (PKCs2) in the 28-32 region (Figure 2). But what about N-terminal PTHrP peptides? While both PTH and PTHrP have very similar 1-20 amino acid sequences (i.e., PKCs1), they have different 28-34 regions and therefore PTHrP may not have the PKCs2 site. But Gagnon et al. [1993] have shown that despite the different primary amino acid sequence PTHrP-(28-34) can also stimulate membrane-associated PKCs activity in ROS 17/2 osteoblasts. Therefore, PTHrP's Domain 1 also has two PKCs-activating sites (Figure 2).

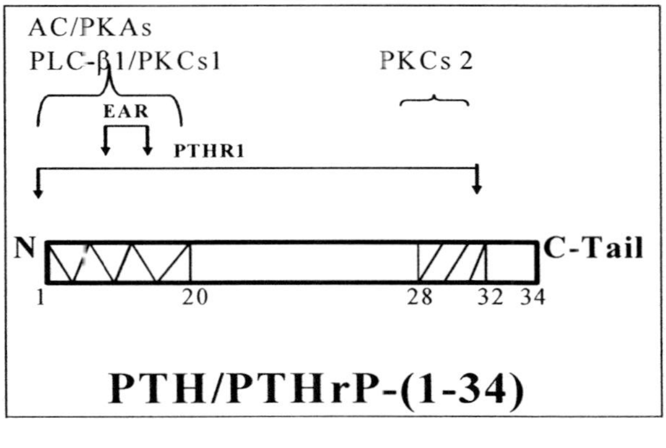

Figure 2. The functional regions of the PTHrP domain-1. Abbreviations; AC, adenylyl cyclase; EAR, Leu^8His^9-Asp^{10}-Lys^{11} endothelin-A receptor- binding sequence; PKCs, protein kinase Cs; PLCβ1, phospholipase Cβ1-activating region; PKCs1, PKCs2, PKCs-stimulating zones;PTHR1, type 1 PTH/PTHrP receptor-binding-activating region.

But there is something else lurking in Domain 1, a sub-domain which when cut out can by itself stimulate one of N-terminal PTHrP's principal functions—bone formation. PTHrP's 8-11 sequence (Leu-His-Asp-Lys) is virtually identical to endothelin-1's residues 6-9 (Leu-Met-Asp-Lys) which means that PTHrP-(8-11) can activate the endothelin A receptor [Mohammad et al., 2003] and thus stimulate adenylyl cyclase and PLC activities [Aramori and Nakanishi, 1992]. Indeed this possibility was suggested 6 and 10 years ago when Schlüter et al [1997, 2001] showed that PTHrP-(7-34) and PTHrP-(1-16) stimulate a cyclic AMP-dependent increase in rat cardiomyocyte contractile activity via endothelin A receptor. As expected from adenylyl cyclase being the initiator of bone-formation, endothelin-1 concentrations as low as 10^{-10} M can indeed stimulate both proliferation and differentiation of endothein-A receptor (EAR)-expressing osteoblastic cells in rat calvarial cell cultures [von Schroeder et al., 2003]. And stimulating the EARs on mouse calvarial cells with either endothelin-1 or PTHrP-(8-11) strongly stimulates bone formation [Mohammad et al., 2003].

B. Examples of Domain-1 Functions

i. PTHrP, Driving Osteoblast Differentiation

Bone formation, for example in response to strain or to fill cracks [reviewed by Martin, 2000; Whitfield, 2007], starts with progeny of multipotent mesenchymal stem cells—the rapidly proliferating "transit amplifying" osteoprogenitor cells (Figure 3).These cells are locked into a program consisting of a limited number growth-division cycles, the ultimate progeny of which irreversibly dismantle their cell cycle machinery and reconfigure their genomes for making bone and thus become mature osteoblasts (Figure 3).

The transition from rapidly proliferating, PTH/PTHrP-unresponsive transit amplifier to proliferatively shutdown bone makers starts with the Runx-2-induced expression of the gene encoding PTHR1, an increasing display of PTHR1s on the cell surface and expressing and constitutively secreting PTHrP to activate them [reviewed by Whitfield, 2007] (Figure 3). The cyclic AMP signals from a mature progenitor's emerging PTHR1s activated by the N-terminal PTHrP constitutively secreted by the more mature pre-osteoblasts and fully mature osteoblasts stop the cell cycling by stimulating the brief appearance of the very labile APRO1 (antiproliferation 1 or TIS21 [mouse]/BTG2[human]/ PC3 [rat]) which is what prevents the ultimate transit-amplifying progenitor from starting a new G_1 build-up to chromosome replication [reviewed by Whitfield, 2007]. This PTHrP-induced cyclic AMP surge also stimulates the expression of Smad 3 which by stopping the cytoplasmic turnover of cytoplasmic β-catenin enables the catenin to surge into the nucleus and combine with Tcf-4 to form a β-catenin•Tcf-4 complex that stimulates the expression of osteoblastic genes such as those for collagen I and alkaline phosphatase [Tobimatsu et al., 2006] (Figure 3). At the same time, the cyclic AMP surge drives Runx-2 into the nucleus which seeks out and stimulates the post-proliferative osteoblast's bone-making genes. Runx-2 also forms a complex with pRb which together with APRO1 suppresses the gene for cyclin D1 and stimulates $p21^{CIP}$ and $p27^{Kip}$ that directly inhibit the cell cycle-starting Cdk4•cyclin D1 and the replication-initiating Cdk2•cyclin E engine kinases [reviewed by Whitfield and Chakravarthy, 2001; Whitfield, 2007].

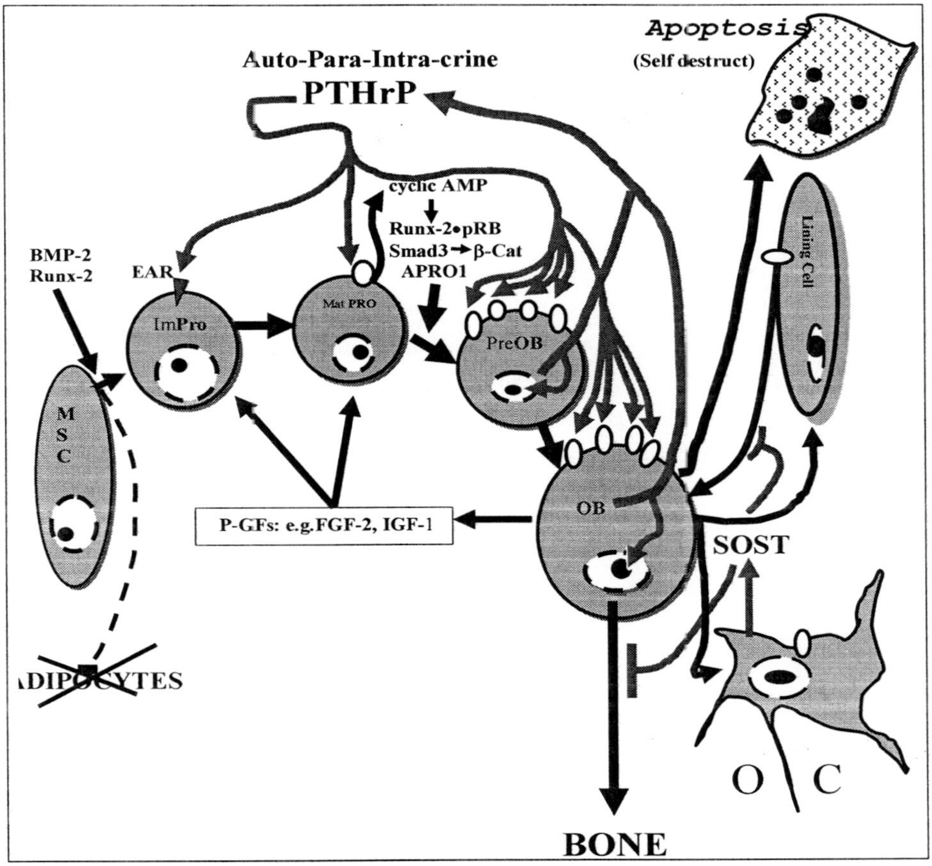

Figure 3. A model of how PTHrP drives the proliferation and maturation of osteoblasts. PTHrP, expressed by PTHR1-expressing maturing preosteoblasts and mature osteoblasts can autocrinely, paracrinely and intracrinely drive the terminal differentiation of transit-amplifying osteoprogenitors into mature bone-building osteoblasts and beyond to non-PTHrP-expressing osteoclasts and bone-lining cells. The mature osteoblasts also secrete paracrine growth factors FGF-2, IGF-1) that drive the proliferation and progression of the transit-amplifying, osteoprogenitors lacking PTHR1s towards osteoblastic maturity and beyond, Although the transit-amplifying progenitors do not yet have PTHR1 receptors, they can still be driven by PTHrP's ability to activate the endothelin-A receptor. When the bone-building is finished some osteoblasts become embedded in the new bone, shut down PTHrP expression and shut down or greatly reduce PTHR1 expression and retool themselves into osteocytes or flat bone-lining cells. It should be understood that we have no idea of which, or even whether, any constituents of the PTHrP chain other than its domain-1 is or are involved in driving bone building. Abbreviations: EAR, endothelin-A receptor; ImPro, immature progenitor (a transit-amplifier); MatPro, mature progenitor (the final transit amplifier); PreOB, preosteoblasts; OB, osteoblast; OC, osteoclast; P-GFs, paracrine growth factors; SOST, sclerostin which is produced by mature osteocytes and prevents hyper-osteogenesis by paracrinely turning off osteoblasts and preventing a possible reversion of lining cells to functioning osteoblasts; 0, PTHr1 receptors that are activated by PTHrP's domain 1.

While the PTHrP from the osteoblasts cannot stimulate the immature progenitors without PTHR1 receptors (Figure 3), the osteoblasts can stimulate them via a set paracrine factors, the "missionary" factors such as IGF-1 and FGF-2 that carry the proliferation message to them [reviewed by Whitfield, 2007]. But maybe the PTHrP from the osteoblasts stimulates them via EAR, the endothelin-A receptor (Figure 3). This seems possible because of von Schroeder et al [2003]'s report that concentrations of endothelin-1 as low as 10^{-10}M can stimulate both the proliferation and differentiation of EAR-bearing osteoblastic cells in rat calvarial cell cultures and PTHrP's 8-11 sequence (Leu-His-Asp-Lys) is virtually identical to endothelin-1's residues 6-9 (Leu-Met-Asp-Lys). Moreover, stimulating the EAR receptors on mouse calvarial cells with either endothelin-1 or PTHrP-(8-11) has been reported by Mohammad et al [2003] to strongly stimulate bone formation. Therefore when the system is set motion the expression of PTHR1 and the expression and constitutive secretion of PTHrP drives an expanding pool of osteoprogenitors. However, when enough bone has been made and the osteogenic signal has faded, most of the now unemployed osteoblasts will obligingly commit apoptotic suicide. However, a few become trapped in the new bone. These are the lucky ones who radically reduce their PTHR1 display, stop making PTHrP and live on to become strain-sensing and response-initiating osteocytes enclosed in their bony cubicles or lacunae, extending processes through canalicular tunnels to contact and form gap junctions with others. Another few will flatten out on the bone surface to become lining cells which retain the ability to reversibly retool themselves into osteoblasts in reponse to signals from their few PTHR1s when triggered by an injected PTH such as hPTHrP-(1-34) [reviewed by Whitfield, 2007] (Figure 3).

ii. PTHrP Drives Long-bone Building

The embryonic femur, for example, starts with the condensation of mesenchymal cells. The mesenchymal cells in an embryo's femur analge are initially separated by matrix and are not interested in each other. But the dispersed cells are soon "velcroized" by expressing N-cadherin, a homophilic cell-cell adhesion protein [Davies, 2005]. As the cells start sticking together, their N-cadherin expression increases and soon a roughly bone-shaped clump of cells appears. The cells in the clump start making the master cartilage-inducing transcription factor known as Sox 9 [de Crombrugghe et al., 2001; Shum and Nuckolls, 2001]. Sox 9 stimulates the expression of the genes for the cell surface components needed for chondrocytic condensation [de Crombrugghe et al., 2001]. It also causes the cells to express L-Sox 5 and 6 which are "architectural" transcription factors that reconfigure nuclear chromatin structures to enable Sox 9 and other transcription factors to turn on chondrocyte-specific genes [de Crombrugghe et al., 2001; Shum and Nuckolls, 2001]. These new chondrocytes lay out a cartilage "model" of the future femur which is surrounded by perichondrial cells. The cells at the center of this "model" stop proliferating, stop making Sox 9 and become swollen hypertrophic cells, which calcify the matrix in which they are embedded to enable it to be resorbed by osteoclasts and replaced by bone. Meanwhile the perichondrium is invaded by capillaries with osteogenic endothelin-1-secreting endothelial cells and changes from a perichondrium into a periosteum. In other words, the perichondrium spawns osteoblasts that deposit bone on the inner surface of the periosteum to make a bony collar or envelope. As this is going on, the hypertrophic cells' matrix calcification reduces their already low oxygen and nutrient supplies which causes them to commit apoptotic suicide. The calcified matrix inside the collar is removed by "chondroclasts" leaving only calcified cores and spicules in the hollowed-out center. Vascular and perivascular cells from the periosteum now invade this space. These invaders produce the marrow sinusoids, and perivascular cells spawn the first osteoblasts that layer onto the calcified cartilage cores to make the first inner bone trabeculae.

As the new bone lengthens, the cartilage layers attached to the inner surfaces of the bony epiphyses at both ends of the growing bone are reduced to thin growth plates. Now the bone has proximal and distal growth plates which contain chondrocyte stem cells that are the engines that drive the lengthening of the bone. The round, moderately sized chondrocytes at the top of a growth plate nearest the epiphysis, the stem cell niche or resting zone, are the stem cells or chondroprogenitor cells [reviewed by Whitfield, 2007].

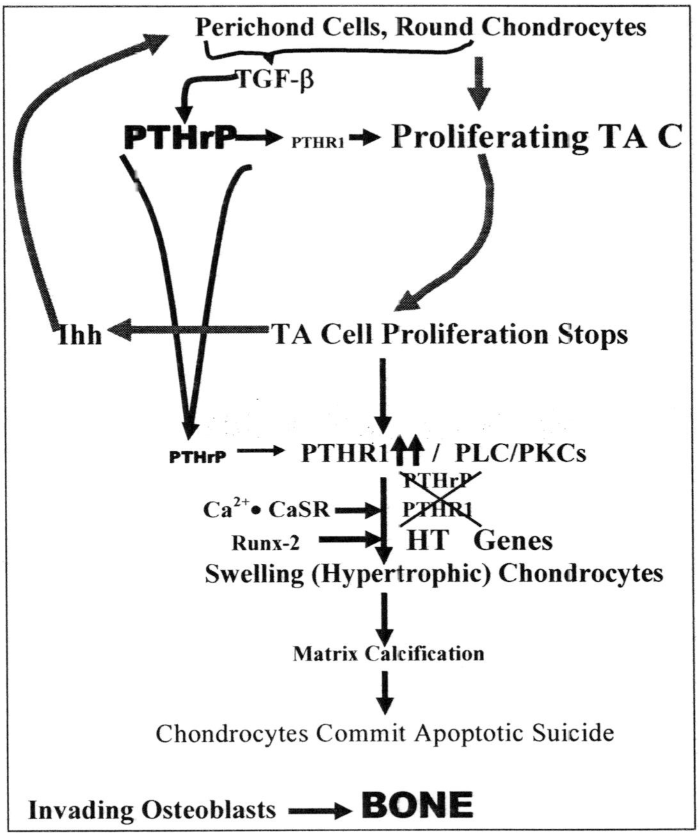

Figure 4. How PTHrP drives the growth of a bone such as the femur. Abbreviations: CaSR, Ca^{2+}-sensing receptor; HT genes, genes, the products of which drive the terminal swelling and apoptotic death of chondrocytes; Ihh, Indian hedgehog; Perichond Cells, perichondral cells; TAC, transit amplifying cells. See text for details.

When a stem cell gets a signal to start its proliferation engine and divide, one of its daughters stays in the stem cell niche while the other leaves the niche to join the parallel columns or stacks of flat or discoid transit-amplifying cells in the proliferative zone where they express the genes for aggrecan core protein, link protein and type II collagen and thus lay down the gel-like permeable matrix through which diffuse oxygen and nutrients from the overlying epiphysis [e.g., Chen, 2004].When they reach the end of the proliferative column they shut down their cell cycle machinery and stop expressing the genes for core protein, link protein and type II collagen and start expressing the gene for CMP (cartilage matrix protein) the specific marker for the cells of the prehypertrophic or maturation zone [Chen, 2004]. As maturation progresses, the Runx-2 transcription factor enters into the process, the cells switch off the CMP gene and start swelling (hypertrophying) 5- to10-fold resorbing adjacent matrix in the process, increasing their expression of alkaline phosphatase, annexin (5), BMP-6, PTHR1 receptors, type X collagen and release Ihh (Indian hedgehog) a very important player we will soon meet below [Balcerzak et al., 2003; Chen, 2004; Zuscik et al., 2002; Kronenberg, 2006] (Figure 4). The purpose of all of this activity driven in the osteoblastic direction by Runx-2 is to lay down a type X cartilaginous matrix in preparation for the calcification it needs for being attacked and removed by invading osteoclasts and ulltimately replaced by bone (Figure 4).

Finally the cells start depositing Ca^{2+}-hydroxyapatite crystals on the type X collagen matrix between the cell columns. The calcification and solidification of the cartilage drives the hypertrophied cells to apoptotic suicide by impeding the diffusion of nutrients and disposal of wastes because of the lack of extensive canalicular networks and the microvasculature that do the jobs for osteocytes locked in rigid impermeable calcified matrix of cortical bone. The dying cells release proteases which shred the cartilaginous matrix in the distal segments of the cell columns, but leave the calcified matrix between the columns alone. The resulting calcified proximal "stalactites" and distal "stalagmites" are targeted by osteoclasts and osteoblasts and become the primary proximal and distal metaphyseal trabeculae. The invasion of these osteoclasts and osteoblasts promoted by the proliferation of blood vessels with endothelial cells firing off stimulators of osteoprogenitor cell proliferation and attractants such as BMP-2, endothelin-1 and VEGF (vascular endothelial growth factor) [reviewed by Whitfield, 2007].

But what is the role of PTHrP in this process? When the proliferating discoid TA (transit-amplifying) chondrocytes stop cycling they start making Ihh which somehow moves upward or downward to start round chondroprogenitors proliferating and replenishing the discoid transit amplifiers [Kronenberg, 2006] (Figure 4). But it also stimulates the expression and secretion of PTHrP by perichondrial cells and by the round cells, possibly a least partly via mediation by TGF-β [reviewed by Kronenberg, 2006 and Whitfield, 2006] (Figure 4). The PTHrP forms a decreasing gradient from the highest at the round chondrocytes level to its lowest at the bottom of the TA discoid cell stacks at the proximal end of the developing femur or the top at the distal end (Figure 4). Above a certain level in the gradient, cyclic AMP signals from the TA cells' relatively small complement of PTHrP-activated PTHR1 receptors keep the TA cells cycling by preventing the expression of $p57^{Kip2}$ which would otherwise prematurely stop the cells cycling and by stimulating the phosphorylation of Sox 9 which increases the activity of this differentiation-restraining protein, and probably prevent the cells from committing apoptotic suicide by stimulating them to make the anti-apoptosis Bcl-2 protein and phosphorylating and inactivating the pro-apoptotic Bad and Bax proteins [Amling et al., 1997; Bellido et al, 2001; deCrombrugghe et al., 2001; Kronenberg, 2006; Shum and Nuckolls, 2001]. However, when the cells reach a point in the stack where the PTHrP gradient is below the level needed to trigger sufficient signaling from the relatively small number of PTHR1 receptors they cannot initiate another cell cycle and proliferatively shut down [Kronenberg, 2006; Whitfield, 2007]. But their proliferative shutdown triggers Ihh expression and secretion (Figure 4). This paracrine Ihh establishes a feedback loop that keeps the flow of discoid TA cells coming down from the proximal, or rising up from, the distal growth plate to replace the cells that are terminally differentiating and about to die (Figure 4).

But they also surprisingly and dramatically increase their display of PTHR1 receptors [Kronenberg, 2006] (Figure 4)! Why? Probably because the signaling intensity is a function of the receptor density especially in the presence of a lower range of PTHrP concentrations. Therefore, although the PTHrP level at this point is too low to trigger proliferation-sustaining proliferogenic signaling from the TA cells' low receptor complement, the dramatic surge of PTHR1 density would raise the signaling volume and enable the differentiation of the proliferatively shut-down cells. As noted in the Introduction, N-terminal PTHrP can trigger PLC and PKCs activities as well as adenylyl cyclase activity [reviewed by Whitfield, 2007] (Figure 1). Apparently the lower PTHrP-driven signaling from the relatively small number of PTHR1s in the cycling discoid cells favors adenylyl cyclase activation and cycling support via the GTP•Gαs transducer, but the signals from the dramatically increased number of PTHR1 receptors at the end of the proliferative zone might favor the activation of the PLC-PKCs mechanism and differentiation by the GTP•Gqα transducer [Bringhurst et al., 1993; Kronenberg, 2006].

But now the cells are in a high-Ca^{2+} zone and entering the terminal prehypertrophic and hypertrophic stages. Ca^{2+}• CaSR signals trigger internal Ca^{2+} surges that finally turn off the PTHrP gene and silence the PTHR1s [reviewed by Whitfield, 2007]. Most importantly, the final silencing of the PTHR1 receptors removes the anti-apoptosis shield and the cells become prone to committing apoptotic suicide. The PTHrP/ PTHR1 phase closes with the opening of the terminal HT (hypertrophic) phase and death of the chondrocytes and their replacement by bone-building osteoblasts [reviewed by Whitfield, 2007] (Figure 4).

iii. PTHrP and Stroke

Neurons in parts of the brain such as the parietal cortex and the striatum make PTHrP [Funk et al., 2003; Weir et al, 1990]. Neurons also have PTHR1 receptors as do the smooth muscle cells of the brain's microvasculature [Funk et al., 2003]. When parts of a "stroked" brain are deprived of blood, both the glial cells and neurons promptly respond by making and secreting the proinflammatory cytokines IL-1β and TNF-α [Liu et al., 1993,1994].These cytokines together stimulate both the endothelial cells of the original blood vessels and local glial cells to make PTHrP [Funk et al, 2001,2003]. This cytokine-PTHrP response is a clever stratagem to get more blood flowing into the ischemic regions [Funk et al., 2003; Whitfield et al., 1997]. The PTHrP from the vascular endothelial cells and associated glial cells binds to PTHR1 receptors on the vascular smooth muscle cells, stimulates a cyclic AMP surge that causes the blood vessels to dilate and the blood flow to increase.

This mechanism is illustrated by experiments reported by Funk et al [2003]. They found that blocking a rat's middle cerebral artery stimulated IL-1β and TNF-α production in the ischemic cerebral hemisphere. These cytokines increased PTHrP by the cerebral vasculature which, by dilating the blood vessels, tripled the flow of blood into the ischemic hemisphere. They also showed that when boluses of PTHrP were delivered into a lateral cerebral ventricle at the rate of 5μl/1-2 min for 30 min before and 90 min after arterial blockage, the infarct was reduced by 34%. Thus, PTHrP and its domain1-activated PTHR1 have the potential of being used to reduce stroke damage if a way could be found to get it into the brain. However, intravenous injection should deliver the peptide (e.g., hPTHrP-[1-34]) to the walls of the blood vessels in the stroke penumbra and cause the vessels to dilate. The cyclicAMP surge caused in blood vessels by PTHrP might also relieve the severe local ischemia caused by the the vasospasm triggered by the NO-binding haemoglobin in the blood released from a burst cerebral blood vessel. But this might make matters worse by dilating the ruptured blood vessel.

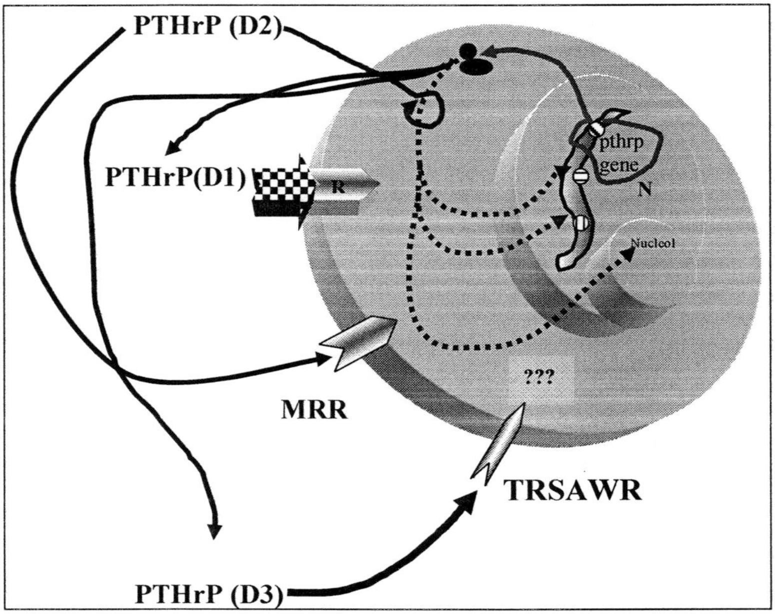

Figure 5. The various pathways that a *pthrp* gene transcript and its processed products can follow. This illustrates the extraordinary versatility of the different products this remarkable chain of cytokines. They may secreted and bind by their domain 1 (D1) to the PTHR1 receptor on the producer cell or a neighboring cell. Or The product may be a domain 2 component, the mid-region peptide, which operates either in the nucleus when attached to the NLS, or is secretd and activtes a mid-region receptor (MMR). Or the product may be be a domain 3 (D3) component which binds to a putative, very high affinity receptor (TRSAWR).

Domain-2

A. The NLS Sub-Region—PTHrP's Intracrine Tool

When the PTHrP mRNA is translated into a protein with a so-called secretory signal sequence it is directed to the Golgi apparatus then further processed and components such as domain 1 or domain 3 put into the secretory machine and secreted. But the mRNA can also be translated from an alternative translation-start site into a protein without a secretory signal sequence [Jans et al., 2003]. This protein is not fed into the secretory mechanism. Instead it binds by its NLS (nuclear localization sequence) to the nucleus-addressed cargo carrier importin-β1 to form a complex that links to a microtubular trackway where it is pulled by a dynein motor to the mouth of a nuclear envelope pore and handed over to the pore channel transport machinery [Lam et al., 1999]. The complex is then ratcheted along the pore channel by a series of dockings to so-called nucleoporins ("nups") lining the pore channel and then dumped into the nucleus where it is separated from the importin carrier when the importin binds avidly to Ran•GTP and homes onto the nucleolus where it can directly affect the nuclear functions such as the ribosome –making machinery [Fried and Kutay, 2003; Jans et al., 2003; Lam et al., 1999, 2002] (Figure 5). In doing this the nuclear PTHrP does its ancient job of coordinating the activity of the protein-making machinery with the signaling from the surface PTHR1s [Amling et al., 1997; Lam et al., 2002; Re, 2005] . However, de Miguel et al (2001) have shown that an NLS-containing peptide does *not* selectively home onto the nucleolus in all cells. Instead it distributes uniformly throughout the nuclei of rat aortic smooth muscle cells. Thus, as illustrated in Figure 5, NLS-bearing PTHrP peptides have different targeting preferences depending on the type of cell.

B. Examples of NLS-Dependent Functions

i. Stimulating Vascular Smooth Muscle Cell Proliferation

PTHrp expression by smooth muscle cells is stimulated by mechanical stretch in various organs such as arteries, bladder and uterus. It is also expressed in the walls of arteries injured by balloon angioplasty. The emerging PTHrP stimulates the vascular smooth muscle cells to proliferate at the site of injury and re-narrow and even occlude the blood vessel (restenosis). And PTHrP's domain 2 is the restenotic culprit.

When the PTHrP gene is activated in response to stretching and injury-induced factors such as proinflammatory cytokines, the secreted PTHR1-activating domain 1 products do not stimulate the initiation of cycling [Fiaschi-Taesch et al., 2006]. Indeed an effective peptide doesn't need domain 1 but it does need domain 2's NLS to carry domain 3 into the nucleus [de Miguel et al, 2001; Fiaschi-Taesch et al., 2006]. It appears that once the domain-3 (with its potent TRSAW region to be discussed further on) has been carried into the nucleus it somehow triggers the proteasomal shredding of $p27^{kip1}$ an inhibitor of the Cdk2•cyclin E cell cycle driver [Fiaschi-Taesch et al., 2006]. The upshot is a striking surge of Cdk2•cyclin E activity [Fiaschi-Taesch et al., 2006] which by hyperphosphorylating, pRb, would unleash the pRb-silenced genes for DNA replication [reviewed by Whitfield and Chakravarthy, 2001]. A possibly relevant clue to what domain 3 might do is its ability to stimulate a PKCs-mediated stimulation of cardiomyocyte protein synthesis and growth which will be discussed further on.

ii. PTHrP, a Maker of Bony Arteries

> *"The emerging view is that plaque calcification represents a meeting of bone biology with chronic plaque inflammation."*—T.M. Doherty et al (2003).

> *"...we see ossification declare itself in precisely the same manner as when an osteophyte forms on the surface of bone ...the osteophytes of the inner table of the skull*

follow the same course of development as the ossifying plates of the internal coats of the aorta and even of the veins... "—R. Virchow [1863].

Carotid and aortic ossification increases the risk of myocardial infarction, heart failure, strokes and death by impairing blood flow [Bostrom and Demer, 2000; Johnson et al., 2006; Towler et al, 2006]. For example, coronary blood flow is normally driven by the diastolic elastic recoiling of the aorta from its systolic ballooning, which, like a second heart, pumps blood into the coronary vascular network. Obviously an ossified aorta can neither balloon nor recoil [Bostrom and Demer, 2000; O'Rourke et al, 2002]. Another danger of vascular ossification is the mechanically unstable seam between the hard ossified and soft parts of an ossified plaque. These seams are sites of high shear strain which in a pulsing blood vessel tear and rupture the plaque which might block the vessel or release bits of tissue and clots that can lethally block distant blood vessels. Therefore the risk of carotid plaque rupture, for example, and the incidence of strokes and transient ischemic attacks should, and does, peak with the number of carotid plaques and seams, but then drops when the carotid's plaques fuse into a seamless stabilizing sheet of bone [reviewed by Whitfield, 2007]. As we are about to see, PTHrP and its domain 2 are major players in this deadly ossification.

Vascular ossification begins with an accumulation of low-density lipoprotein (LDL) complexes in an injured patch of arterial wall where their lipids are oxidized and their apolipoproteins are glycated [reviewed by Whitfield, 2007] (Figure 6). The modified LDLs cause endothelial cells to display molecules such as E-selectin to snare passing monocytes and T-lymphocytes which collect in the vessel wall. There the monocytes mature into macrophages which, feasting on the altered LDLs, become fat globule-packed "foam cells" (Figure 6). The foam cells produce pro-inflammatory cytokines that stimulate T-cells and, most importantly in the present context, the VSMCs.

The VSMCs in the "shoulder region"—the inflammation action center—of human carotid atherosclerotic plaques overexpress PTHrP and the PTHR1 receptor [Martin-Ventura et al., 2003]. The cyclic AMP signals from the PTHR1 receptors stimulate the VSMCs to make MCP-1 chemokine to stimulate the migration of circulating monocytes across the vascular endothelium and expand the sub-endothelial pool of foam cells [Charo and Taubman, 2004; Martin-Ventura et al, 2003] (Figure 6). Therefore, the VSMCs' overexpressed PTHrPs load the plaque's intima with proinflamatory and osteoinductive factors such as BMP-2 from the accumulating foam cells.

The *pthrp* gene transcript in a VSMC has alternative translation initiation sites, some of which if used can produce a peptide without a secretion-enabling signal sequence but has a NLS in the 86-106 region of its domain 2 [de Miguel et al., 2001; Fiaschi-Taesch et al., 2006; reviewed by Whitfield,2007] (Figure 1). This emerging full-length peptide's NLS is grabbed and shipped into the nucleus where it stimulates proliferation with its attached domain-3 which, as said above, promotes cell cycling by increasing the activity of Cdk2•cyclin E and the destruction of the $p27^{kip1}$ cycling-inhibitor [Fiaschi-Taesch et al., 2006]. These proliferating cells are potentially equivalent to the TA osteoprogenitor cells in a bone.

The conversion of the proliferating VSMCs into mature osteoblasts is driven by the BMP-2 from the cytokines-stimulated endothelial cells inducing Msx2 which stimulates Wnt secretion and ultimately the surging of β-catenin into the nucleus which stops proliferation and and stimulates a cluster of osteoblast-specific bone-building genes [reviewed by Whitfield, 2007] (Figures 3 and 6).

To summarize, only non-secretable PTHrP peptides with intact domains 2 and 3 can drive the proliferation of VSMCs and their conversion to functioning osteoblasts. Secreted PTHR1-binding PTHrPs (and injected N-terminus-intact PTHs) cannot promote VSMC proliferation and actually prevent BMP-2-driven VSMC-osteoblast conversion (Figure 6).

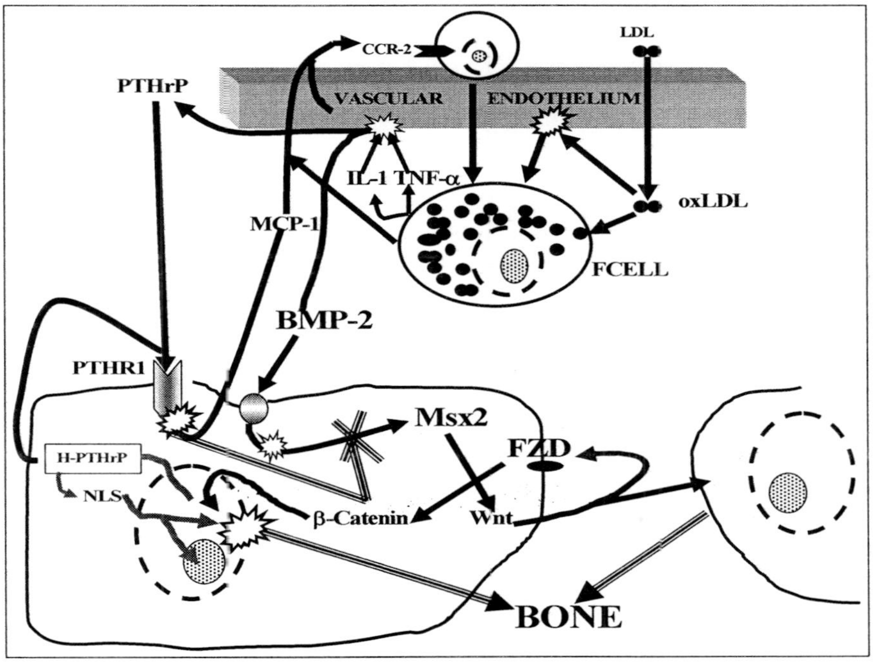

Figure 6. The involvement of PTHrP and the PTHR1 receptor in vascular ossification. Vascular bone formation starts with the influx of LDL (low-density lipoprotein) particles through the endothelium into the intima of a lesion-prone region of an arterial wall to start an inflammatory process. There the LDLs are modified by oxidation (oxLDL) and cause the endothelial cells to express surface molecules that grab passing mononuclear cells. The snared mononuclear cells are induced to move across the endothelium by diapedesis when the MCP-1 chemoattractant chemokine binds to their CCR-2 receptors. In the subendothelial intima the mononuclear cells cells transform into macrophages that feed on LDLs to become foam cells (FCELLs) which produce several cytokines, chemokines (including MCP-1) and growth factors (IL-1, TNF-α). One of the effects of the many factors from the endothelial cells and macrophages, particularly the osteogenic BMP-2, is to cause the endothelial cells to make PTHrP and the vascular smooth muscle cells to express both PTHrP and the PTHR1 receptor. The full-length PTHrP (H-PTHrP, holo PTHrP) made by the cells gets into the nucleus via its NLS (nuclear localization signal sequence). Meanwhile BMP-2 stimulates the expression of Msx2, which, in turn, activates the Wnt mechanism that is promoted by the PTHrP and stimulates bone formation by β-catenin-activation of osteoblast-specific genes. However, the cell's own secreted PTHrP, or an injected N-terminal PTHrP fragment (e.g., hPTHrP-(1-34) that cannot get into the cell nucleus because it lacks the NLS only activates the cells PTHR1s, the signals from which prevent the smooth muscle cell from becoming an osteoblast by stopping BMP-2 from stimulating Msx2 and the Wnt mechanism. But the PTHR1's cyclic AMP signaling also stimulates the expression of MCP-1 which further drives the migration of mononuclear cells into the vascular wall and with this the atheromatous process. Additional abbreviation: FZD, "frizzled", the Wnt receptor.

B. Domain-2's Mid-Region

i. Placental Ca^{2+} Pumping

PTHrP's highly conserved mid-region was the first of the functionally active post-N-terminal parts of the chain to be defined. Seventeen years ago in 1990, Care et al reported that PTHrP-(67-86)NH_2, PTHrP-(75-86)NH_2, and PTHrP-(75-84)NH_2 did something that N-terminal PTHrP fragments did not; they all rapidly stimulated the placental transport of Ca^{2+} and Mg^{2+} by fetal sheep placenta. Since PTHrP-(67-86)NH_2 was the most active of the three peptides they suggested that it was a part of the PTHrP mid-region containing the 67-86 sequence that drives the placental Ca^{2+}pump.

ii. Driving Cancer Cell Proliferation

Domain 2 indeed appears to contain another important and intensely conserved sub-domain, the 67-86 region, with its own, still uncharacterized "mid-region" receptor [Kumari et al, 2006; Orloff et al, 1996; Wu et al, 1996]. This mid-region is cut out of the nascent PTHrP chain in the Golgi apparatus or in secretory granules and then, depending on the type of cell, secreted by the regulated mechanism or by the constitutively operating mechanism [Orloff et al, 1996; Plawner et al, 1995; Soifer et al., 1992]. In SqCC/Y1 squamous carcinoma cells, the activated receptor stimulates PLC activity with the release of Ca^{2+} from internal stores [Orloff et al, 1996]. But the receptor can trigger a transient Ca^{2+}surge in breast cancer cells without activating PLCs which suggests that it operates by increasing the inward flow of external Ca^{2+} instead of mobilizing Ca^{2+} from internal stores [Kumari et al, 2006].

According to Kumari et al [2006] hPTHrP-(67-86) is unable to stimulate breast cancer cells' proliferative activity despite its ability to cause an internal Ca^{2+} surge probably via the "mid-region" receptor (Figure 5). On the other hand when the mid-region was extended to include the residues 87-101 and thus the NLS, the resulting hPTHrP-(67-101) peptide was transported into the cell nucleus and stimulated proliferation (Figure 5). In other words, activating the "mid-region" receptor was not enough to trigger proliferation. Instead the peptide had to be carried from the cytoplasm into the nucleus. This is very different from the stimulation of VSMC proliferation, which, as we have seen above, requires the NLS to carry the C-terminal domain 3 into the nucleus.

DOMAIN-3

A. TRSAW Receptor Signaling

One of the mature PTHrP molecule's invitations to endoproteases is the multibasic K(Lys)^{102} K^{103}K^{104}R(Arg)^{105} R^{106} domain (Fenton et al., 1991 a,b,; Orloff et al., 1994). This indicates that some cells might, and in fact do, cut out and secrete a peptide such as PTHrP-(107-139). Indeed Fenton et al [1991a, 1991b, 1993, 1994] have shown that this peptide or just its T(Thr)^{107}R(Arg)^{108}S(Ser)^{109}A(Ala) ^{110}W(Tryp)^{111} portion inhibits rat osteoclastic bone resorption with an incredibly low EC_{50} value of 10^{-15}M! Hence, Anna Fenton and her colleagues named it "osteostatin". This clearly indicated that this remarkable peptide operates through its own very high-affinity receptor, the TRSAW receptor [Cuthbertson et al., 1999; Whitfield, 2007], because rat osteoclasts do not display PTHR1 receptors and, as expected, PTHR1 activators such as hPTHrP-(1-34) do not affect rat osteoclast activity. Neither does it activate the putative 67-86 "mid region" receptor because hPTHrP-(1-108) also does not affect the osteoclasts [Fenton et al., 1991a]. Indeed calling the receptor the TRSAW receptor is appropriate because the EC_{50} for hPTHrP-(107-141) is much higher, 10^{-11}M, than that the 10^{-15}M for TRSAW (Fenton et al., 1991a). The extremely high affinity for this putative receptor has also been reported by Whitfield et al [1996] who found that hPTHrP-(107-111)'s EC_{50} for reducing DNA replication by primary human skin keratinocytes (as indicated by ^{3}H-thymidine uptake) was about 10^{-14}M.

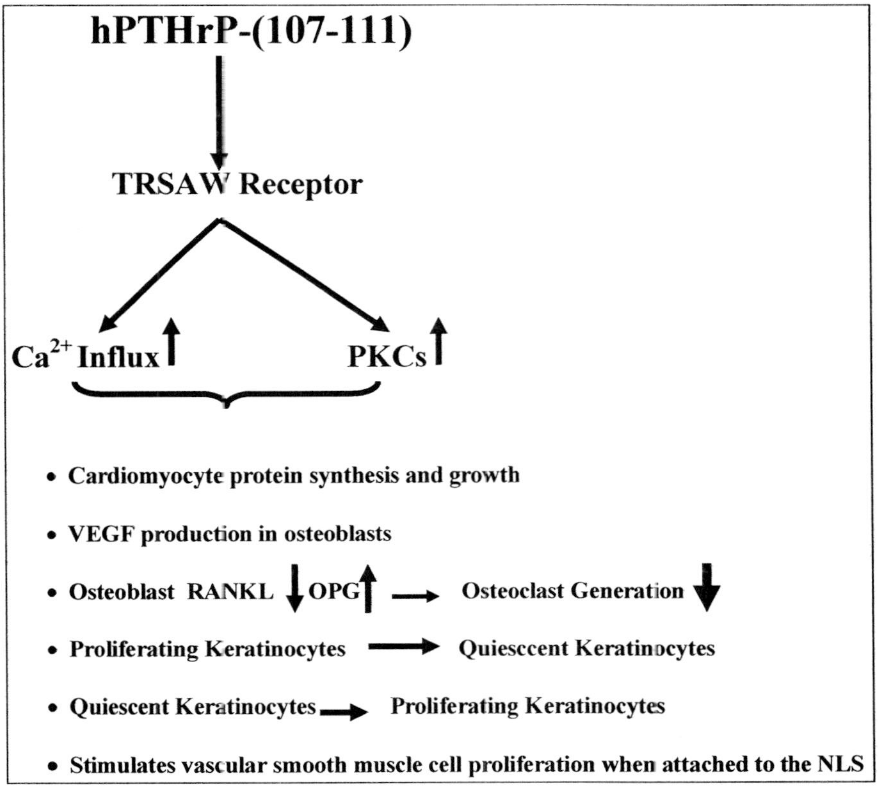

Figure 7. The signals from the putative, very high affinity TRSAW receptor and the known effects of this signaling. Abbreviations: RANKL, receptor-activator for nuclear factor-κB ligand, a stimulator of osteoclastogenesis; OPG, osteoprotegerin, an inhibitor of osteoclastogenesis.

What signals would this putative TRSAW receptor send into a cell? Various studies using inhibitors suggested that the various TRSAW receptor-induced functions are mediated by PKCs [de Gortazar et al, 2006; Esbrit et al, 2000; Schlüter et al, 1997; Valin et al., 1991,2001]. However, Gagnon et al [1993] were the first actually to show that hPTH-(107-111) actually does stimulate membrane-associated PKC activity in ROS 17/2 osteosarcoma cells. Moreover, Whitfield et al [1994] showed that hPTHrP-(107-111) and hPTHrP-(107-139) could stimulate membrane-associated PKC activity in rat spleen lymphocytes at concentrations between 10^{-15} and 10^{-8}M. They also proved that it was the TRSAW region that did the stimulating by showing that hPTHrP-(120-139) did not affect the lymphocytes'membrane-associated PKC activity. Then Whitfield et al [1996] reported that hPTH-(107-111) and hPTHrP-(107-139) strongly stimulated membrane-associated PKC activity in murine BALB/MK-2 keratinocytes within 10 minutes, but they could not activate adenylyl cyclase although the cells were equipped to do so as indicated by a strong response of their adenylyl cyclase to forskolin (Figure 7). It also appeared that the activated TRSAW receptor directly stimulated PKCs that were already resident in the cell membrane because there was no transfer of enzymes from the cytosol to the membrane as happened when the cells were stimulated by 12-O-tetradecanoyl phorbol-13-acetate (TPA). In other words, the BALB/MK-2 keratinocytes had pre-loaded inactive, TRSAW-stimulable PKCs in their membranes.

Along with this membrane action is the PKCs-independent transient opening (activation) of L-type Ca^{2+} channels induced in UMR 106 osteosarcoma cells by hPTHrP-(107-111) with an EC_{50} of 10^{-13} M [Valin et al, 2001] which could activate several mechanisms such as those driven by Ca^{2+}• calmodulin.

B. Examples of Domain-3's TRSAW-Driven Functions

i. Keratinocytes

Both the differentiation-competent keratinocytes of the murine BALB/MK-2 line and primary human keratinocytes are responsive to very low concentrations of hPTHrP-(107-111) and hPTHrP-(107-139). When EGF-driven cultures of the murine keratinocytes were exposed to 10^{-8}M hPTHrP-(107-111) for just 30 minutes they stopped replicating DNA and proliferating despite the presence of EGF for at least the next 4 or 5 days [Whitfield et al, 1996]. Similarly, exposing primary human keratinocytes to concentrations of hPTHrP-(107-111) as low as 10^{-14} or 10^{-13}M also suppressed DNA replication [Whitfield et al., 1996].This prolonged suppression of replication could have been due to the TRSAW–triggered Ca^{2+} signals (Figure 7) triggering the Ca^{2+}-driven proliferative shut-down that is part of the keratinocyte's apoptosis-like terminal differentiation program ("diffpoptosis") [Whitfield and Charavarthy, 2001; Whitfield et al, 1996].

By contrast single-daily 30-minute pulses of 10^{-8}M hPTH-(107-111) stimulated quiescent-EGF-deprived murine BALB/MK-2 keratinocytes to resume cycling without EGF [Whitfield et al., 1996]. Similarly, 10^{-11}-10^{-8}M hPTH-(107-11) could also stimulate the resumption of DNA replication by EGF-deprived primary human keratinocytes. In other words the signals from the putative TRSAW receptor can replace the cycle-driving signals from the EGF receptor.

Parenthetically, these observations should serve as a warning that the proliferative responses of cells to the TRSAW peptides is a function of their initial proliferative status and can produce opposite yet correct views of the peptides' functions.

Upon detaching from the basal lamina and entering the suprabasal spinous layer, skin keratinocytes start making PTHrP [reviewed by Whitfield and Chakravarthy, 2001; Whitfield 2007]. But the keratinocytes do not have conventional PTHR1 receptors that would enable this autocrine/paracrine PTHrP's domain-1 to stimulate adenylyl cyclase [reviewed by Whitfield and Chakravarthy, 2001]. Is it possible that as keratinocytes lift off the proliferative zone on the basal lamina they produce autocrine/paracrine PTHrP–(107-111) to stop cycling and start the terminal progression to cornified cadaver? Is it also possible that NLS-linked TRSAW operates independently from the membrane receptor to drive the diffpoptosis program?

ii. Cardiomyocytes

PTHrP is expressed in the heart and it appears its TRSAW-containing peptides could affect the cardiomyocyte structure and function Exposing rat ventricular cardiomyocytes to hPTHrP-(107-111) stimulates p42 MAP kinase, creatine kinase BB isoform, protein synthesis and cell growth without affecting contractile activity [Schlüter et al, 1997]. And the peptide operated by its ability to stimulate PKC activity as suggested by the inhibition of the responses by bisindolylmaleimide [Schlüter et al, 1997].

iii. Bone

hPTHrP-(107-111) and hPTHrP-(107-139), but not hPTHrP-(120-139), stimulate the proliferation of cultured fetal rat osteoblasts [Cornish et al,1999]. And hPTHrP-(107-111) stimulates bone nodule formation by cultured MG-63 human osteoblastic osteosarcoma cells [de Gortazar et al,2004]. Intermittent, but not continuous, exposure to 10-100 nM hPTHrP-(107-139) has more recently been shown to stimulate MG-63 human osteosarcoma cells and human trabecular bone osteoblasts via PKC to express the master osteoblast differentiation controller, Runx-2, and the osteoblast-specific alkaline phosphatase and osteocalcin. The cells also expressed VEGF (vascular endothelial growth factor) receptor 2 [de Gortazar et al, 2006]. And Esbrit et al [2000] had earlier shown that the TRSAWs can indeed stimulate osteoblast maturation and functions among which is the expression of VEGF which drives the angiogenesis needed for bone formation and microcrack repair [reviewed by Whitfield, 2007].

But theTRSAWs can also indirectly promote bone formation by attacking the bone-resorbing osteoclasts. In fact, the domain-3/TRSAW story began in 1991 with Fenton et al's report that femtomolar concentrations of hPTHrP-(107-111) and hPTHrP-(107-139) inhibited osteoclast generation and activity [Fenton et al, 1991a, 1991b]. And then Zheng et al [1994] reported that PTH-(107-111) (with an EC_{50} of about 10^{-13}M) strongly reduced osteoclast tartrate-resistant acid phosphatase secretion and stimulated the rapid cellular retraction of both human and rat osteoclasts. The deGortazar et al [2006] experiments cited above have now shown how the TRSAW peptides can operate against osteoclasts. Intermittent exposures to hPTHrP-(107-139) induce osteoblasts to express osteoprotegerin, the physiological inhibitor of osteoclastogenesis while inhibiting the expression of RANKL, the physiological promoter of osteoclast generation and function. Another example of the TRSAW's anti-osteoclast activity has been provided by Rihani-Basharat and Lewinson [1997] who showed that hPTHrP-(107-111) could stop hPTHrP-(1-34) –induced bone resorption in neonatal mice. And Cornish et al [1997] reported that single daily injections of 4 x 10^{-13}, 4 x 10^{-11} or 4 x 10^{-9} M PTHrP-(107-139) over the hemi-calvaria of adult male mice reduced osteoclast number, osteoclast perimeter, and eroded perimeter by as much as 50-70%.

Conclusion

We have now seen the many known and likely functions of the widely expressed string of cytokines that was named PTHrP because of its PTH-like ability to cause hypercalcemia in cancer patients and its PTH-like N-terminal domain-1. But despite the endoproteolytic processing of the pro-PTHrP into at least three secreted components, we still only know in any depth domain-1 and the signals from the PTHR1 receptor it shares with N-terminal PTH fragments and analogs one of which, hPTH-(1-34) (Forteo™), is now being used to treat osteoporosis [reviewed by Whitfield, 2007]. The separately acting domain-2 mid-region and a specific "mid-region" receptor for driving the placental Ca^{2+} pump and breast cancer cell proliferation remain largely uncharacterized. Finally, despite the striking indications of the impressive functional variety and potency of the TRSAW region of domain-3, an apparently very high-affinity TRSAW receptor has not yet been demonstated and characterized, although the skin keratinocyte might be a good place to look because the TRSAW is reportedly produced and secreted by human foreskin keratinocytes [K.H.Yang et al, 1994]. When we shift our focus from the currently pharmaceutically exciting N-terminus of PTH to the post-N-terminal components of this ancient string of cytokines we will certainly expand our knowledge of a physiologically significant group of signalers and perhaps find some novel drugs.

References

Amling, M., Neff, L., Tanaka, S., Inoue, D., Kuida, K., Weir, E., Philbrick, W.M., Broadus, A.E., & Baron, R. (1997). Bcl-2 lies dpwnstream of parathyroid hormone-related peptide ina signaling pathway that regulates chondrocyte maturation during skeletal development. *J. Cell. Biol. 136*, 205-213.

Aramori, I. & Nakanishi, S. (1992). Coupling of two endothelin receptor subtypes to differing signal transduction in transfected Chinese hamster ovary cells. *J. Biol. Chem. 267*, 12468-12474.

Balcerzak, M., Hamade, E., Zhang, L., Pikula, S., Azzar, G., Radisson, J., Bandorowicz-Pikula, J., & Buchet, R. (2003). The roles of annexins and alkaline phosphatase in mineralization process. *Acta Biochim. Pol. 50*, 1019-1038.

Bellido, T., Plotkin, L.I., Davis, J. (2001). Prtien kinase A-dependent phosphorylation and inactivation of he pro-apoptotic protein Bad mediates the anti-apoptotic effect of PTH on osteoblastic cells. *J. Bone Miner. Res. 16*, S203.

Bostrom, K. &Demer, L.L. (2000). Regulatory mechanisms in vascular calcification. *Crit. Rev. Eukaryotic Gene Express. 12*,151-158.

Bringhurst, F. R., Jüppner, H., Guo, J., Urena, P., Potts, J.T. Jr., Kronenberg, H. M., Abou-Samra, A. B., & Segre, G.V. (1993). Cloned, stably expressed parathyroid hormone (PTH)/PTH-related peptide receptors activate multiple messenger signals and biological responses in LLC-PK1 kidney cells. *Endocrinology 132*, 2090-2098.

Care, A. D., Abbas, S.K., Pickard, D.W., Barri, M., Drinkhill, M., Findlay J.B., White, I.R., & Caple, I.W. (1990). Stimulation of ovine placental transport of calcium and magnesium by mid-molecule fragments of human parathyroid hormone-related protein. *Exp.Physiol.74*, 605-608.

Charo, I.F. & Taubman, M.B. (20040. Chemokines in the pathogenesis of vascular diseases. *Circ. Res. 95*, 858-866.

Chen, Q. Mechanotransduction pathways in cartilage. In: Massaro, E.J., Rogers, J.M. editors. *The Skeleton*. Totowa: Humana Press; 2004; 89-98.

Clemens, T.L., Cormier, S., Eichinger, A., Endlich, K., Fiaschi-Taesch, N., Fischer, E., Friedman, P.A., et al. (2001). Parathtyroid hormone-related protein and its receptors: nuclear functions and roles in the renal and cardiovascular systems, the placental trophoblasts and the pancreatic islets. *Brit. J. Pharmacol. 134*, 1113-1136.

Cornish, J., Callon, K.E., & Nicholson, G.C. (1997). Parathyroid hormone–related protein-(107-139) inhibits bone resorption *in vivo*. *Endocrinology 138*, 1299-1304.

Coenish, J., Callon, K.E., Lin, C., Xiao, C., Moseley, J.M., & Reid, I.R. (1999). Stimulation of osteoblast proliferation by C-terminal fragments of parathyroid hormone-related protein. *J. Bone Miner. Res. 14*, 915-922.

Cuthberston, R.M., Kem, B.E., & Barden, J.A. (1999). Structure of osteostatin PTHRp[thr 107] (107-139). *Biochim. Biophys. Acta 1432*, 64-72.

Davies, J.A. *Mechanisms of Morphogenesis: The Creation of Biological Form*. Burlington, MA: Elsevier Academic Press; 2005.

Doherty, T.M., Asotra,K., Fitzpatrick, L.A., Qiao,,J.H.,Wilkin, D.J., Detrano, R.C., Dunstan, C.R., Shah, P.K., & Rajavashisth, T. B. (2003). Calcification in atherosclerosis: bone biology and chronic inflammation at the arterial crossroads. *Proc. Natl. Acad. Sci. USA 100*, 11201-11206.

de Crombrugge, B., Lefevre, V., & Nakashima, K. (2001). Regulatory mechanisms in the pathways of cartilage and bone formation. *Curr. Opin. Cell Biol. 13*, 721-727.

de Gortazar, A.R., Alonso, V., Alvarez-Arroyo, M.V., & Esbrit, P. (2006). Transient exposure to PTHrP (107-139) exerts anabolic effects through vascular endothelial growth factor receptor 2 in human osteobastic cells in vitro. *Calcif. Tissue Int. 79*, 360-369.

de Miguel, F., Fiaschi-Taesch, N., Lopez-Talavera, J.C., Takane, K.K., Massfelder, T., Helwig, J.-J., & Stewart, A.F. (2001). The C-terminal region of PTHrP, in addition to the nuclear localization signal, is essential for the stimulation of proliferation in vascular smooth muscle cells. *Endocrinology 142*, 4096-4105.

Esbrit, P., Alvarez-Arroyo, M. V., De Miguel, F., Martin, O., Martinez, M.E., & Caramelo, C. (2000). C-terminal parathyroid hormone-related protein increases vascular endothelial growth factor in human osteoblastic cells. *J. Am. Soc. Nehrol. 11*, 1085-1092.

Fenton, A.J., Kemp, B.E., Hammonds, R.G. Jr., Mitchelhill, K., Moseley J.M., Martin, T.J., & Nicholson, G.C. (1991a). A potent inhibitor of osteoclastic bone resporption within a highly conserved pentapeptide region of parathyroid hormone-related protein; PTHrP[107-111]. *Endocrinology 129*, 3424-3426.

Fenton, A.J., Kemp, B.E., Kent, G.N., Moseley, J.M., Zheng, M.H., Rowe, D.J., Britto, J.M., Martin, T.J., & Nicholson, G.C. (1991b). A carboxyl-terminal peptide from the parathyroid hormone-related protein inhibits bone resorption by osteoclasts. *Endocrinology 129*, 1762-1768.

Fenton, A. J., Martin, T.J., & Nicholson, G.C. (1993). Long-term culture of disaggregated rat osteoclasts: inhibition of bone resorption and reduction of osteoclast-like cell number by calcitonin and PTHrP[107-139]. *J. Cell. Physiol 155*, 1-7.

Fenton, A. J., Martin, T.J., & Nicholson, G.C. (1994). Carboxy-terminal parahthyroid hormone-related protein inhibits bone resorption by isolated chicken osteoblasts. *J. Bone Miner. Res. 9*, 515-519.

Fiaschi-aeschh, N., Sicari, B.M., Ubriani, K., Bigatel, T., Takane, K. K., Cozar-Castellano, I., Bisello, A., Law, B., & Stewart, A. F. (2006). Cellular mechanism through which parathyroid hormone-related protein induces proliferation in arterial smooth muscle cells: definition of an arterial smooth muscle PTHrP/p27^{kip1}pathway. *Circ. Res. 99*, 933-942.

Fried, H. & Kuttay, U. (2003). Nucleocytoplasmic transport; taking an inventory. *Cell. Mol. Life Sci. 60*, 1659-1688.

Funk, J.l., Migliati, E., Chen, G., Wei, H., Wilson, J., Downey, K. J., Mullarky, P. J.,, Coull, B.M., McDonagh, P. F., & Ritter, L. S. (2003). Parathyroidhormone –related protein induction in focal stroke: a neuroprotective vascular peptide. *Am. J. Physiol. Regula. Integr. Comp. Physiol. 284*, R1021-1030.

Gagnon, L., Jouishomme, H., Whitfield, J.F., Durkin, J.P., MacLean, S., Neugebauer, W., Willick, G., Rixon, R.H., & Chakravarthy, B. (1993). Protein kinase C-activating domains of parathyroid hormone-related protein. *J. Bone Mine. Res. 8*, 497-503.

Hull, K., Marler, R., & Harvey, S. (2006). Neual calcitropic peptides: Immunoreactive characterization in fish and invertebrates. *Neurosci. Lett. 404*,15-19.

Hull, K.L., Fathimani, K., Sharma, P., & Harvey, S. (1998). Calcitropic peptides: neurap perspectives. *Compp. Biochem. Physiol. C 119*, 389-410.

Ingleton, P.M. (2002). Parathyroid hormone-related protein in lower vertebrates. *Comp. Biochem. Physiol. B Biochem. Mol. Biol. 132*, 87-95.

Jans, D.A., Thomas, R.J., & Gillespie, M.T. (2003). Parathyroid hormone-related protein: A nucleoplasmic shuttling protein with distinct paracrine and intracrine roles. *Vitamins and Hormones 66*, 345-384.

Janulis, M., Wong, M.S., & Favus, M.J. (1993). Structurefunction requirements of parathyroid hormone for stimulation of 1,25-dihydroxyvitamin D_3 production by rat renal proximal tubules. *Endocrinology 133*, 713-719.

Johnson, R.C., Leopold, J.A., & Loscalzo, J. (2006). Vascular calcification: pathological mechanisms and clinical implications. *Circ. Res. 99*, 1044-1059.

Jouishomme, H., Whitfield, J.F., Chakravarthy, B., Durkin, J.P., Gagnon, L., Isaacs, R.J., MacLean, S., Neugebauer, W., Willick, G., & Rixon, R.H. (1992). The protein kinase-C activation domain of the parathyroid hormone. *Endocrinology 130*, 53-60.

Kronenberg, H.M. (2006). PTHrP and skeletal development. Ann. N.Y. Acad. Sci. 1068, 1-13.

Kumari, R., Roberston, J.F., & Watson, S.A. (2006). Nuclear targeting of a mid-region PTHrP fragment is necessary for stimulating growth in breast cancer cells. *Int. J. Cancer. 119*, 49-59.

Lam, M.H.C., Briggs, L.J., Wei, H., Martin, J., Gillespie, M.T., & Jans, D.A. (1999). Importin β recognizes parathyroid hormone-related protein with high affinity and mediates its nuclear import in the absence of importin α. *J. Biol. Chem. 274*, 7391-7398.

Lam, M.H.C., Thomas, R.J., Loveland, K.L., Schilders, S., Gu, M., Martin, J., Gillespie, M.T., & Jans, D.A. (2002). Nuclear transport of parathyroid hormone (PTH)-related protein is dependent on microtubules. *Mol. Endocrinol. 16*, 390-401.

Liu, T., Clark, R.K., McDonnell, P.C., Young, P.R., White, R.F., Barone, F.C., & Feuerstein, G.Z. (199$). Tumor necrosis factor-α expression in ischemic neurons. *Stroke 25*, 1481-1488.

Liu, T., McDonnell, P.C., Young, P.R., White, R.F., Siren, A.L., Hallenbeck, J.M., Barone, F.C., & Feuerstein, G.Z. (1993). Interleukin-1β mRNA expression in ischemic rat cortex. *Stroke 24*, 1746-1750.

Martin, R.B. (2000). Toward a unifying theory of bone remodeling. 26,1-6.

Martin-Ventura, J. L., Ortego, M., Esbrit, P., Hernandez-Presa, M.A., Ortega, L., & Egido, J. (2003). Possible role of parathyroid hormone–related protein asa proinflammatory cytokine in atherosclerosis. *Stroke 34*, 1783-1789.

Mohammad, K.S., Guise, T.A., & Chirgwin, J.M. (2003). PTHrP timulates new bone formation by molecular mimicry of endothelin-1. *J. Bone Miner. Res. 18*, S26.

Orloff, J.J., Ganz, M.B., Nathanson, M.H., Moyer, M.S., Kats, Y., Mitnick, M., Behal, A., Gasalla-Herraiz, J., & Isales, C.M. (1996). A midregion of parathyroid hormone-related peptide mobilizes cytosolic calcium and stimulates formation of inositol trisphosphate in a sqaumous carcinoma cell line. *Endocrinology 137*, 5376-5385.

Orloff,J. J., Reddy, D., de Papp, A.E., Yang, K. H., Soifer, N.E., & Stewart,A. F. (1994). Parathyroid hormone-related protein as a prohormone: posttranslational processing and receptor interactions. *Endocrine Rev. 15*, 40-60.

O'Rourke, M.F., Staessen, J.A., Vlachopoulos, C., Duprez, D., & Plante, G.E. (2002). Clinical applications of arterial stiffness: definitions and refernce values. *Am. J. Hypertens. 15*, 426-444.

Re, R.N. & Cook, J.L. (2005). The intracrine hypothesis: An update. *Regul. Pept. 133*, 1-9.

Philbrick, W.M., Wysolmerski, J.J., Galbraith, S., Holt, E., Orloff, J.J., Yang, K.H., Vasavada, R.C., Weir, E.C., Broadus, A.E., & Stewart, A.E. (1996). Defining the roles of parathyroid hormone-related protein in normal physiology. *Physiol. Rev. 76*, 127-173.

Plawner, L.L., Philbrick, W.M., Burtis, W.J., Broadus, A.E., & Stewart, A.E. (1995). Cell type-specific secretion of parathyroid hormone-related protein via the regulated *versus* the constitutive secretory pathway. *J. Biol. Chem. 270*, 14078-14084.

Rihani-Basharat, S. & Lewinson, D. (1997). PTHrP(107-111) inhibits in vivo resporption that was stimulated by PTHrP(1-34) when applied intermittently to neonatal mice. *Calcif. Tissue Int. 61*, 426-428.

Schlüter, K.D., Katzer, C., & Piper, H.M. (2001). AN-terminal PTHrP peptide fragment void of a PTHrP-receptor bnding domain activates cardiac ET(A) receptors. *Br. J. Pharmacol. 132*, 427-432.

Schlüter, K.D., Weber, M., & Piper, H.M. (1997). Effects of PTHrP(107-111) and PTHrP-(7-34) on adult cardiomyocytes. *J. Mol. Cell. Cardiol. 29*, 3057-3065.

Shum, L.& Nuckolls, G. (2001). The life cycle of chondrocytes in the developing skeleton. *Arthritis Res. 4*, 94-106.

Soifer, N.E., Dee, K.E., Insogna, K.L., Burtis, W.J., Matovcik, L.M., Wu, T.L., Milstone, L.M., Broadus, A.E., Philbrick, W.M., & Stewart, A.F. (1992). Parathyroid hormone-related protein. Evidence for secretion of a novel mid-region fragment by three different cell types. *J. Biol. Chem. 267*, 18236-18243.

Stewart, A.F. (1996). PTHrP(1-36) as a skeletal anabolic agent for the treatment of osteoporosis. *Bone 19*, 303-306.

Takasu, H., Gardella, T.J., Luck, M.D., Potts, J.T. Jr., & Bringhurst, F.R. (1999). Amino-terminal modifications of human parathyroid hormone (PTH) selectively alter phospholipase C signalling via the type 1 PTH receptor; implications for design of signal-specific PTH ligands. *Biochemistry 38*, 13453-13460.

Tobimatsu, T., Kaji, H., Sowa, H., Naito, J., Canaff, L., Hendy, G.N., Sugimoto, T., & Chihara, K. (2006). Parathyroid hormone increases β-catenin levels through smad-3 in mouse osteoblastic cells. *Endocrinology 147*, 2583-2590.

Towler, D.A., Shao, J.-S., Cheng, S.-L. Pingsterhaus, J.M., & Loewy, A.P. (2006). Osteogenic regulation of vascular calcification. *Ann. N.Y.Acad. Sci. 1068*, 327-333.

Valin, A., Garcia-Ocana, A., De Miguel, F., Sarasa, J.L., Esbrit, P. (1997). Antiproliferative effect of the C-terminal fragments of parathyroid homone-related protein, PTHrP-(107-111) and (107-139), on osteoblastic osteosarcoma cells. *J. Cell. Physiol. 170*, 209-215.

Valin, A., Guillen, C., & Esbrit, P. (2001). C-terminal parathyroid hormone-related protein (PTHrP) (107-139) stimulates intracellular Ca^{2+} through a receptor different from the type 1 PTH/PTHrP receptor in osteoblastic osteosaroma UMR 106 cells. *Endocrinology 142*, 2752-2759.

Virchow R. *Cellular Pathology: As Based Upon Physiological and Pathological Histology*. New York: Dover; 1863/1971.

von Schroeder, H.P., Veillette, C. J., Payandeh, J., Qureshi, A., & Heersche, J.N. (2003). Endothelin-1 promotes osteoprogenitor proliferation and differentiation in fetal rat calvarial cell cultures. *Bone 33*, 673-684.

Weir, E.C., Brines, M. L., Ikeda, K., Burtis, W. J., Broadus, A.E., & R. J. Robbins (1990. PTHrP gene is expressed in the mammalian central nervous system. *Proc. Natl. Acad. Sci. USA 87*, 108-112.

Whitfield, J.F., (2006a). Parathyroid hormone: a novel tool for treating bone marrow depletion in cancer patients caused by chemotherapeutic drugs and ionizing radiation. *Cancer Lett. 244*, 8-15.

Whitfield, J.F. (2006b). Osteoporosis-treating parathyroid hormone peptides: What are they? What do they do? How might they do it? Curr. Opin.Investig. *Drugs 7*, 349-359.

Whitfield, J.F. *Growing Bone*, Second Edition. Georgetown, TX: Landes Bioscience; 2007

Whitfield, J. F. & Chakravarthy, B. *Calcium: The Grand Master Cell Signaler*. Ottawa: NRC Research Press; 2001.

Whitfield, J.F., Isaacs, R. J., Chakravarthy, B.R., Durkin, J.P., Morley, P., Neugebauer, W., Williams, R.E., Willick, G., & Rixon, R.H. (1994), C-terminal fragments of parathyroid hormone-related protein , PTHrP-(107-111) and (107-139), and the N-terminal PTHrP-(1-40) fragment stimulate membrane-associated protein kinase C activity in rat spleen lymphocytes. *J. Cell. Physiol. 158*, 518-522.

Whitfield, J.F., Isaacs, R.J., Chakravarthy, B., MacLean, S., Morley, P., Willick, G., Divieti, P., & Bringhurst, F.R. (2001). Stimulation of proteinkinase C activity in cells expressing human parathyroid hormone receptors by C-and N-terminally truncated fragments of parathyroid hormone 1-34. *J. Bone Miner. Res. 16*, 441-447.

Whitfield, J. F., Isaacs, R. I., Jouishomme, H., MacLean, S., Chakravarthy, B. R., Morley, P., Barisoni, D., Regalia, E., & Armato, U. (1996). C-terminal fragments of parathyroid hormone-related protein, PTHrP-(107-111), stimulates membrane-associated protein kinase C activity and modulates the proliferation of human and murine skin keratinocytes. *J.Cell. Physiol. 166*, 1-11.

Whitfield, J.F., Morley, P., Ross, V., Preston, E., Soska, M., Barbier, J.-R., Isaacs, R.J., MacLean, S., Ohannessian-Barry, L., & Willick, G.E. (1997). The hypotensive action of osteogenic and non-osteogenic parathyroid hormone. *Calcif. Tissue Int. 60*, 302-308.

Whitfield, J.F., Morley, P., Willick, G. E., Ross, V., Langille,R., MacLean, S., Barbier, J.-R., Isaacs, R.J., & Ohannessian-Barry, L. (1997). Comparison of the abilities of human parathyroid hormone (1-31)NH_2 and human parathyroid hormone-related protein (1-31)NH_2 to stimulate femoral trabecular bone growth in ovariectomized rats. *Calcif. Tissue Int. 61*, 322-326.

Yang, D., Guo, J., Divieti, P., & Bringhurst, F.FR. (2005). Parathyroid hormone activates PKC-δ via a PLC-independent pathway. *Bone 38*, 485-496.

Yang, K.H., de Papp, A.E., Soifer, N.E., Dreyer, B.E., Wu, T.L., Porter, S.E., Bellatoni, M., et al. (1994). Parathyroid hormone-related protein: evidence for isoform- and tissue-specific posttranslational processing. *Biochemistry 33*, 7460-7469.

Zheng, M.H., McCaughan, H.B., Papadimitriou, J.M., Nicholoson, G.C., & Wood, D.J. (1994). Tartrate-resistant acid phosphatase activity in rat cultured osteoclasts is inhibited by a carboxyl terminal peptide (ostestatin) from parathyroid hormone-related protein. *J. Cell. Biochem. 54*, 145-153.

In: Novel Aspects of PTHrP Physiopathology
Editor: Claudio Luparello, pp. 27-40
ISBN: 978-1-60021-857-6

Chapter II

PARATHYROID HORMONE AND RELATED PEPTIDES IN FISH: FROM SEQUENCE TO FUNCTION

Adelino V.M. Canário, Juan Fuentes, Pedro M. Guerreiro and Deborah M. Power
Centre of Marine Sciences, CIMAR- Associate Laboratory, University of Algarve, Gambelas, 8005-139 Faro, Portugal.

ABSTRACT

Parathyroid hormone related protein (PTHrP) was the first member of the parathyroid family to be identified in fish. Comparative genome and protein sequence analysis reveals fundamental features preserved throughout the vertebrates and allows the understanding of function conservation and evolution. Extending the analysis at the level of tissue expression and physiology suggests that the peptide may perhaps function as an endocrine factor in teleost fishes, while a paracrine/autocrine function may be a feature in more advanced vertebrates. Recently, duplicated genes for parathyroid hormone (PTH) and PTHrP have been identified in teleost fish, as well as a novel gene encoding for a peptide, PTH-L, with hybrid characteristics. In teleosts fishes PTHrP and PTH-L appear to be involved in calcium regulation while PTH seems to have acquired other functions. The diversity of PTH peptides suggests wide ranging functions. Since all these peptides appear to share common receptors, understanding their interactions will be an important research focus.

INTRODUCTION

Studies in the 1970s identified parathyroid hormone (PTH)-like immunoreactive material in the pituitary gland of teleost fish [1]. However, over 20 years lapsed before the genes encoding parathyroid hormone related protein [PTHrP; 2,3] and PTH [4,5] were isolated from fish. The relatively long delay before these genes were cloned was most likely a consequence of their low abundance, unknown tissue distribution and in the case of PTH the absence of a parathyroid gland. Moreover, it was generally considered that as fish mostly inhabit calcium rich environments hypercalcaemic hormones, such as PTH, were unlikely to be important. The significant progress in sequencing the genomes of a number of model teleosts such as zebrafish (*Danio rerio*), fugu puffer fish (*Takifugu rubripes*) and green spotted puffer fish (*Tetraodon nigrividris*), also commonly referred to as tetraodon, greatly facilitated the identification and isolation of PTHrP and later PTH. *In silico* analysis of the fugu and tetraodon genome has recently led to the identification of multiple genes encoding PTH and PTHrP [6].

Comparative analysis of PTH and PTHrP genes with representatives of most vertebrate groups has revealed that duplicate PTH and PTHrP genes exist in fugu and tetraodon which is perhaps unsurprising taking into consideration the proposed teleost specific whole genome duplication [7-10]. The most surprising observation is the identification of a novel gene encoding a protein, PTH-L, with sequence and functional qualities hybrid between PTH and PTHrP. Considerable debate surrounds the origin of PTH/PTHrP in vertebrates and initial proposals based upon analysis of the genes in terrestrial vertebrates suggest that PTHrP localised on human chromosome 12 was more like the ancestral gene than PTH on chromosome 11. However, the availability of sequences for PTH, PTHrP and PTH-L in teleosts has permitted much more robust phylogenetic analysis and resulting tree topology suggests PTH-L is most like the ancestral gene [6]. So far it has not been possible to identify PTH-L in mammals despite extensive *in silico* analysis of their fully sequenced genomes suggesting that the gene has been lost in the lineage leading to mammals.

Characteristics of PTH, PTHrP and PTH-L Gene and Protein in Fish

The organisation of the genes for PTH and PTHrP in teleosts and their mammalian counterparts indicates they are generally well conserved [3,6]. The PTH gene in vertebrates has the simplest organisation. It is composed of 3 exons, the first contains most of the 5'UTR, the remainder is encoded together with most of the signal peptide on the second exon and the third exon encodes the remaining signal peptide, the mature protein and the 3'UTR. The PTHrP gene is more divergent in vertebrates, in teleosts the organisation is identical to PTH [3], but in chicken and mammals it contains 4 and 8 exons, respectively, and in humans through alternative promoter usage and alternative splicing several transcripts arise [4,5,11]. The gene organisation of piscine PTH-L is most like PTH [6].

The amino acid sequence identity between fish, human and chicken PTH is around 20-25%, although amino acid similarity is 40%. Comparison of the N-terminal region of PTH (1-34) reveals higher conservation and 10/24 amino acids are identical or similar [6]. Moreover, a number of amino acids crucial for interaction with the receptor and signal transduction have been highly conserved. The length of teleost PTHs is variable and in zebrafish zPTH1 and zPTH2 are 68 and 67 amino acids, respectively [5], while in pufferfish pPTHA and pPTHB are 80 and 62 amino acids [4,6,12]. PTH-L resembles PTH in length but contains the MHD motif characteristic of PTHrP. Puffer fish PTH-L shares 36% and 30% sequence similarity with pPTHA and pPTHB, but in the N-terminal (1-34) region share 58% and 52% similarity, respectively [6,12].

Mature PTHrP is longer than PTH and comparison of the amino acid sequence of piscine and mammalian PTHrP reveals low overall amino acid sequence identity (36%), although the N-terminal region (1-34) shares 60% identity. However, if similarity between piscine and mammalian PTHrP is assessed using the physicochemical nature of the amino acids, the mature protein shares 50% similarity and for the N-terminal region (1-34) this rises to 85%. Several additional regions of PTHrP are well conserved across vertebrates and correspond to the arginine rich RNA binding region (87-106 in human) and the nuclear transporter region (70-84 in human) [13,14]. Additional conserved characteristics of PTHrP from all species is the presence of basic amino acid repeats which may represent potential sites of posttranslational cleavage and the presence of consensus sequences for glycosylation and amidation [15]. In puffer fish, sea bream (*Sparus aurata*) and European flounder (*Platichthys flesus*) PTHrPA is 126, 125 and 126 amino acids, respectively, and they share 90% sequence similarity which rises to over 95% if only the N-terminal region (1-34) is considered. The recently identified pufferfish (p)PTHrPB is 161 amino acids and shares 63% sequence similarity with pPTHrPA and less than 58% similarity with tetrapod PTHrPs [6].

The tissue distribution of PTH and PTHrP in fish has recently been extensively reviewed [12] and it is clear considerable work will be required to fully characterise the localisation of the PTH/PTHrP family of genes and proteins. The absence of a parathyroid gland in fish means that PTH may be localised in a number of different tissues. For example, in zebrafish embryos 24 hours post fertilisation, *in situ* hybridisation reveals transcripts of zPTH1 in the posterior portion of the lateral line and in a discrete group of cells immediately dorsal to the notochord and by 4 days post fertilisaton (dpf) expression is restricted to the midline of the neural tube [16]. In contrast, in zebrafish embryos of a similar age zPTH2 transcript has a bilateral distribution in cells on either side of the midline. Immunohistochemical studies with zebrafish (3-4 dpf) reveals the zPTH1 protein in neuromast cells and in cells in the anterior region of the dental apparatus [16]. In juvenile pufferfish transcripts of PTH have been identified using RT-PCR in pituitary, brain, kidney, ultimobranchial gland, and spinal chord [6]. PTHrP has a widespread tissue distribution in larval and adult teleosts. In general, PTHrP protein and (or) mRNA expression are principally associated with the pituitary gland, nerve tissue, skeletal tissue and epithelia having important roles in ion exchange [reviewed by 12]). So far no reports describing the localisation of PTH-L exist.

Characterisation of PTH/PTHrP Receptors

The actions of PTH and PTHrP in target tissues are mediated by transmembrane G-protein coupled receptors that belong to the secretin receptor family. In terrestrial vertebrates two PTH receptors have been identified and are designated PTH1R and PTH2R. These receptors have different tissue distribution and affinity for the ligands [17-19]. PTH1R has similar affinity for PTH and PTHrP and is highly expressed in bone and renal tissue where it mediates the classical actions of these hormones on calcium and phosphate homeostasis. This receptor is also expressed at low levels in a range of other tissues and probably mediates local autocrine or paracrine actions of PTHrP. In contrast, PTH2R is mainly restricted to the hypothalamus and is activated by tuberoinfundibular peptide 39 (TIP39), although it also binds PTH; the physiological relevance of these interactions is still unclear [18,20,21].

Several studies exist about the evolution of the secretin family of GPCRs [22-24], although specific studies of PTH and PTHrP receptors in lower vertebrates are scarce. In teleost fish, in addition to PTH1R and PTH2R, a third receptor type has been identified, PTH3R, which appears to be a paralogue of PTH1R [25,26]. The amino acid sequence identity between PTH1R and PTH3R is only 56% in the zebrafish, and 50% in fugu, but is higher than the amino acid sequence identity (42%) between PTH3R and PTH2R within each species (Table 1). The relatively low amino acid sequence conservation between the three PTHRs suggests they have divergent functions.

Table 1. Comparisons of the amino acid sequences of the mature protein from different PTH receptors identified in vertebrates. Values are %-Identity / %-Similarity

		PTH1R				PTH2R		PTH3R		
		Fish	Frog	bird	human	fish	human	fish	frog	bird
PTH1R	fish	***								
	frog	76/85	***							
	bird	78/89	87/93	***						
	human	60/73	66/75	69/78	***					
PTH2R	fish	**49/66**	50/67	50/67	45/59	***				
	human	49/66	49/66	52/68	**44/58**	58/74	***			
PTH3R	fish	**53/67**	53/67	55/70	48/62	**42/58**	43/59	***		
	frog	52/66	**52/67**	53/67	47/61	41/57	43/58	57/79	***	
	bird	53/67	53/67	**55/68**	50/61	43/59	44/62	58/67	57/67	***

Values in bold indicate comparisons of the different receptor types in the same taxonomic group.

The N-terminal ligand binding domain of the 3 PTHRs contain conserved motifs which include six cysteine residues and N-linked glycosylation sites. Moreover, the highly conserved N-terminal amino acid sequences in teleost PTH and PTHrP [6,12] which interact with the receptors suggest they probably have overlapping receptor binding and activation profiles [see 17], although this remains to be established. Based upon sequence analysis and the results of the few functional studies that exist, it seems likely that there has been conservation of ligand binding and activation sites throughout the vertebrates [6,27].

In juvenile sea bream RT-PCR studies show that PTH1R is in general a low abundance transcript that is most highly expressed in liver and gonad and weakly expressed in skin, brain and pituitary [28]. PTH1R is also expressed in scales [29,30] and kidney (unpublished results) and both PTH1R and PTH3R are expressed in the interrenal glands where it seems to modulate PTHrP action via at least two signalling pathways [31]. PTH3R has also been detected in enterocytes [32] and region specific differences in the magnitude of PTHrP-induced calcium transport across the intestinal wall occur [33] although it remains to be determined if this is due to the number and types of receptors. In zebrafish PTH2R has been isolated from kidney and liver RNA [25,26] and subsequently identified in the developing CNS by whole-mount *in situ* hybridization [34]. There is still no information about the localisation of PTH1R and PTH3R in zebrafish.

The structure/activity profile of fish PTH1R is similar to the human receptor [18,35]. Zebrafish zPTH1R expressed in COS-7 cells binds human (h)PTH and hPTHrP with higher affinity than pPTHrPA but the two human peptides are equipotent to zPTH1 in inducing cAMP production and more potent than zPTH2 [18,25]. In contrast, zPTH1 and zPTH2 are equipotent with hPTH and hPTHrP in inducing cAMP production when bound to hPTH1R [18]. The divergent activation profile of piscine PTHs has been taken to suggest they may have distinct functions in fish.

In vitro assays with sea bream scales have shown that pPTHrPA induces PTH1R signalling through both the adenylyl cyclase (AC)-protein kinase A (PKA) and phospholipase C – protein kinase C (PLC-PKC) pathways [30]. Human and bovine (b)PTH, but not hPTHrP, also induce cAMP production in scales, but pPTH1, pPTH2, and pPTHrPB have no effect. Interestingly, pPTH-L stimulates cAMP with equal potency to pPTHrPA in scales [6] although the specific amino acids essential for receptor activation have not yet been defined. However, truncated N-terminal forms of pPTHrPA (2-34; 3-34 and 7-34) do not stimulate cAMP release in scales but do stimulate IP3 accumulation with similar potency to the intact peptide [30]. This indicates that the N-terminal amino acids are essential for AC-PKA transactivation.

Zebrafish PTH2R is activated preferentially by TIP39 and human TIP39 slightly more effective in inducing cAMP accumulation than zTIP39 [34]. Human TIP39 and hPTH have the same EC_{50} on binding to rat PTH2R and the zPTH2R, although the maximal response to hPTH is only 35% of that induced by hTIP39 [27].

The zPTH3R is apparently selective for pPTHrP rather than hPTHrP and it is equipotent with zPTH1 in stimulating cAMP accumulation [26,27]. In sea bream enterocytes PTH3R has a K_d of 2.59 nM for pufferfish [^{125}I]PTHrP(1-35Tyr^{35}) [32], which is in the same order of magnitude as zPTH1R and zPTH3R when pufferfish [^{125}I]PTHrP(1-36Tyr^{36}) is used to displace human [^{125}I]PTHrP(1-36Tyr^{36}) from transfected COS-7 cells [26]. In sea bream enterocytes and scales, there is no difference in specific binding between the intact and N-terminal truncated forms but only pPTHrP(1-34) stimulates cAMP accumulation [30,32]. However, none of the intact or truncated peptides stimulate the PLC-PKC pathway which constitutes an important difference from PTH1R.

In sea bream interrenal tissue, which expresses both PTH1R and PTH3R, pPTHrP(1-34) stimulates the production of cAMP and IP_3 and results in a dose-dependent increase in cortisol release [31]. Administration of either AC or PLC inhibitors in the presence of pPTHrP(1-34) does not affect cortisol release, although the combination of inhibitors block the stimulatory effect of pPTHrP(1-34). The preceding observations appear to suggest that convergent signalling pathways exist between the receptors and stimulation alone or in combination may elicit different functions.

In the last decade evidence has arisen suggesting receptors may exist for the C-terminus of PTH which mediate functions distinct from those attributed to the amino-terminal [for a review, see 36]. So far no specific receptors have been isolated, although ligand binding affinities and the intracellular signalling pathways activated have recently been reported [37,38]. Whether these receptors also exist in fish is entirely unknown. However, the domains responsible for receptor binding and transactivation (hPTH[Arg^{25}-Lys^{26}-Lys^{27}] and [Lys^{53}-Lys^{54}]) [37,39] are absent from piscine PTHs or PTHrPs [6,12]. It will be important to establish if receptors binding other regions of PTH and PTHrP also exist in fish.

Functional Aspects of PTH/PTHrP Proteins

PTH/PTHrP in Calcium Regulation

Functional characterisation of PTH/PTHrP peptides in lower vertebrates such as fish [40], amphibians [41] and birds [42,43] has focussed mainly on their effect on calcium transport. The source of calcium in fish differs from that of terrestrial vertebrates as hypercalcaemic endocrine factors in addition to mobilising internal stores and increasing dietary uptake may also stimulate uptake from the surrounding water. Initial experiments with sea bream larvae exposed to increasing doses of water-borne piscine PTHrPA(1-38) showed a dose-dependent increase in calcium uptake and a reduction in calcium loss which leads to an increase in available calcium [40]. In the same bioassay PTH-L is also hypercalcaemic [44].

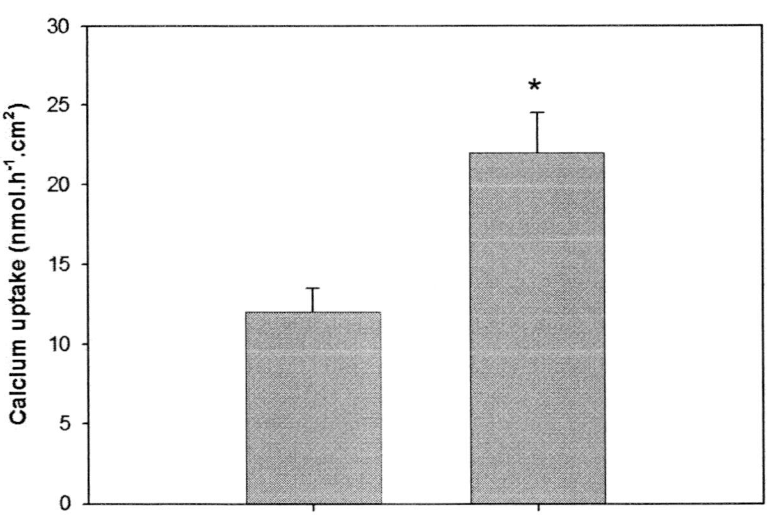

Figure 1. Total calcium in blood plasma of the killifish *(Fundulus heteroclitus)* in response to a single intra peritoneal injection of saline (control) or pPTHrP(1-34) (1μg/g body weight). Mean±SEM, n=5 for control and n=8 for pPTHrP(1-34). * denotes significantly different values ($p<0.05$) from the control (Student's t-test).

More recent evidence strongly support PTHrP as a hypercalcemic factor in teleost fish. Injection of pPTHrPA(1-34) increases plasma calcium levels in the teleosts sea bream [45] and killifish (Figure 1) Furthermore, administration of the PTH/PTHrP receptor antagonist PTHrP(7-34) suppresses hypercalcemia and hyperphosphatemia induced by estradiol-17β in sea bream [45]. This is strongly supportive of a role for PTHrP and/or related peptides in calcium and phosphate regulation and in the process of vitellogenesis, when calcium and phosphate are in high demand. A role for PTHrP in vitellogenesis was indicated by synergistic effects of E_2 and PTHrP on vitellogenin production *in vitro* by hepatocytes [46].

There is also evidence that PTHrP has a hypercalcemic role in cartilaginous fish, the presence of which presence is supported by immunochemical evidence [47]. In the sturgeon (*Acipenser nacarii*) pPTHrP(1-34) increases calcium influx and decreases calcium efflux in epithelia, and causes a rapid rise in plasma calcium only 4 hours after peptide injection [48]. It appears that calcium regulation is a general feature of this family of peptides across the vertebrates.

To date, the mechanism or combination of ion transporting mechanisms responsible for calcium transport across epithelia in fish is largely uncharacterised. However, calcitropic hormones may act on specialised cells, the chloride cells or ionocytes, which are responsible for transcellular calcium movements in fish gills [49]. The intestine may also be important in calcium uptake as it is the entry point for calcium in the diet and drinking water [50,51]. Seawater fish have high drinking rates and live in a medium containing 10-12 mmol l^{-1} calcium. The fish kidney may also be a site at which calcitrophic hormones act and this organ is important in secretion/resorption of divalent ions in seawater fish. Results from *in vitro* studies using sea bream operculum and intestine are in general agreement with results from whole body *in vivo* studies. Basolateral (but not apical) application of pPTHrPA(1-34) to sea bream intestine mounted in Ussing chambers increases calcium entry and decreases epithelial calcium efflux [33]. It seems likely that this action is brought about by PTH3R which is expressed in the enterocytes [32]. Similar results have been observed with sea bream opercular skin *in vitro* and basolateral application of pPTHrPA(1-34) enhances calcium uptake (Figure 2). The function of PTHrP on calcium handling in the fish kidney remains to be elucidated, but preliminary experiments suggest it has a calcium preserving action (authors unpublished results).

In keeping with the action of PTHrPA on calcium fluxes *in vivo* and *in vitro*, a recent study [30] with sea bream scales has shown that pPTHrP(1-34) stimulates tartrate-resistant acid phosphatase activity indicating osteoclast activity and probably calcium mobilisation. Such studies suggest that scales can act as an internal calcium store from where it is mobilised by PTHrPA thus reinforcing the notion that this peptide is hypercalcemic. The relative importance to calcium homeostasis of calcium mobilisation from scales and calcium transport across epithelia remains to be established in teleosts and may be dependent on the physiological status of the animals.

The mechanism by which PTH/PTHrP influences epithelial calcium transport has yet to be demonstrated but it is likely they act on established pathways. The pathways which influence transcellular calcium uptake in vertebrates include; i) apical calcium channels (ECAC) which are the rate limiting factor for Ca^{2+} entry into the cell, ii) Na^{+}/Ca^{2+} exchanger which regulates basolateral Ca^{2+} transport and iii) plasma membrane Ca^{2+}-ATPase which regulate Ca^{2+} movements to the extracellular fluid [52].

Studies with confluent proximal tubule cell monolayers of the chick (*Gallus domesticus*) reveal that PTH/PTHrP may influence other mechanisms. PTH stimulates short circuit current at the nanomolar level and this effect is blocked by both EIPA (an inhibitor of Na^+/H^+ exchangers) and 5-nitro-2-(3-phenylpropylamino) benzoic acid (Cl^- channel blocker). Such observations suggest PTH controls the Na^+/H^+ exchanger and Cl^- channels [53]. In addition, in primary culture monolayers of chick proximal tubules PTH inhibits Pi reabsorption probably by regulation of the Na^+-Pi cotransporter NaPi-IIa [54]. In fish and in particular the American flounder (*Pseudopleuronectes americanus*) PTHrP stimulates Pi secretion across fish proximal tubule cells in culture [55].

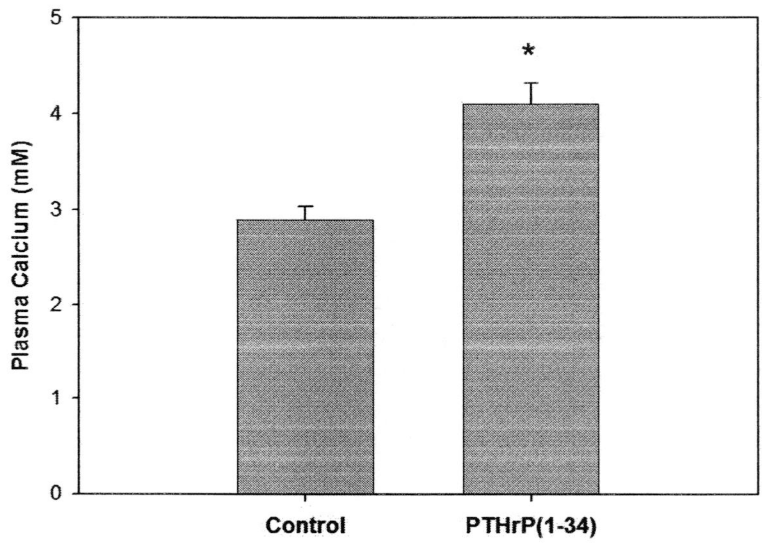

Figure 2. The effect of pPTHrP(1-34) (100ng/ml) in mucose to serose calcium flux in the opercular skin of the sea bream mounted in an Ussing chamber, before (control) and after addition of the peptide to the basolateral side. Mean±SEM, n=4. * denotes significantly different values ($p<0.05$) from the control (paired Student's t-test).

Interaction of PTH/PTHrP with other Endocrine Factors

In sea bream pPTHrP(1-34) also has a corticosteroidogenic activity on interrenal tissue *in vitro* [31] and a cross-regulatory mechanism has been shown between cortisol and PTHrP *in vivo* [56]. The physiological relevance of this relationship remains to be established. However, in mammals this interaction also occurs and glucocorticoids have been found to regulate PTHrP gene expression and secretion in a number of different experimental models including uterus and bone cells [57-60].

pPTHrP(1-34) administered to intact sea bream and tilapia, *Oreochromis mossambicus* (Figure 3) causes hypercalcemia but also reduces drinking [40]. The way in which PTHrP influence drinking has yet to be elucidated but could involve the rennin-angiotensin system (RAS) which in fish has an important role in sustaining the drinking response [50]. The interaction between the PTH/PTHrP family and RAS seems to be common to other vertebrates and the main bioactive factor, angiotensin II, regulates the expression of PTHrP and PTH1R in the kidney of rats [61,62] and modulates PTHrP expression in vascular smooth muscle cells in culture [63,64]. Further evidence for the involvement of PTH/PTHrP family in water handling comes from the inhibitory action of PTH on vasopressin- and cyclic AMP-stimulated water transport in the toad and turtle bladder [65].

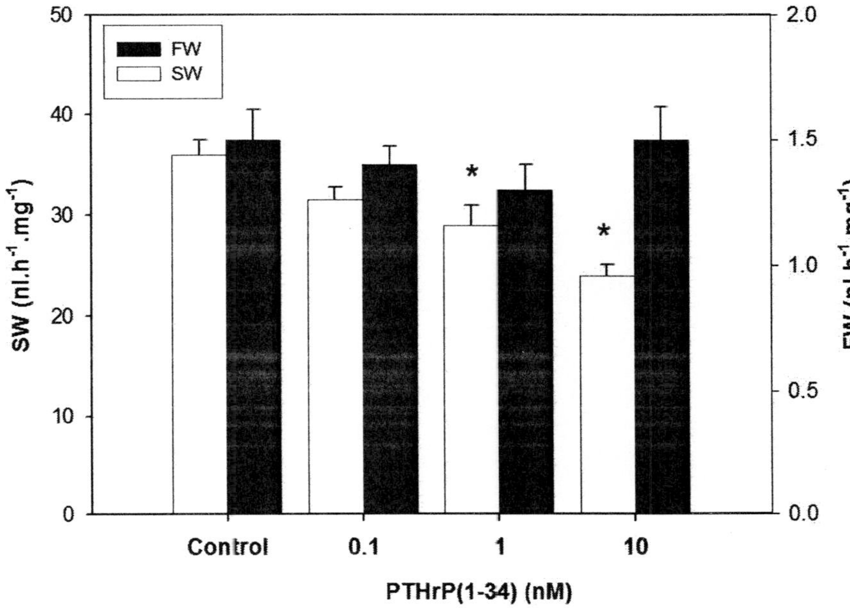

Figure 3. Drinking rate of freshwater (FW) and seawater (SW) adapted tilapia in response to increasing doses of water-borne pPTHrP(1-34). Each column represents the mean±SEM of 30-35 fish. * denotes significantly different values ($p<0.05$) from the corresponding control (One-way ANOVA).

Conclusion

Current evidence points to the PTH family of peptides, PTH, PTHrP and PTH-L, having first evolved in the vertebrate lineage. However, considering the high homology of the N-terminal region of the three peptides and their well conserved calciotropic activity an ancestral protein in invertebrates with a role in calcium metabolism cannot be ruled out. Unlike, higher vertebrates, fish do not possess a parathyroid gland and until now it has not been established if any of these factors are secreted. However, blood levels of PTHrP are relatively high suggesting that a glandular tissue, perhaps diffuse, may be present in fish. Of the three peptides, only PTHrP and PTH-L appear to be calciotropic in fish, and although they activate PTH/PTHrP receptors no specific biological effect has been found for fish PTHs. PTH-L appears to be at least as active as PTHrP in calcium transport raising the possibility of coordinated actions for these factors. The availability of peptide specific antisera and recombinant proteins should help answer some of these and other questions.

Acknowledgements

Supported by European Social Fund and National funds under Portuguese National Science Foundation (FCT) projects POCTI/CVT/48946/ 2002 and POCTI/CVT/ /61052/2004. PMG is funded by the Ministry of Science, Portugal through fellowship SFRH/BPD/9464/02.

References

[1] Parsons J; Gray D; Rafferty B; Zanelli J. Evidence for a hypercalcaemic factor in the fish pituitary immunologically related to mammalian parathyroid hormone. In: Copp D; Talmage R, eds. *Endocrinology of Calcium Metabolism*. Amsterdam: Elsevier 1978:111-14.

[2] Flanagan JA; Power DM; Bendell LA; Guerreiro PM; Fuentes J; Clark MS; Canario AV; Danks JA; Brown BL; Ingleton PM. Cloning of the cDNA for sea bream (*Sparus aurata*) parathyroid hormone-related protein. *Gen Comp Endocrinol*, 2000, 118, 373-82.

[3] Power DM; Ingleton PM; Flanagan J; Canario AV; Danks J; Elgar G; Clark MS. Genomic structure and expression of parathyroid hormone-related protein gene (PTHrP) in a teleost, *Fugu rubripes*. *Gene*, 2000, 250, 67-76.

[4] Danks JA; Ho PM; Notini AJ; Katsis F; Hoffmann P; Kemp BE; Martin TJ; Zajac JD. Identification of a parathyroid hormone in the fish *Fugu rubripes*. *J Bone Miner Res*, 2003, 18, 1326-31.

[5] Gensure RC; Ponugoti B; Gunes Y; Papasani MR; Lanske B; Bastepe M; Rubin DA; Juppner H. Identification and characterization of two parathyroid hormone-like molecules in zebrafish. *Endocrinology*, 2004, 145, 1634-9.

[6] Canario AVM; Rotllant J; Fuentes J; Guerreiro PM; Teodosio HR; Power DM; Clark MS. Novel bioactive parathyroid hormone and related peptides in teleost fish. *FEBS Lett*, 2006, 580, 291-99.

[7] Meyer A; Van de Peer Y. From 2R to 3R: evidence for a fish-specific genome duplication (FSGD). *Bioessays*, 2005, 27, 937-45.

[8] Taylor JS; Braasch I; Frickey T; Meyer A; de Peer YV. Genome duplication, a trait shared by 22,000 species of ray-finned fish. *Genome Res*, 2003, 13, 382-90.

[9] Taylor JS; Van de Peer Y; Meyer A. Revisiting recent challenges to the ancient fish-specific genome duplication hypothesis. *Curr Biol*, 2001, 11, R1005-R07.

[10] Wittbrodt J; Meyer A; Schartl M. More genes in fish? *Bioessays*, 1998, 20, 511-15.

[11] Ingleton PM. Parathyroid hormone-related protein in lower vertebrates. *Comp Biochem Physiol B*, 2002, 132, 87-95.

[12] Guerreiro PM; Renfro JL; Power DM; Canario AV. The parathyroid hormone family of peptides: structure, tissue distribution, regulation, and potential functional roles in calcium and phosphate balance in fish. *Am J Physiol Regul Integr Comp Physiol*, 2007, 292, R679-96.

[13] Aarts MM; Levy D; He B; Stregger S; Chen T; Richard S; Henderson JE. Parathyroid hormone-related protein interacts with RNA. *J Biol Chem*, 1999, 274, 4832-8.

[14] Aarts MM; Rix A; Guo J; Bringhurst R; Henderson JE. The nucleolar targeting signal (NTS) of parathyroid hormone related protein mediates endocytosis and nucleolar translocation. *J Bone Miner Res*, 1999, 14, 1493-503.

[15] Orloff JJ; Reddy D; de Papp AE; Yang KH; Soifer NE; Stewart AF. Parathyroid hormone-related protein as a prohormone: posttranslational processing and receptor interactions. *Endocr Rev*, 1994, 15, 40-60.

[16] Hogan BM; Danks JA; Layton JE; Hall NE; Heath JK; Lieschke GJ. Duplicate zebrafish *pth* genes are expressed along the lateral line and in the central nervous system during embryogenesis. *Endocrinology*, 2005, 146, 547-51.

[17] Gardella TJ; Juppner H. Molecular properties of the PTH/PTHrP receptor. *Trends Endocrinol Metab*, 2001, 12, 210-7.

[18] Gensure RC; Gardella TJ; Juppner H. Parathyroid hormone and parathyroid hormone-related peptide, and their receptors. *Biochem Biophys Res Commun*, 2005, 328, 666-78.

[19] Mannstadt M; Juppner H; Gardella TJ. Receptors for PTH and PTHrP: their biological importance and functional properties. *Am J Physiol*, 1999, 277, F665-75.

[20] Clemens TL; Cormier S; Eichinger A; Endlich K; Fiaschi-Taesch N; Fischer E; Friedman PA; Karaplis AC; Massfelder T; Rossert J; Schluter KD; Silve C; Stewart AF; Takane K; Helwig JJ. Parathyroid hormone-related protein and its receptors: nuclear functions and roles in the renal and cardiovascular systems, the placental trophoblasts and the pancreatic islets. *Br J Pharmacol*, 2001, 134, 1113-36.

[21] Usdin TB. Evidence for a parathyroid hormone-2 receptor selective ligand in the hypothalamus. *Endocrinology*, 1997, 138, 831-4.

[22] Cardoso JCR; Pinto VC; Vieira FA; Clark MS; Power DM. Evolution of secretin family GPCR members in the metazoa. *BMC Evol Biol*, 2006, 6.

[23] Cardoso JC; Clark MS; Viera FA; Bridge PD; Gilles A; Power DM. The secretin G-protein-coupled receptor family: teleost receptors. *J Mol Endocrinol*, 2005, 34, 753-65.

[24] Fredriksson R; Lagerstrom MC; Lundin LG; Schioth HB. The G-protein-coupled receptors in the human genome form five main families. Phylogenetic analysis, paralogon groups, and fingerprints. *Mol Pharmacol*, 2003, 63, 1256-72.

[25] Rubin DA; Hellman P; Zon LI; Lobb CJ; Bergwitz C; Juppner H. A G protein-coupled receptor from zebrafish is activated by human parathyroid hormone and not by human or teleost parathyroid hormone-related peptide. Implications for the evolutionary conservation of calcium-regulating peptide hormones. *J Biol Chem*, 1999, 274, 23035-42.

[26] Rubin DA; Juppner H. Zebrafish express the common parathyroid hormone/parathyroid hormone-related peptide receptor (PTH1R) and a novel receptor (PTH3R) that is preferentially activated by mammalian and fugufish parathyroid hormone-related peptide. *J Biol Chem*, 1999, 274, 28185-90.

[27] Hoare SR; Rubin DA; Juppner H; Usdin TB. Evaluating the ligand specificity of zebrafish parathyroid hormone (PTH) receptors: comparison of PTH, PTH-related protein, and tuberoinfundibular peptide of 39 residues. *Endocrinology*, 2000, 141, 3080-6.

[28] Hang XM; Power D; Flik G; Balment RJ. Measurement of PTHrP, PTHR1, and CaSR expression levels in tissues of sea bream (*Sparus aurata*) using quantitative PCR. *Ann N Y Acad Sci*, 2005, 1040, 340-4.

[29] Redruello B; Estêvão MD; Rotllant J; Guerreiro PM; Anjos LI; Canario AV; Power DM. Isolation and characterization of piscine osteonectin and downregulation of its expression by PTH-related protein. *J Bone Miner Res*, 2005, 20, 682-92.

[30] Rotllant J; Redruello B; Guerreiro PM; Fernandes H; Canario AVM; Power DM. Calcium mobilization from fish scales is mediated by parathyroid hormone-related protein via the parathyroid hormone type 1 receptor. *Regul Pept*, 2005, 132, 33-40.

[31] Rotllant J; Guerreiro PM; Anjos L; Redruello B; Canario AV; Power DM. Stimulation of cortisol release by the N terminus of teleost parathyroid hormone-related protein in interrenal cells *in vitro*. *Endocrinology*, 2005, 146, 71-6.

[32] Rotllant J; Guerreiro PM; Redruello B; Fernandes H; Apolónia L; Anjos L; Canario AVM; Power DM. Ligand binding and signalling pathways of PTH receptors in sea bream (*Sparus auratus*) enterocytes. *Cell Tissue Res*, 2006, 323, 333-41.

[33] Fuentes J; Figueiredo J; Power DM; Canario AVM. Parathyroid hormone-related protein regulates intestinal calcium transport in the sea bream (*Sparus auratus*). *Am J Physiol Regul Integr Comp Physiol*, 2006, 291, R1499-R506.

[34] Papasani MR; Gensure RC; Yan YL; Gunes Y; Postlethwait JH; Ponugoti B; John MR; Juppner H; Rubin DA. Identification and characterization of the zebrafish and fugu genes encoding tuberoinfundibular peptide 39. *Endocrinology*, 2004, 145, 5294-304.

[35] Juppner H. Receptors for parathyroid hormone and parathyroid hormone-related peptide: exploration of their biological importance. *Bone*, 1999, 25, 87-90.

[36] Murray TM; Rao LG; Divieti P; Bringhurst FR. Parathyroid hormone secretion and action: Evidence for discrete receptors for the carboxyl-terminal region and related biological actions of carboxyl-terminal ligands. *Endocr Rev*, 2005, 26, 78-113.

[37] Banerjee S; Selim H; Suliman G; Geller AI; Juppner H; Bringhurst FR; Divieti P. Synthesis and characterization of novel biotinylated carboxyl-terminal parathyroid hormone peptides that specifically crosslink to the CPTH-receptor. *Peptides*, 2006, 27, 3352-62.

[38] Selim AA; Mahon M; Juppner H; Bringhurst FR; Divieti P. Role of calcium channels in carboxyl-terminal parathyroid hormone receptor signaling. *Am J Physiol Cell Physiol*, 2006, 291, C114-C21.

[39] Divieti P; Geller AI; Suliman G; Juppner H; Bringhurst FR. Receptors specific for the carboxyl-terminal region of parathyroid hormone on bone-derived cells: Determinants of ligand binding and bioactivity. *Endocrinology*, 2005, 146, 1863-70.

[40] Guerreiro PM; Fuentes J; Power DM; Ingleton PM; Flik G; Canario AVM. Parathyroid hormone-related protein: a calcium regulatory factor in sea bream (*Sparus aurata* L.) larvae. *Am J Physiol Regul Integr Comp Physiol*, 2001, 281, R855-R60.

[41] Stiffler DF; Yee JC; Tefft JD. Responses of frog skin, Rana pipiens, calcium ion transport to parathyroid hormone, calcitonin, and vitamin D3. *Gen Comp Endocrinol*, 1998, 112, 191-9.

[42] Zhou LX; Nemere I; Norman AW. A parathyroid-related peptide induces transcaltachia (the rapid, hormonal stimulation of intestinal Ca^{2+} transport). *Biochem Biophys Res Commun*, 1992, 186, 69-73.

[43] Packard MJ; Clark NB; Erickson JP. The effect of calcium-regulating hormones on transport of calcium across the chorioallantoic membrane of the chicken embryo. *Comp Biochem Physiol A-Mol Integr Physiol*, 1998, 119, 547-52.

[44] Canario AVM; Rotllant J; Fuentes J; Guerreiro PM; Teodosio HR; Power DM; Clark MS. Novel bioactive parathyroid hormone and related peptides in teleost fish. *Febs Letters*, 2006, 580, 291-99.

[45] Fuentes J; Guerreiro PM; Modesto T; Rotllant J; Canario AVM; Power DM. A PTH/PTHrP receptor antagonist blocks the hypercalcemic and hyperphosphatemic response to estradiol-17β. *Am J Physiol Regul Integr Comp Physiol*, 2007, 293, R956 - R960.

[46] Bevelander GS; Hang X; Abbink W; Spanings T; Canario AVM; Flik G. PTHrP potentiating estradiol-induced vitellogenesis in sea bream (*Sparus auratus*, L.). *Gen Comp Endocrinol*, 2006, 149, 159-65.

[47] Trivett MK; Walker TI; Macmillan DL; Clement JG; Martin TJ; Danks JA. Parathyroid hormone-related protein (PTHrP) production sites in elasmobranchs. *J Anat*, 2002, 201, 41-52.

[48] Fuentes J; Haond C; Guerreiro PM; Silva N; Power DM; Canario AVM. Regulation of calcium balance in the sturgeon (*Acipenser naccarii*): a role for PTHrP. *Am J Physiol Regul Integr Comp Physiol*, 2007, 293, R884 - R893.

[49] Perry SF. The chloride cell: Structure and function in the gills of freshwater fishes. *Annu Rev Physiol*, 1997, 59, 325-47.

[50] Fuentes J, Eddy, F.B. Drinking in freshwater, euryhaline and marine teleosts. In *"Ionic Regulation in Animals"* N Hazon, FB Eddy and G Flik (Eds) Springer-Verlag ISBN 3-540-61083-9 pp135-149, 1997.

[51] Abbink W; Bevelander GS; Rotllant J; Canario AVM; Flik G. Calcium handling in *Sparus auratus*: effects of water and dietary calcium levels on mineral composition, cortisol and PTHrP levels. *J Exp Biol*, 2004, 207, 4077-84.

[52] Hoenderop JGJ; Nilius B; Bindels RJM. Calcium absorption across epithelia. *Physiol Rev*, 2005, 85, 373-422.

[53] Laverty G; McWilliams C; Sheldon A; Arnason SS. PTH stimulates a Cl^--dependent and EIPA-sensitive current in chick proximal tubule cells in culture. *Am J Physiol Renal*, 2003, 284, F987-F95.

[54] Dudas PL; Villalobos AR; Gacek-Sutterlin G; Laverty G; Renfro JL. Regulation of transepithelial phosphate transport by PTH in chicken proximal tubule epithelium. *Am J Physiol Regul Integr Comp Physiol*, 2002, 282, R139-R46.

[55] Guerreiro PM; Canario AVM; Power DM; Renfro JL. Parathyroid hormone (PTH)-related protein stimulates Pi secretion across fish proximal tubule cells. *J Exp Zool Part A*, 2006, 305A, 130.

[56] Guerreiro PM; Rotllant J; Fuentes J; Power DM; Canario AVM. Cortisol and parathyroid hormone-related peptide are reciprocally modulated by negative feedback. *Gen Comp Endocrinol*, 2006, 148, 227-35.

[57] Schilling T; Pecherstorfer M; Blind E; Kohl B; Wagner H; Ziegler R; Raue F. Glucocorticoids decrease the production of parathyroid hormone-related protein *in vitro* but not *in vivo* in the Walker carcinosarcoma 256 rat model. *Bone*, 1996, 18, 315-19.

[58] Kasono K; Isozaki O; Sato K; Sato Y; Shizume K; Ohsumi K; Demura H. Effects of glucocorticoids and calcitonin on parathyroid hormone-related protein (PTHrP) gene expression and PTHrP release in human cancer cells causing humoral hypercalcemia. *Jpn J Cancer Res*, 1991, 82, 1008-14.

[59] Paspaliaris V; Petersen DN; Thiede MA. Steroid regulation of parathyroid hormone-related protein expression and action in the rat uterus. *J Steroid Biochem Mol Biol* 1995, 53 259–65.

[60] Walsh CA; Birch MA; Fraser WD; Lawton R; Dorgan J; Walsh S; Sansom D; Beresford JN; Gallagher JA. Expression and secretion of parathyroid hormone-related protein by human bone-derived cells *in vitro*: effects of glucocorticoids. *J Bone Miner Res*, 1995, 10, 17-25.

[61] Welsch S; Schordan E; Coquard C; Massfelder T; Fiaschi-Taesch N; Helwig JJ; Barthelmebs M. Abnormal renovascular parathyroid hormone-1 receptor in hypertension: Primary defect or secondary to angiotensin II type 1 receptor activation? *Endocrinology*, 2006, 147, 4384-91.

[62] Lorenzo O; Ruiz-Ortega M; Esbrit P; Ruperez M; Ortega A; Santos S; Blanco J; Ortega L; Egido J. Angiotensin II increases parathyroid hormone-related protein (PTHrP) and the type 1 PTH/PTHrP receptor in the kidney.. *J Am Soc Nephrol*, 2002, 13, 1595-607.

[63] Pirola CJ; Wang HM; Kamyar A; Wu S; Enomoto H; Sharifi B; Forrester JS; Clemens TL; Fagin JA. Angiotensin II regulates parathyroid hormone-related protein expression in cultured rat aortic smooth muscle cells through transcriptional and post-transcriptional mechanisms. *J Biol Chem*, 1993, 268, 1987-94.

[64] Noda M; Katoh T; Takuwa N; Kumada M; Kurokawa K; Takuwa Y. Synergistic stimulation of parathyroid hormone-related peptide gene expression by mechanical stretch and angiotensin II in rat aortic smooth muscle cells. *J Biol Chem*, 1994, 269, 17911-7.

[65] Sabatini S; Kurtzman NA. Effect of parathyroid-hormone on transport by toad and turtle bladder. *Am J Physiol*, 1987, 252, R63-R68.

In: Novel Aspects of PTHrP Physiopathology
Editor: Claudio Luparello, pp. 41-71
ISBN: 978-1-60021-857-6

Chapter III

PTHrP Function in the Skin: Probing Beneath the Surface

John Foley[1,2,3,*], A. Godwin Diamond[1], Ryan M. Gonterman[1], Carlos D. Offutt[1] and Yong-Mee Cho[1]

[1]Medical Sciences, Indiana University School of Medicine, Bloomington, IN 47405, USA;

[2]Department of Dermatology, Indiana University School of Medicine, Indianapolis, IN 46202, USA;

[3]Institute for Molecular Biology, Indiana University, Bloomington, IN 47405, USA.

Abstract

In 1986, Arthur Broadus and Andy Stewart's group reported that cultured primary epidermal keratinocytes were the first non-tumor derived cell type to produce substantial parathyroid hormone-like factor. This finding coupled with the completion of sequencing of parathyroid hormone-like/related protein/peptide prompted speculation that this calcitropic factor was a central modulator of proliferation and differentiation of the epidermis. In the early 90s, this concept was supported by the studies with cultured keratinocytes. However, by the millennium, a substantial revision of the peptide's physiological function within the integument has occurred. At this point, the most well established function for PTHrP is that of a classical developmental inductive factor required to establish the specialized epidermis of the nipple. Also, accumulating evidence indicates that PTHrP may be a regulator of the hair cycle. Surprisingly, very little evidence supports the concept that PTHrP regulates the proliferation and differentiation within the undisturbed epidermis. This review details the cellular and molecular mechanism of PTHrP function within the skin by integrating data from gene expression reports, cell culture studies, as well as knockout and transgenic mouse phenotypes. In

* Correspondence concerning this article should be addressed to: John Foley, Associate Professor Anatomy & Cell biology and Dermatology Medical Sciences, Indiana University School of Medicine, Jordan Hall Bloomington, IN 47405. Phone: 812-855-3189; E-mail: jgfoley@indiana.edu.

addition, some of the short-comings of past experimental approaches are discussed and consideration is given to how this has colored the field. Finally, other potential integument related physiological roles for the protein are discussed as well as its influence on skin pathologies contemplated.

Keywords: PTHrP, PTH/PTHrP receptor, gene expression, nipple, hair cycle, angiogenesis, skin diseases and psoriasis.

Introduction to the Cellular Components of the Skin

The skin is the largest organ of the body consisting of two main layers. It provides protection against ultraviolet light as well as a barrier against mechanical, chemical, and thermal insults. The surface is relatively impermeable which prevents dehydration and acts as a physical barrier against invasion by microorganisms (Chu *et al.*, 2003; Elias *et al.*, 2003). The skin also has specialized epithelial appendages such as hair follicles, sebaceous glands, nails, sweat glands and mammary glands which arise as down growths of the epidermis into the dermis during embryological development (Chu *et al.*, 2003).

The epidermis is a layer of stratified squamous epithelium that rests on top of a basement membrane, which separates it and its appendages from the underlying mesenchymally derived dermis. The epidermis appears to be maintained by stem cells of the deepest epidermal layer, the stratum basale. Most cells within the basal layer are the rapidly dividing progeny of stem cells (Jones *et al.*, 1995). These transiently amplifying cells undergo a limited number of divisions before they withdraw from the cell cycle, commit to terminal differentiation, detach from the basement membrane and begin there journey towards the surface of the skin (Barrandon and Green, 1987). The next layer is known as the stratum spinosum and is one cell thick in mice and several cells thick in human skin. These cells contain a weblike system of high molecular weight keratins that span their cytosol to attach to desmosomes (Elias *et al.*, 2003). The keratinocytes of this layer begin to flatten and appear irregular in shape. The stratum granulosum ranges from one to five layers of keratinocytes in mammals. These cells continue to flatten due to the disintegration of their nuclei and the organelles and the cytoplasm begins to accumulate keratohyaline and lammellar granules (Elias *et al.*, 2003). The filaggrin in the keratohyaline bundles keratins and the lamellar granules contain a waterproofing glycolipid that is spewed into the extracellular space and is a major factor in slowing water loss across the epidermis (Elias *et al.*, 2003). The outer keratinized layer of the epidermis is shed continuously and is replaced by the progressive movement and maturation of cells from the germinal layer (stratum basale); thus all of the cells of this lineage that will eventually become metabolically inactive, enucleated cells of the outer stratum corneum (Elias *et al.*, 2003).

The dermal layer of the skin provides a flexible but robust base for the epidermis and contains the vascular supply for the metabolic support of the avascular epidermis and skin appendages (Chu *et al.*, 2003). The dermis is divided into two sub-layers defined by the density of its collagen. The very fine, interlacing collagen fibrils of the superficial, thin, papillary dermis contains venules, arterioles, and capillary loops, as well as lymphatics and fine nerve endings from sensory nerves (Chu *et al.*, 2003). The deeper and wider reticular dermis consists of coarse, irregularly situated bundles of collagen within which are the blood vessels that join the plexus of vessels in the papillary dermis. The cellular component of the dermis is mainly the fibroblasts which are responsible for the production of collagen and other forms of extracellular matrix (Chu *et al.*, 2003).

The subcutaneous tissue just deep to the skin is known as the hypodermis. The hypodermis is not necessarily part of the skin but shares some of the skins special protective functions. It is composed of primarily adipose tissue and some areolar connective tissue that acts as a shock absorber and an insulator that prevents heat loss from the body (Chu *et al.*, 2003).

Skin appendages include hair follicles, sebaceous glands, sweat glands, nails and mammary glands. Appendage formation begins in embryonic life based upon signaling between the ectoderm and the underlying mesoderm. Early in development, specific foci of the ectoderm become competent to produce a skin appendage. It is still unclear whether the signal which initiates appendage formation is generated by the ectoderm or mesenchyme and it may be different in specific appendages (Botchkarev *et al.*, 1999; Hardy, 1992; Kratochwil *et al.*, 1996; Millar, 2002). In mammals, the hair follicle and the associated sebaceous gland is the most abundant appendage and it covers the entire body with the exception of patches of specialized epidermis such as palm/sole/foot pad, lips, nipples and regions of the genitals (Sengel, 1976; Mahler *et al.*, 2004). One unique characteristic of hair is that it undergoes a regenerative cycling to maintain pelage throughout the lifetime of a mammal. Interestingly, stem cells within the bulge region of the hair follicle can produce progeny that not only differentiate into hair, but into sebocytes and interfollicular epidermis as well (Cotsarelis *et al.*, 1990; Oshima *et al.*, 2001).

PTHrP/PPR EXPRESSION STUDIES

PTHrP

In 1986 Andy Stewardt, Arthur Broadus and colleagues published a manuscript in *Science* reporting that conditioned media from primary human foreskin keratinocytes stimulated cAMP production in a rat osteosarcoma line (Merendino *et al.*, 1986). The adenyl cyclase stimulating activity of the conditioned media was blocked by the synthetic PTH receptor antagonist based upon bovine PTH 3-34 but not PTH antibodies (Merendino *et al.*, 1986). These bio-assay characteristics and other biochemical features were similar to the PTH-like humoral hypercalcemia factor previously characterized by this group. After the human PTHrP cDNA had been cloned (Mangin *et al.*, 1988; Suva *et al.*, 1987) keratinocytes were found to have a northern blot hybridization pattern that was similar to HHM producing tumor cell lines (Ikeda *et al.*, 1989; Insogna *et al.*, 1988; Kremer *et al.*, 1991). Thus, keratinocytes became a model system to study PTHrP gene expression, leading to findings that epidermal growth factor (EGF), and calcium induced differentiation increased PTHrP protein expression (Kremer *et al.*, 1991; Heath *et al.*, 1995), whereas this was repressed by 1,25 dihydroxy vitamin D3 (Kremer *et al.*, 1996).

These observations were followed up with a series of immunohistochemical studies using a variety of antibodies generated against N-terminal and midregion PTHrP (Atillasoy *et al.*, 1991; Danks *et al.*, 1989; Hayman *et al.*, 1989; Rosol *et al.*, 1993; Sharpe *et al.*, 1998) (Kitazawa *et al.*, 1991; Zabel *et al.*, 1999; Moniz *et al.*, 1990; Blomme *et al.*, 1999; Juhlin *et al.*, 1992) There was controversy about the specific epidermal layers that labeled with PTHrP antibodies and this lead to an exchange of letters between the Melbourne and New Haven groups published by the Journal of Investigative Dermatology (Danks *et al.*, 1991). Nevertheless, in all of the studies, the interfollicular epidermis and epidermal hair follicle components were labeled with these antibodies, but for the most part staining was observed in the spinous and granular layers (Danks *et al.*, 1989; Hayman *et al.*, 1989; Rosol *et al.*, 1993; Sharpe *et al.*, 1998; Zabel *et al.*, 1999; Kitzazowa *et al.*, 1990; Blomme *et al.*, 1999; Moniz *et al.*, 1990). In addition, squamous cell carcinomas of the skin, melanomas and tumors derived from the matrix of the hair follicle labeled with PTHrP antibodies, but not basal cell carcinomas (Danks *et al.*, 1989; Hayman *et al.*, 1989). These findings helped solidify the notion that PTHrP might be a regulator of epidermal differentiation and proliferation.

Once the **various human and rodent** PTHrP genes had been cloned, the tools were in place to detect PTHrP mRNA expression. *In situ* hybridization technology provided the basis of a seminal paper by K. Lee, H. Kronenberg and colleagues describing PTHrP and PPR gene expression during rat embryonic development (Lee *et al.*, 1995). These findings provided the starting point from which most of the current models of physiological PTHrP-PPR signaling were built upon. In the developing skin, PTHrP transcripts were localized to the developing hair follicle and the PPR was enriched in the surrounding mesenchyme (Lee *et al.*, 1995). PTHrP transcripts did not appear to be present in the interfollicular epidermis; however, the study was terminated at birth and there is considerable skin development that occurs in early postnatal life of the rodent.

We followed up this study with an *in situ* hybridization evaluation of PTHrP transcripts in the developing and adult skin up to 2-years of age. We reconfirmed the findings of J. Wysolmerski, M.Dunbar and colleagues (Dunbar *et al.*, 1999; Wysolmerski *et al.*, 1998) that early in development (E-12) the invaginated mammary epithelium expressed very high levels of PTHrP transcripts (Cho *et al.*, 2003). At later times, we observed intense labeling of PTHrP transcripts in hair follicle placodes, the outer portion of the distal end of the down growing follicles and large portions of the outer root sheath of mature shaft producing follicles (Cho *et al.*, 2003). At all points in postnatal life, PTHrP transcripts were observed in the isthmus of the hair follicle (Cho *et al.*, 2003). In the older mice, the intensity of PTHrP transcript expression decreased; however, the spatial pattern was not altered, and specific labeling was not observed in the interfollicular epidermis (Cho *et al.*, 2003).

The single example of *in situ* hybridization performed on human skin indicated a low level of transcripts in the suprabasal layers of the epidermis (Danks et a., 1995). The trunk skin of rodents lacks extensive suprabasal epidermal layers; therefore, we evaluated PTHrP transcript expression in the thickened specialized epidermis of the murine footpad and nipple. Again, very little hybridization of antisense PTHrP probes was localized to any epidermal layer of these structures (Cho *et al.*, 2003) (see Figure 5).

Along with our *in situ* hybridization studies, we had performed immunohistochemistry on corresponding mouse skin sections with PTHrP antibodies. These antibodies diffusely labeled the entire hair follicle and intensely labeled the interfollicular epidermis. The lack of correspondence between *in situ* hybridization and immunohistochemistry suggested that these antibodies might be non-specific. We tested this hypothesis performing immunohistochemistry on E-20 wild type and PTHrP knockout fetuses using the following affinity purified PTHrP antibodies: a chicken polyclonal raised against human PTHrP 1-36 (Rosol *et al.*, 1993) a rabbit polyclonal raised against human PTHrP 1-34 (rb 1-34) (Peninsula Labs, San Carlos, CA); and a rabbit polyclonal raised against human PTHrP 34-53 (Calbiochem, San Diego, CA). As shown in figure 1, all antibodies labeled the interfollicular epidermis of the littermates and the PTHrP knockout, whereas the hair follicles were minimally labeled. Recently a novel PTHrP knockout mouse was developed where the PTHrP coding gene and 3' sequences had been replaced by a β-galactosidase sequence (PTHrP-β-gal knockin) (Chen *et al.*, 2006). In mice bearing this gene, the enzyme is under control of PTHrP regulatory sequences and its presence can be detected by a colorometric reaction. Here again β-galactosidase colormetric activity was restricted to the hair follicles and absent in the developing interfollicular epidermis (Chen *et al.*, 2006). Taken together these findings suggest it is unlikely that the murine interfollicular epidermis is a substantial source of PTHrP.

To determine if the human epidermis was an authentic source of high levels of PTHrP gene expression, RNase protection and a quantitative real time reverse transcriptase polymerase chain reaction (QRTPCR) assays were used to measure PTHrP transcripts in intact skin samples (90% of mRNA from skin is derived from the epidermis) and cultured keratinocytes derived from these samples. PTHrP transcripts could not be detected in intact skin by RNase protection and were at the limit of detection of the QRTPCR assay (Cho *et al.*, 2004). In contrast, the cultured primary keratinocytes expressed abundant PTHrP transcripts (Cho *et al.*, 2004). Unlike the epidermis, cultured keratinocytes lack a basement membrane, an underlying dermis and the interactions stemming from stratification (Freedberg *et al.*, 2001; Jiang *et al.*, 1993) The keratinocyte culture system is designed to maximize proliferation resulting in a large fraction of cells expressing markers of hyperproliferation usually associated with wound healing or preneoplastic conditions (Freedberg *et al.*, 2001; Jiang *et al.*, 1993). One aspect of the hyperproliferative or "activated" state is the production of endogeneous EGF-related growth factors (transforming growth factor-alpha, heparin binding-EGF and amphiregulin) that can signal their receptor, the epidermal growth factor receptor (EGFR) establishing an autocrine loop (Marques *et al.*, 1999; Piepkorn *et al.*, 1998). Treatment of the cultured human keratinocytes with the specific EGFR inhibitor, PD153035 and neutralizing antibodies to the EGFR ligand, ampiregulin, reduced PTHrP mRNA levels by 70- 85% in rapidly growing keratinocytes (Cho *et al*, 2004). Amphiregulin and other EGFR ligands are not expressed in the non-pathological epidermis (Freedberg *et al.*, 2001; Jiang *et al.*, 1993).); therefore, the high level of PTHrP mRNA and protein expression observed in cultured keratinocytes appears to be an anomaly generated by culture conditions.

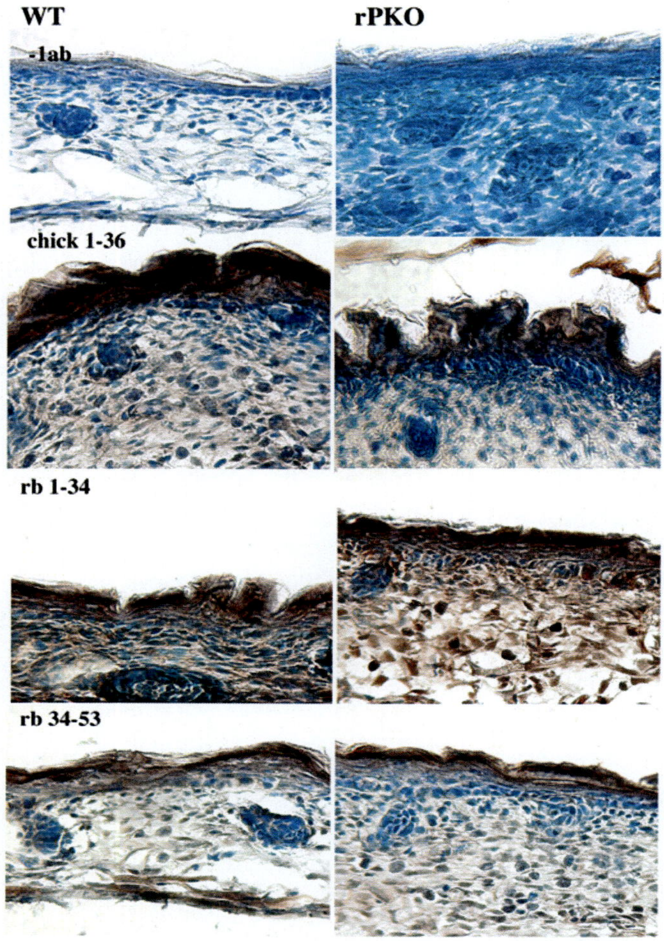

Figure 1. PTHrP antibody labeling of E-20 wild-type and PTHrP-knockout fetuses. The top row of micrographs represents the negative control with primary antibody omitted. The following affinity purified PTHrP antibodies and dilutions were used: a chicken polyclonal raised against human PTHrP 1-36 1 to 100 (chick 1-36) (Rosol *et al.*, 1993); a rabbit polyclonal raised against human PTHrP 1-34 1 to 1000 (rb 1-34) (Peninsula Labs, San Carlos, CA); and a rabbit polyclonal raised against human PTHrP 34-53 1 to 5000 (rb 34-53) (Calbiochem, San Diego, CA). Immunohistochemistry was performed on frozen paraformaldehyde fixed tissues using standard directions from a Vectastain kit (Vector labs, Burlingame, CA). Even though a wide range of dilutions was used for each antibody (up to 1 to 10,000) staining was observed in the interfollicular epidermis of the PTHrP-knockout mice. High dilutions of the chick 1-36 antibody failed to label either wild type (WT) or PTHrP-knockout skins but labeled both at low dilutions. This observation leads us to conclude that the antibodies were not specific reagents for detecting PTHrP in murine skin.

PPR

Expression of the PTH/PTHrP receptor (PPR) has generally been monitored by RNA based technologies. Again, cultured skin cells proved useful for PPR expression studies. Repeated Northern analysis as well as RT-PCR failed to detect PTH/PTHrP receptor (PPR) transcripts in poly (A)+ RNA isolated from cultured keratinocytes (Hanafin *et al*, 1995; Sharpe *et al*, 1998). Northern analysis, detected the appropriate 2.5 kb and 2.3 kb bands in poly (A)+ RNA isolated from cultured human fibroblasts and this was confirmed by RT-PCR (Hanafin *et al.*, 1995; Sharpe *et al.*, 1998). These findings were consistent with reports that primary dermal fibroblasts bound PTH and produced cAMP in response to this agonist (Wu *et al.*, 1987). Using intact organs, Urena et al demonstrated PPR transcripts in many non-classical PTH target organs and tissues, including the skin (Urena *et al.*, 1993). Using *in situ* hybridization, PPR expression in the skin was found to be abundant in the E15 and E16 rat dermis surrounding the developing hair follicles and vibrissae as well as underneath the interfollcular epidermis (Lee *et al.*, 1995). We found that the high PPR transcript levels underneath the epidermis and around the hair follicles both in the dorsal and ventral skin in E13 and E16 fetuses; however, the transcript labeling gradually diminished during development and early postnatal life (Cho *et al.*, 2003). At postnatal day 7, PPR mRNA receptor expression was still found in the upper dermis, but mainly surrounding the proximal region of the hair follicle along the dermal sheath (Cho *et al.*, 2003). In mice greater than 3-weeks of age, PPR transcripts were not detectable above background in the dermis except as punctuate foci in the dermal sheath of growing hair follicles (Cho *et al.*, 2003).

There have been a limited number of studies investigating PPR expression in the skin using immunodetection methods. PPR immunoreactivity was reported in cultured dermal papilla and dermal sheath fibroblasts detected by western blots (Thomson *et al.*, 2003). Another group reported substantial PPR antibody labeling of the interfollicular epidermis and hair follicles as well as cells in the dermis of the neonatal rat (Errazahi *et al.*, 2003). Using RT-PCR this group also detected PPR transcripts in 1-day-old neonatal rat keratinocyte cultures, but not in older cultures (Errazahi *et al.*, 2003). We have used four commercially available PPR polyclonal antibodies (Convance) under multiple fixation and tissue processing immunohistochemistry schema, but the resulting labeling did not correspond to our *in situ* hybridization findings. Using one of these commercial antibodies we found that the PPR-knock out epidermis could be labeled with dilutions recommended for immunohistochemistry. Thus, some controversy remains as to the precise cellular localization of PPR within or human skin. In part, this is due to the limitations of the *in stitu* hybridization technique. Adult rodent skin is a heavily keratinzed tissue and provides many surfaces for non-specific binding of probes. Also the traditional radioactive labeling of the *in situ* probes did not provide the sensitivity and discrimination necessary to identify specific cell types expressing low levels of PPR mRNA expressed. The precise location of the PPR in adult mouse skin will not be completely established until a transgenic line on the order of a PPR-β-gal knockin mouse is developed or better detection reagents become available.

Other PTHrP Receptors

Over the years, additional PTH/PTHrP receptors have been proposed by many groups. In some squamous cell lines and keratinocytes (Orloff *et al.*, 1992), insulinoma cells (Gaich *et al.*, 1993) and lymphocytes, (McCauley *et al.*, 1992) the signaling mechanism seemed to differ from the cloned PPR. Orloff and colleagues had shown an induction of intracellular calcium in response to amino terminal PTH and PTHrP but no significant cAMP accumulation in response to either peptide in squamous cells and normal human keratinocytes (Orloff *et al.*, 1992). Northern blots using various PPR probes failed to detect a 2.3 kb band in mRNA derived from the squamous cell lines; however, smaller and larger bands were observed. The most prominent band in the squamous cell line and normal human keratinocyte RNA was 1 kb (Orloff *et al.*, 1992). Interestingly, squamous carcinoma cells stably transfected with the PPR displayed sensitive intracellular cAMP responses to PTHrP and PTH, indicating that these cells express functional G proteins necessary to signal through adenyl cyclase (Orloff *et al.*, 1995).

In addition, Orloff *et al.*, had demonstrated that the mid-region of PTHrP (67-86) activates phospholipase C-dependent pathways in SqCC/Y1 cells through a receptor distinct from the squamous PTH/PTHRP receptor (Orloff *et al.*, 1996). It is still not clear whether some of the skin phenotypes revealed by the PTHrP transgenic mice might be due to signaling of these alternative receptors.

Summary of Gene Expression Studies

The PTHrP and PPR expression surveys do not support the concept that this signaling system plays a major role in regulating events in the interfollicular epidermis. The focal expression of PTHrP in the mammary bud, hair follicle, developing footpad and nail bed suggest a role for this signaling peptide in the development and cycling of epidermal appendages. In fact, highest levels of PPR transcripts appear very early in skin development prior to hair follicle formation in regions that will form glabrous skin, possibly reflecting a central role of this ligand-receptor pair in the creation of specialized epidermis in place of hair contiang skin. The EGFR-mediated activation of PTHrP gene expression in cultured epidermal cells raises the possibility that the peptide could play a role in various pathologies in which the "activated" keratinocyte is observed. From this prospective we will consider the studies that address the function of PTHrP in the skin.

Physiological Functions of PTHrP in the Skin

Models

From studies of long bone, lung and tooth, the physiological function of PTHrP can be generalized as a developmental regulatory protein. PTHrP-PPR signaling is part of an integrated cascade of molecular pathways that control cell fate decisions in tissues undergoing morphogenesis. Given this complexity, transgenic knockout mouse models have provided the greatest insight into the function of PTHrP-PPR signaling in the skin. These include the classical PTHrP (Karaplis *et al.*, 1994) and PPR (Lanske *et al.*, 1996) knockouts as well as the keratin 14 promoter driven PTHrP (K14-PTHrP) transgenic mouse (Wysolmerski t al., 1994). However, there are limitations to the insights these mice provide for skin physiology. In the case of the PTHrP and PPR knockouts these mice die at birth before skin development is complete. The K14-PTHrP mouse is technically not an overexpression model but a missexpression model because it constantly produces the peptide in the basal layer of the interfollicular epidermis as well in the outer root sheath of the hair follicle. To address concerns of developmental defects masking roles of PTHrP in adult physiology a series of inducible transgenic or knockout mice have been developed. A keratin 14 driven tetracycline transactivator bitransgenic tetracycline-off PTHrP mouse (K14-tTA and Tet_o-PTHrP) (Foley *et al.*, 2001) and floxed knockout for PTHrP has been generated (He *et al.*, 2001). In addition, cultured skin cells as well as normal and mutant mouse strains continued to be used to identify functions for the various PTHrP fragments. Together these research approaches have established an interesting niche for PTHrP in skin development and physiology.

Cell Culture Studies

PTHrP as an Autocrine Regulator of Keratinocytes in Culture

The impact of PTHrP on keratinocyte growth and differentiation has been intensively studied; however, the many cell types, culture conditions and poliferation/differentiation assays have failed to generate true consensus of the role of the protein in this experimental model. Antisense-mediated decreases in PTHrP expression in a human papilloma virus immortalized keratinocyte cell line increased proliferation and impeded the expression of high calcium and serum induced differentiation marker expression, suggesting a non-PPR-mediated autocrine or intracrine role for some portion of the peptide (Kaiser *et al.*, 1992; Kaiser *et al.*, 1994). Treatment of primary human foreskin keratinocytes with N-terminal PTHrP 1-34 and PTH 1-34 grown over 7 days in serum free low calcium media produced a dose dependent reduction (~30%) in the number of cells with basal morphological characteristics, which was interpreted to be consistent with an antiproliferative role for these peptides (Holick *et al.*, 1994). In addition, C-terminal PTHrP fragments 107-111 and 107-139 were reported to activate protein kinase C (PKC) in primary mouse keratinocytes (Whitfield *et al.*, 1996). This modulation of PKC inhibited proliferation in rapidly dividing murine or human keratinocytes and activated proliferation in quiescent cells (Whitfield *et al.*, 1996). Using the freshly isolated keratinocytes from neonatal rats that expressed low levels of PPR mRNA, Errazahi *et al.* found human PTHrP 1-34 increased $[^3H]$thymidine incorporation by 50% over 24 hours and this could be blocked by the antagonist, PTH 7-34, and PPR antibodies (Errazahi *et al.*, 2003). Curiously, a potent PTH agonist, bovine PTH 1-34, failed to increase proliferation of these freshly isolated rat keratinocytes (Errazahi *et al.*, 2003). Despite these most recent findings, the keratinocytes, primary or immortialized, used in the other studies did not express detectable levels of PPR, indicating that PTHrP peptides exerted their effects through other receptors or signaling mechanisms. Given that keratinocyte culture is poor model of the intact epidermis, these studies provide little insight into the role of the peptide in skin physiology, but may provide insight into cutaneous diseases.

PTHrP as a Paracrine Regulator of Dermal Fibroblast Function

The partitioning of ligand to the epidermal structures and receptor to the dermis suggests that PTHrP-PPR signaling participates in epithelial mesenchymal interactions (Lee *et al.*, 1995). N-terminal PTHrP and PTH stimulate both the cyclic AMP and the phospholipase C mediated signaling pathways in dermal fibroblasts (Hanafin *et al.*, 1995; Pun and Tam, 1995). Addition of various doses of PTHrP 1-40 to primary human dermal fibroblasts resulted in a dose-dependent inhibition of proliferation (Maioli *et al.*, 2002). Stimulation of cAMP production has long been recognized to be an antiproliferative signal for mesenchyme derived cell types such as fibroblasts (Maioli *et al.*, 2002). However, PTHrP 1-40 had no effect on type I collagen synthesis evaluated by [^{3}H]-proline incorporation or by radioimmunoassay for the carboxy-terminal fragments (Maioli *et al.*, 2002). Nevertheless, the gelatinase, matrix metalloproteinase-2 (MMP-2), was increased by N-terminal PTHrP treatment of dermal fibroblasts (Maioli *et al.*, 2002). Also, N-terminal PTHrP increased IGF-1 production by primary dermal fibroblasts *in vitro* (Shin *et al.*, 1997). Taken together, these studies suggest fibroblasts respond to PTHrP-PPR signaling by withdrawing from the cell cycle and producing proteases that cleave proteoglycans and glycoproteins as well as IGF-1 a growth factor that promotes proliferation and resistance to apoptosis in the epidermis. PTHrP-IGF-1 signaling appears to be part of the tumor cell-ostoeblast paracrine relationship involved in bone metastasis (Yoneda 2001) and provides an appealing hypothesis explaining epidermal-mesenchyme interactions that might be governed by the peptide.

Of course there are several limitations to the approach of using cultured dermal fibroblasts as assay to model *in vivo* PTHrP-PPR signaling. First, the appropriate targets of PTHrP signaling in the skin appear to be very specialized mesenchymal cells associated with epidermal appendages rather than the general dermal fibroblasts that produces the type I collagen. Most primary dermal fibroblast cultures are derived from human foreskins or neonatal trunk skin of mice, which tend to be enriched in the collagen producing cells of the reticular dermis (Sorrell and Caplan, 2004). Second, culturing mesenchymal cells in monolayers with serum leads to the loss of the ability of these cells to direct specific types of epidermal differentiation (Kishimoto *et al.*, 2000). Thus, it is not clear whether the results of these *in vitro* studies reflect PTHrP-PPR driven epithelial-mesencymal interactions *in vivo*.

Epidermis and Dermis in Animal Models

In the 1990s, there was a general expectation that modulation of PTHrP expression or function in mice would result in an alteration of the interfollicular epidermis. Consistent with this notion, Holick and colleagues observed a ~60% decrease in the incorporation of [^{3}H]thymidine into epidermal DNA of SKH-1 hairless mice after receiving intraperitoneal injections of 0.5 μg of PTH 1-34 daily for 3 days (Holick *et al.*, 1994). A similar degree of inhibition was observed with a daily dose of 0.1 μg of 1,25 $(OH)_2D_3$ for 3 days (Holick *et al.*, 1994). The PPR antagonist PTH 7-34 caused a dose-dependent increase in the incorporation of [^{3}H]thymidine into epidermal DNA (Holick *et al.*, 1994). A 100% increase in BrdU incorportion was observed when PTH 7-34 was delivered topically in liposomes composed of synthetic lipids (novasomes) (Safer *et al.*, 2006). These experiments did not report any alterations in the dermis. In contrast, overexpression of PTHrP driven by the K14 promoter in basal keratinocytes produced a slight increase in the cellularity of the epidermis and a thickening of the dermal collagen layer (Wysolmerski *et al.*, 1994). The presence of epidermal and dermal phenotypes were not reported in either of the original PTHrP and PPR knockout papers (Karaplis *et al.*, 1994; Lanske *et al.*, 1996). On an outbred CD-1 background, it is possible for PTHrP and PPR knockout mice to survive to birth. After examination of H&E stained skin sections from neonatal PTHrP and PPR knockouts, we failed to identify any abnormalities (Figure 2). However many aspects of murine skin development, including hair follicle development, sebaceous gland morphogenesis as well as epidermal and dermal maturation occur over the first three weeks of postnatal life. The perinatal lethality of the PTHrP and PPR knockout mice prevented complete evaluation of the skin phenotype in these mice.

The first attempt to characterize the adult PTHrP-null skin involved the replacement (or rescue) of PTHrP gene expression in the chondrocytes of knockout mice with a procollagen II-PTHrP transgene (col II-PTHrP/PTHrP-/- mice). This cross produced a viable but fragile animal that lacked the peptide in all tissues except cartilage (Philbrick *et al.*, 1998; Wysolmerski *et al.*, 1998). These rescued PTHrP-knockout mice displayed a number of defects in ectodermally-derived structures including failure of mammary development beyond the bud stage and absence of tooth eruption (Philbrick *et al.*, 1998; Wysolmerski *et al.*, 1998). The skin abnormalities included a matted greasy coat, thinning of the hair with age, malformed nails, and flattened footpads (Foley *et al.*, 1998). From about 3-weeks-old the skin of the rescued PTHrP-knockout progressively atrophied, resulting in a thin epidermis with a hyperkeratotic cornified layer, hypoplastic sebaceous glands, and a fibrotic dermis that lacked adipose tissue (Foley *et al.*, 1998). Crossing in the K14-PTHrP transgene to produce a K14/col II-PTHrP/PTHrP-/- mouse (double rescue) that provided the peptide to cartilage and most stratified epithelia, restored teeth and mammary glands phenotypes along with ameliorating the skin phenotype in 2 and 3 month old animals with the exception of the nail defect (Foley *et al.*, 1998). It should be noted that the constellation skin defects of the rescued PTHrP mouse were not consistent with the peptide acting as an anti-proliferation and pro-differentiation factor in the epidermis as had been expected based upon keratinocyte culture experiments or the antagonist treatments of the SKH-1 hairless mice.

Due to the lack of teeth and dermal fat, the rescued PTHrP-knockout mice required careful husbandry including a liquid diet and 30°C cage temperature. The mice were very inactive and required help grooming to remove accumulated food and body secretions. The col II-PTHrP/PTHrP-/- as well as the K14/col II-PTHrP/PTHrP-/- mice grew to about 30% the size of transgenic and PTHrP +/- littermates. We began to question whether the atrophy-like skin and the mild hair loss phenotype of the col II-PTHrP/PTHrP-/- animals might be related to a pathology in another organ system rather than a skin-specific defect. Consistent with this conclusion, microscopic examination of hair follicles plucked from the rescued PTHrP-knockout mice were squared at the base (not shown), which has been reported for malnourished mammals of many types, including rodents (Mathur and Doe, 1976). Also, the oldest (6 to 7 month) K14/col II-PTHrP/PTHrP-/- mice developed an atrophied skin phenotype similar to the col II-PTHrP/PTHrP-/- mice. To test the hypothesis that the skin phenotype of the rescued PTHrP-knockout mouse was due to systemic rather than a cutaneous defect in PTHrP-PPR signaling, we grafted the trunk skin of E-18.5 traditional PTHrP and PPR knockouts onto athymic nude mice. As shown in figure 3, grafts of both PTHrP and PPR-knockouts skins produced hair shafts. Also, the histology of 10-week-old

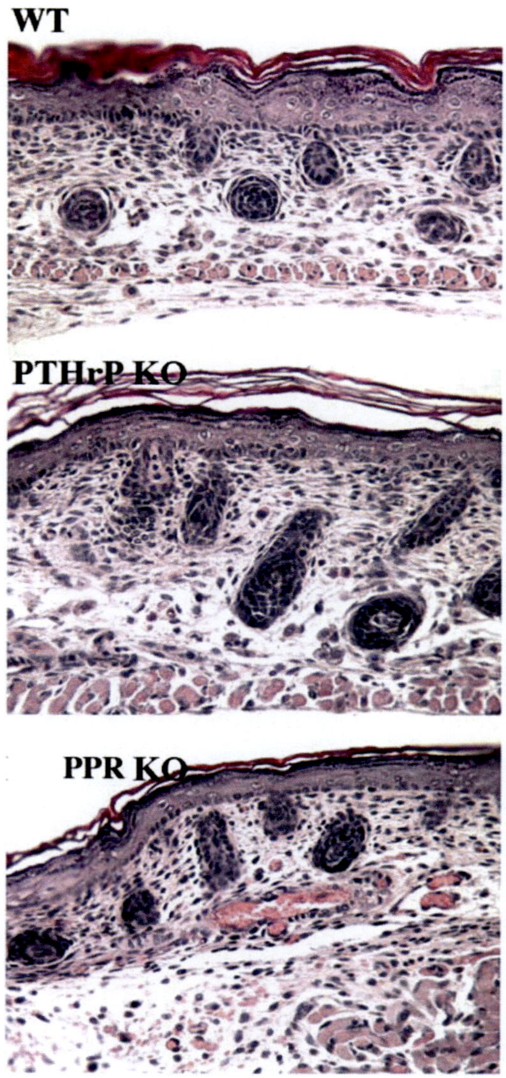

Figure 2. Skin histology of the neonatal PTHrP or PPR knockout mice. Trunk skin from new born wild-type PTHrP and PPR knockouts stained with hematoxylin and eosin. The genotype is indicated in the left hand corner of the micrograph. Note presence of normal appearing epidermis and hair follicles in all images.

grafts was indistinguishable from those from wild type and heterozygous littermates, and did not manifest any aspect of the severe skin phenotype exhibited by the col II-PTHrP/PTHrP-/- mice. Thus, it is likely that much of the trunk skin phenotype of the rescued PTHrP mouse was due to byproduct of systemic disease caused by lack of the peptide in other tissues. Moreover, it appears that PTHrP and the PPR are not required for the development of the general interfollicular epidermis and dermis in the trunk skin of the mouse, consistent with the lack of discernable expression of PTHrP mRNA in this region at any point in the development of the skin. Nevertheless, the high levels PTHrP gene expression observed in developing footpads and nails of the PTHrP-β-gal knockin mice suggest that the defects in these epidermal appendages exhibited by the col II-PTHrP/PTHrP-/- mouse may indicate a genuine role for the peptide in regulating the growth of these structures (Chen *et al.*, 2006).

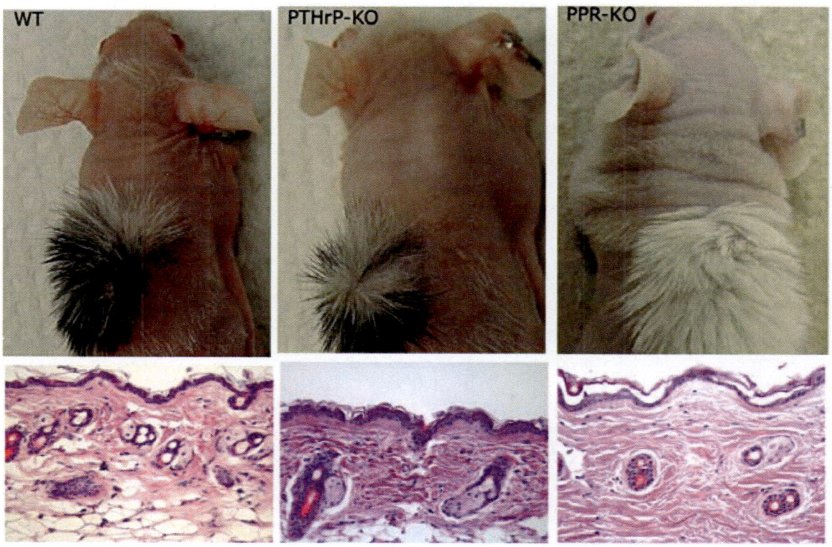

Figure 3. Lack of PTHrP or PPR does not interfere with hair follicle development and hair shaft production in grafted skin. a-c) Trunk skin from E18.5 fetal mice 5 weeks after engraftment onto athymic nude mice. The genotype of the skin is indicated in the right hand corner of a-c: rpKO= PTHrP-knockout RKO=PPR-knockout . d-f) H&E stained skin section of the respective grafts. Note presence of normal appearing epidermis and hair follicles in all the grafts.

Hair

The Hair Cycle and Structure of the hair Follicle

The hair follicle undergoes a life-long cyclic transformation from the resting phase (telogen) to the growth phase (anagen) and then to the apoptosis driven regression phase (catagen) (Chase, 1954; Hardy, 1992; Paus and Cotsarelis, 1999) (see schematic in Figure 4). Anagen encompases two distinct process: 1) in the initial srages of anagen, there is a rapid proliferation and down growth of epidermal cells from the permanent portion of the hair follicle (the upper portion that extends from the epidermis to the insertion point of the arrector pili muscle) to create the hair bulb and matrix where the hair shaft will form. 2) In the latter portion of anagen, proliferation continues in the matrix while the hair shaft is produced and pushed up through the hair follicle and above the epidermis. This latter part of anagen lasts for 5 to 7 days in the mouse and in some cases several years in the human scalp. The duration of late anagen determines the length of the hair shaft (Chase, 1954; Hardy, 1992). Like all epidermal appendages, the hair follicle is composed of dermal and epithelium-derived cell populations that exchange signals to coordinate development and post natal growth. The mesenchyme-derived component consists of fibroblast-like cells of the dermal papilla (a strip of connective tissue enclosed by the epithelia of the hair bulb at the base of the late anagen hair follicle and the fibroblasts that form the dermal sheath surrounding the entire epithelial hair follicle component (Paus and Cotsarelis, 1999) (see Figure 4). Signaling by dermal papilla cells controls the cell dynamics of the epidermal component (hair cycle) and the overall physical properties of the hair follicle and shaft (Chase, 1954; Chuong, 1998; McElwee and Hoffmann, 2000).

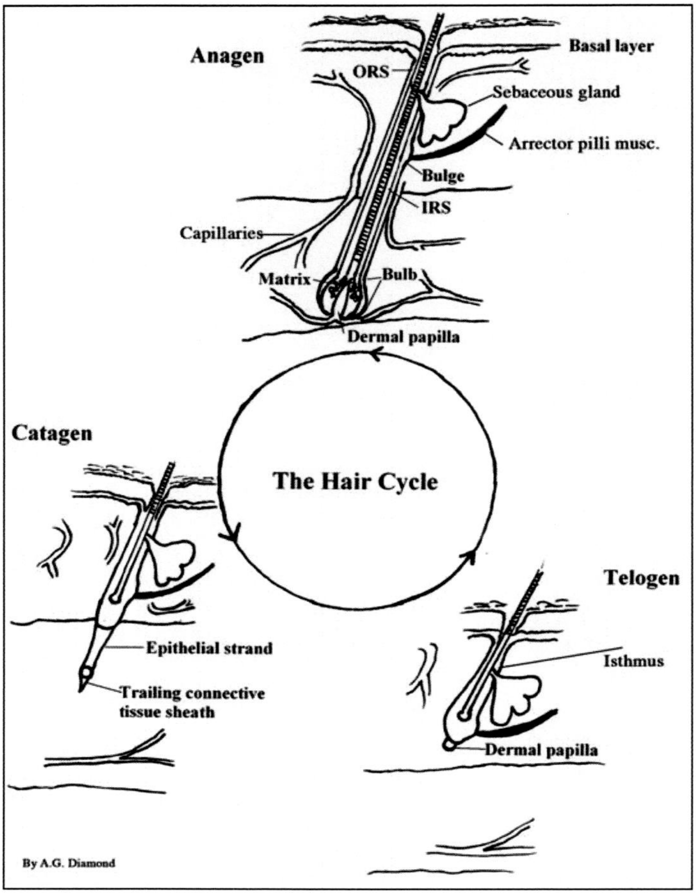

Figure 4. The Hair follicle and the hair cycle. The drawing illustrates the different layers of the hair follicle and how it appears during different phases of the hair cycle.

The epithelial hair follicle compartments consist of concentric cylinders: one to two layers of the outer root sheath cells (ORS), three layers of the inner root sheath (IRS), as well as the cuticle, cortex and medulla that make up the actual hair shaft. All of these cylinders represent a distinct lineage of epithelial differentiation and display characteristic structural proteins (e.g., hair keratins, trichohyolin), adhesion and matrix molecules as well as enzyme activities (Langbein *et al.*, 2001). The ORS, IRS, hair matrix (part of the bulb that contains undifferentiated cells that rapidly proliferate during anagen) all arise from the progeny of epithelial stem cells located in the bulge region of the hair follicle (site of arrector pili muscle attachment). The epithelial stem cells remain in the bulge region throughout life and are responsible for generating the ORS by producing transiently amplifying cells that rapidly proliferate to populate the structure.

The anagen hair bulb contains the actual hair shaft *factory* (Paus and Foitzik, 2004; Paus *et al.*, 1999; Paus and Cotsarelis, 1999). The rapidly proliferating keratinocytes of the matrix initiate their terminal differentiation to become the hair shaft and IRS just above the dermal papilla. Cells of the inner root sheath become only lightly keratinized and disintegrate at the level of the sebaceous gland ducts leaving a space into which sebum is secreted into the maturing hair (Paus and Foitzik, 2004; Paus *et al.*, 1999; Paus and Cotsarelis, 1999).

Like the interfollicular epidermis, hair follicles are avascular and cyclic hair growth is dependent upon induction of angiogenesis to meet the increased nutritional needs of the hair follicles during the growing stage of rapid cell proliferation. Increases in diameter, length, and proliferating endothelial cells have been associated with the anagen stage of the hair cycle (Mecklenburg *et al.*, 2000; Yano *et al.*, 2001). Inhibiting angiogenesis *in vivo* by the intraperitoneal application of a fumagillin derivative inhibits the experimentally induced anagen development in mice (Mecklenburg *et al.*, 2000).

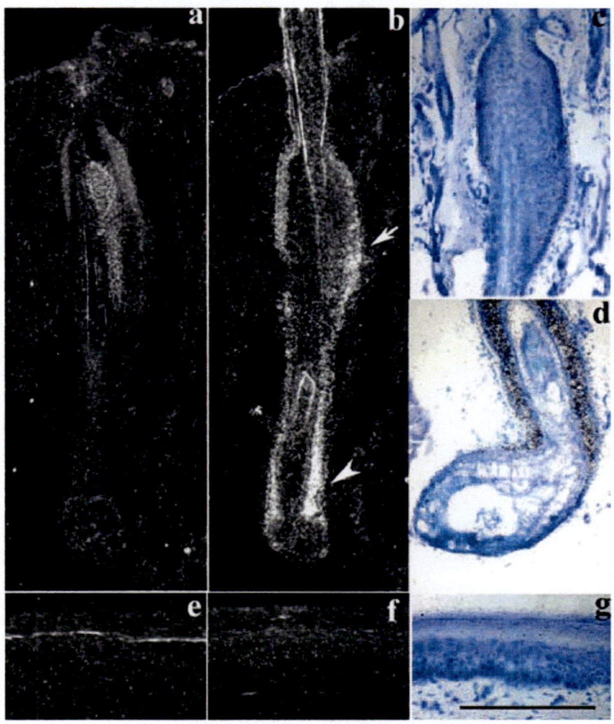

Figure 5. PTHrP mRNA expression detected by *in situ* hybridization in the footpad and vibrissa of the adult mice. Vibrissae and footpad skin from a 4 month-old mouse subjected to *in situ* hybridization. PTHrP sense probe (left column), antisense probe middle column and right antisense probe plus methylene blue counter stain. a – d) In the vibrissa hair follicle, PTHrP transcripts are strongly expressed in the ORS. They are especially abundant in the peripheral portion of bulge (arrow) and proximal ORS (arrow head). c and d are high magnification of distal and proximal portions of a vibrissa, respectively. e – g) High levels of PTHrP mRNA expression were not apparent in the foot pad skin, which has thick epidermal layer. Bar represents 162 μm in (a, b), 65 μm in (c, d), and 100 μm in (e – g).

PTHrP and PPR Expression over the Hair Cycle

Depilation of 7-week-old mice by wax-rosin to synchronize the hair cycle beginning with the growing stage (anagen) was employed to further elucidate the expression of PTHrP and its receptor during the hair cycle. In early anagen, PTHrP transcripts were at their lowest levels weakly expressed in the isthmus of the hair follicle (Cho *et al.*, 2003). At late anagen, PTHrP transcripts were at their greatest levels in the isthmus, throughout the entire outer root sheath including the bulge, and slightly over background in the matrix (Figure 5 shows vibrissa which is in late anagen). During catagen induction at day-19 post-depilation, PTHrP mRNA expression was still found in the isthmus but was not apparent in the regressing hair follicle. Telogen showed weak expression of PTHrP transcripts in the isthmus (Cho *et al.*, 2003). The lone point at which PPR transcripts were distinguishable by *in situ* hybridization was early anagen. At this point they appeared to be punctate clusters along the dermal sheath (Cho *et al.*, 2003). Thus, there appears to be a reciprocal expression pattern between PTHrP in the ORS and the PPR in the dermal sheath during early and late anagen (Cho *et al.*, 2003) Stimulation by N-terminal PTHrP or PTH results in down regulation of the PPR receptor mRNA (Okano *et al.*, 1994). Whether the reciprocal expression pattern during anagen indicates productive signaling between PTHrP and the PPR in the hair follicle remains to be established.

PTHrP and Hair Shaft Length

The first reports that PTHrP might influence the hair cycle stem from the initial characterization of the K14-PTHrP mouse. The human K14 promoter missexpress PTHrP over the entire ORS throughout hair follicle development and cycling. This mouse had a very striking hair phenotype: the ventral surface of the female mouse failed to develop hair follicles (Wysolmerski *et al.*, 1994), but as will be discussed later, this had little to do with the peptides role in the hair cycle. In comparison, the changes of the dorsal skin of the K14-PTHrP mouse were surprisingly mild, consisting of what appeared to be a decrease in the density of hair follicles. At birth, these transgenic mice were indistinguishable from their wild-type littermates but by 6 days of life there was a delay of hair eruption on the dorsal surface (Wysolmerski *et al.*, 1994). Follow up studies indicated that the three main types of hair found on dorsal surface of mice were shorter on both male and female K14-PTHrP animals (Cho *et al.*, 2003). When the adult hair cycle was synchronized by depilation, delayed hair eruption was not observed in the transgenics; however the K14-PTHrP mice entered catagen two days earlier than wild-type littermates (Cho *et al.*, 2003). The premature termination of anagen accounted for the 32-40% decrease in the length of the hair shafts in the K14-PTHrP mice relative to wild-type littermates (Diamond *et al.*, 2006). Further scrutiny of the K14-PTHrP hair shafts and follicles revealed that the both were 20-30% thinner in the latter part of anagen and this was preceded by decreased proliferation of keratinocytes in the matrix of the transgenic follicles (Diamond *et al.* 2006). Correlated with these findings was a decrease in capillary size and density around the late anagen hair follicles of K14-PTHrP mice as compared to that of wild-type littermates (Diamond *et al.*, 2006). The expression of other positive and negative angiogenesis factors was not reduced in the K14-PTHrP mice; therefore, we concluded that PTHrP may act directly as an inhibitor of proangiogenic behaviors by targeting the PPR expressing capillary endothelial cells (Diamond et al 2006;

Bakre *et al.*, 2002). Thus, the over expression of PTHrP in the epidermis and hair follicles leads to shorter and thinner hair shafts as the result of decreased proliferation in the matrix of the hair follicle and premature entrance into catagen, all of which are consistent with reduced capillary support of the hair follicle (Diamond et al 2006).

The hair cycle findings from the K14-PTHrP mouse have been supported by a series of studies that have used PPR agonists and antagonists to manipulate hair growth using inbred mice as well as those with hair follicle defects. The initial antagonist studies used the SKH-1 hairless mouse. The SKH-1 hairless mouse has a disruption of the *hairless* gene which encodes a transcription corepressor required for catagen progression and initiation of anagen (Beaudoin *et al.*, 2005; Panteleyev *et al.*, 1999). As a result the SKH-1 hairless mouse loses most of its hair shafts after the catagen phase of the first hair cycle at 3 weeks after birth and majority of hair follicles form cysts (Panteleyev *et al.*, 1999). Five to six-week-old SKH-1 hairless mice treated with intraperitoneal injections of the antagonist, PTH 7-34, for 7 days were notably more hairy when compared with the control group (Holick *et al.*, 1994). There was a 246% increase in number residual hair shafts on these mice and 180% increase in the length of the shafts (Holick *et al.*, 1994). PTH 1-34 injections did not affect these parameters in the SKH-1 hairless mouse (Holick *et al.*, 1994). Recently more dramatic increases in hair length (300%) were observed when PTH 7-34 was delivered topically in novasomes (Safer *et al.*, 2006). In 24-day-old C57BL/6 mice naturally synchronized in telogen at the termination of the first hair cycle, injections of PTH 7-34 caused a premature entry into anagen (Schilli *et al.*, 1997). By 14 days of treatment, more than 99% of the hair follicles were in anagen while 100% of the hair follicles of the control group were still in telogen (Schilli *et al.*, 1997). These antagonists injections delayed catagen in the spontaneous or depilation induced hair cycle in the C57BL/6 mice (Schilli *et al.*, 1997). The antagonists PTH 7-34 and PTHrP 7-34 also reduced hair loss in adult mice treated with the chemotherapy agent cyclophosphamide, whereas application of the PPR agonist PTH 1-34 increased the loss (Peters *et al.*, 2001). Interestingly, PTHrP 7-34 was far more effective in preventing cyclophosphamide-induced catagen than PTH 7-34 (Peters *et al.*, 2001). Taken together, the PPR agonists appear to lead to premature initiation of anagen and prolong anagen by conferring a resistance to catagen.

On the basis of the hair phenotype of the K14-PTHrP and the antagonist experiments one would expect that hair follicles that lacked PTHrP would prematurely initiate anagen, have a prolonged anagen and possibly fail to undergo a proper catagen transition, preventing further hair cycles. PTHrP and PPR knockout had normal hair follicles at birth, which is not unexpected because the morphogeneis of the follicle is just being completed at that time (Figure 2). As indicated in Figure 3, we have grafted both the PTHrP and the PPR knockout skins onto nude mice to study postnatal skin and hair follicle development. As shown in figure 3, grafts of both PTHrP and PPR knockouts skins produced hair shafts that were similar in density to that of controls. The length of hair shafts plucked from PTHrP and PPR-knockout grafts was not different than those of controls (not shown). After hair emerged on the grafts, it was clipped and regrowth occurred in knockout and control grafts indicating a second hair cycle had occurred. Thus, it appears that PTHrP expression in the hair follicle and presence of the PPR in dermal components are not required for hair follicle morphogenesis, control of hair shaft growth or hair cycling. The absence of any hair phenotype in fetal or grafted PTHrP and PPR knockout skins raises questions about physiological relevance of the antagonist application findings and the K14-PTHrP mouse model.

However, some caution should be taken in considering the implications of these grafting experiments. In order for the grafts to take, host endothelial cells must invade the tissue and either link with existing vasculature or form new capillaries. Endothelial cells have been shown to express the PPR (Isales *et al.*, 2000), and we speculate that his may be the actual target of PTHrP during the hair cycle. In fact, the E-18.5 PTHrP and PPR knockout skins had increased size and density of capillaries along the epidermis (Diamond *et al.*, 2006). Another confounding issue with these experiments is that wounds associated with placement of the graft could lead to activation of PTHrP production by keratinocytes that surround the graft as well as macrophages directed by tissue damage entering the graft (Blomme *et al.*, 1999). On the basis of these considerations, it is clear that the precise role of PTHrP and in the hair cycle will only be established by the generation of an epidermis targeted inducible Cre/floxed PTHrP mouse by Karaplis and colleagues.

Nipple

The biological significance of the striking hairless ventral skin phenotype of the K14-PTHrP mouse remained obscure until careful examination of the traditional PTHrP and PPR-knockout fetuses. These mice lacked mammary glands and nipples (Wysolmerski *et al.*, 1998). As in the formation of other epithelial organs, development of embryonic mammary glands depends on reciprocal and sequential exchanges of information between the developing epithelium and the mammary mesenchyme (Sakakura, 1987). Extensive work by J. Wysolmerski's group has established that PTHrP mRNA was highly expressed in the invaginated mammary bud (E-11 to E-12) and signaling to the PPR on the surrounding condensed mesenchyme differentiates this layer to primary mammary mesenchyme (Wysolmerski *et al.*, 1998; Dunbar *et al.*, 1999; Dunbar *et al.*, 1998). This PTHrP-PPR signal is a key event in the acquisition of primary mammary markers such as tenascin C, androgen receptor and LEF-1 (Dunbar *et al.*, 1999).

It is well known that the primary mammary mesenchyme directs the down growth and branching of the mammary epithelium, but it also leads to the formation of the thickened epidermis of the nipple sheath at ~E-17 (Sakadura 1987). The missexpression of PTHrP in the developing ventral epidermis by the human K14 promoter leads to the differentiation of the entire underlying dermis to primary mammary mesenchyme expressing the markers of the androgen receptor, LEF-1 and tenascin C (Dunbar *et al.*, 1999; Foley *et al.*, 2001). These observations suggest that the hairless ventral skin of the adult K14-PTHrP mouse is actually nipple epidermis. Consistent with this conclusion the epidermis of the adult female K14-PTHrP mouse is substantially thicker with additional spinous and granular layers similar to the nipple (Foley *et al.*, 2001; Mahler *et al.*, 2004) This epidermis expresses keratins 2e and 6 as well as a cytoskeletal protein epiplakin that are present in the nipple but are absent in the interfollicular epidermis (Mahler *et al.*, 2004; Eastwood *et al.*, 2006). The ventral dermal matrix of the K14-PTHrP mouse contains smaller collagen bundles, increased elastic fibers and glycosaminoglycan content similar to nipple connective tissue (Abdalkhani *et al.*, 2002).

Likewise, ventral K14-PTHrP dermis contained increased vasculature, melanocytes, mast cells and smooth muscle all of which distinguish nipple connective tissue from the surrounding dermis (Abdalkhani *et al.*, 2002).

The formation of mammary mesenchyme in the ventral surface of the K14-PTHrP mouse also explains sexual dimorphism observed in this transgenic line. The male K14-PTHrP mice have considerably more hair on their ventral surface, a thinner epidermis and less cellular dermis (Abdalkhani *et al.*, 2002) Male mice lack nipples and mammary glands and this is due to androgen directed apoptosis of both the primary mammary mesenchyme and the epithelia at E 13.5 (Sakakura 1987; Dunbar *et al.*, 1999) Both PTHrP and the PPR are required for androgen receptor expression in the mammary mesenchyme and the male knockouts fail to undergo destruction of the mammary bulb (Dunbar *et al.*, 1999). Treatment of mothers with high levels of testosterone eliminated the sexual dimorphism between the ventral skin phenotypes of the male and female K14-PTHrP mice (Abdalkhani *et al.*, 2002).

The acquisition of the nipple-like skin phenotype of the K14-PTHrP mouse is dependent on the correct temporal and spatial epidermal overexpression of peptide. The K14-tTA and Tet_o-PTHrP mice were used to control the overexpression of PTHrP at different times of development by manipulating tetracycline consumption. Formation of the ventral nipple-like skin required PTHrP overexpression during embryonic development, whereas transgene expression post-weaning produced normal hairy ventral skin (Foley *et al.*, 2001). Mammary gland development in the mouse begins at E10 to E11 (Sakakura, 1987). This is well before pelage begins to develop dorsal region, (E13.5). In the whole embryo, the dorsal dermis arises from the somitic dermomyotome (Sengel, 1976). It has been proposed that the dorsal mesenchyme is preprogrammed to produce generalized epidermal appendages in vertebrates such as hair, feathers and scales by exposure to a Wnt that is produced by the dorsal neural tube (Olivera-Martinez *et al.*, 2001). As a result hair follicles initially develop on the dorsal surface of the embryo and over time follicle formation proceeds in a wave-like fashion towards the ventral surface (Olivera-Martinez *et al.*, 2001; Sengel, 1976). In contrast, we believe that the mammary mesencyme is derived from the ventral dermis that arises from the somatic lateral plate mesoderm (Sengel, 1976), and is likely to be influenced by BMP signaling (Hens et al., 2007). We speculate that since the ventral mesenchyme develops apart form the neural tube, and it would not be preprogrammed to participate in generalized epidermal appendage formation. The PTHrP-PPR responisvenenss of the ventral mesenchymal cells is probably limited to a developmental window (E11 to E13) prior to the acquisition of competence of these cells to participate in hair follicle morphogenesis (E14). We believe the combination of the unique cellular characteristics of the ventral mesencymal cells and the absence of hair follicle initiation signals permits these cells to be uniquely responsive to PTH-PTHrP signaling and differentiate into the primary mammary mesenchyme.

What other signaling cascades cooperate with PTHrP-PPR signaling to produce the primary mammary mesenchyme and generate the unique hairless epidermis of the nipple? Wnt signaling is clearly required for placode formation and LEF-1, a transcription factor downstream of the canonical Wnt pathway has been reported to be required for maintenance of mammary epithelial buds (Chu *et al.*, 2004; Kratochwil *et al.*, 1996). At the time of nipple sheath formation, an indicator of wnt signaling, nuclear Lef1, is lost in the epidermal portion, whereas the underlying primary mammary mesencyhme has acquired this marker (Foley *et al.*, 2001). Work from Wysolmerski's group suggests that PTHrP signaling augments BMP 4-induced SMAD 1, 5 and 8 phosphorylation in the mammary mesenchyme in the transgenic lines as well as mesenchymal cell lines *in vitro* (Hens et al., 2007). PTHrP and BMP signaling apparently upregulate MSX2 expression in the mammary mesenchyme that inhibits hair follicle formation (Hens et al., 2007). Unlike hair and teeth, the early developing mammary gland lacks detectable hedgehog signaling, and a repressor of this pathway, Gli3, is required for the induction of mammary placodes (Hatsell and Cowin, 2006). It is clear that unlike the developing long bone (Vortkamp *et al.*, 1996), hedgehog does not activate PTHrP gene expression in the mammary bud (Hatsell and Cowin, 2006; Widelitz *et al.*, 2007). Taken together, PTHrP signaling appears to reduce hair follicle stimulating Wnt signaling in the epidermis while augmenting BMP-4 signaling in the dermis, which has been reported to limit hair follicle induction (Botchkarev and Sharov, 2004; Plikus *et al.*, 2004). In combination, these signals would be expected to result in a glaborous nipple sheath. One important aspect that remains to be established is identification the signaling pathway/s that activate PTHrP gene expression in the developing mammary epithelium.

Sebaceous Gland

Sebaceous glands are holocrine glands derived from the epidermis and located within the dermis and are connected via a short duct to the distal, permanent portion of the hair follicle near the isthmus, where upon which the gland secretes its product, sebum (Chu *et al.*, 2003). The most peripheral gland cells are contiguous with the outer root sheath of the hair follicle, which is an extension of the basal layer of the epidermis. This peripheral layer represents the germinative layer from which cells divide and differentiate into sebocytes (Chu *et al.*, 2003). The sebocytes produce the lipids, wax esters, cholesterol and triglycerides that make up the sebum which accumulate in the cytoplasm as the cells move upward, toward the excretory duct, where they lyse and release their contents (Thiboutot, 2004). Sebum is believed to play a role in epidermal desquamation and separation of the hair shaft from the internal root sheath by breaking the sheath down before it reaches the isthmus as well as conferring a water repellant quality to the hair shaft (Chu *et al.*, 2003).

PTHrP expression near the sebaceous gland is located at the isthmus, a complex region where keratinocyte progenitor cells can be incorporated either into sebaceous glands or the ORS (Niemann *et al.*, 2003). The human K14 promoter drives expression in the germinative peripheral layer of the gland. The sebaceous glands of the K14-PTHrP mouse appeared hyperplastic and had increased numbers of sebocytes (Foley *et al.*, 1998). Further study will be required to determine if PTHrP influences proliferation and differentiation of the adult sebaceous gland or whether the phenotype of the K14-PTHrP mouse results from a developmental patterning defect (Grachtchouk *et al.*, 2005).

SKIN PATHOLOGY

Roles for PTHrP in skin pathologies have not been systematically explored. This will require sensitive mRNA based detection methods to establish the expression of PTHrP and the PPR in various pathologies. A start in this area has been made by the Melbourne group in following up the original skin tumor PTHrP antibody labeling studies with an *in situ* hybridization report, using a colorometric detection methodology (Danks *et al.*, 1995). Not surprisingly, squamous cell carcinomas of the skin stained intensely with the PTHrP antisense probes labeled above the low level of normal epidermis (Danks *et al.*, 1995). Squamous cell carcinomas of the skin frequently have activated EGFR signaling or ras mutations both of which have been found to activate PTHrP gene expression (Aklilu *et al.*, 1997; Cho *et al.*, 2004; Yuspa *et al.*, 2000). Interestingly, basal cell carcinomas did not hybridize with the PTHrP probes and these tumors are almost never associated with hypercalcemia of malignancy (Danks *et al.*, 1995). A large fraction of basal cell carcinomas are initiated by aberrant hedgehog signaling (Callahan and Oro, 2001; Quinn and Epstein, 2003), and the lack of PTHrP gene expression may possibly indicate that this pathway does not activate peptide expression in cells of the keratinocyte lineage. Thus far, the expression studies have not pointed towards a specific role for PTHrP in skin tumor progression. We speculate that in skin cancers, as in neoplasms of other organs, PTHrP will both inhibit and facilitate disease progression in a microenvironment dependent fashion similar to how TGF-β influences tumor growth (Bierie and Moses, 2006).

The successful treatment of psoriasis with PTH 1-34 (Holick *et al.*, 2003) provides one of most encouraging yet perplexing arenas to consider PTHrP function. Psoriasis, in part, is an autoimmune disease driven by activated TH2 cells present in the dermis of psoriatic lesions (Nickoloff *et al.*, 2006). It is thought that cytokines from the T cells trigger a form of "activated keratinocyte" phenotype where proliferation is increased and many of the epidermal differentiation-specific proteins associated with the cornifed layer are not produced leading, to the silver, flaky plaques that characterize the disease (Freedberg *et al.*, 2001; Nickoloff *et al.*, 2006). As part of the psoriatic keratinocyte phenotype amphiregulin is produced and the EGFR is activated (Bhagavathula *et al.*, 2005; Cook *et al.*, 1997; Cook *et al.*, 1992). Since amphiregulin-EGFR signaling appears to be activated in the psoriatic keratinocytes, PTHrP would be expected to be produced and in the disease.

Most evidence suggests that PTHrP is not produced in psoriasis. Julin *et al.*, used PTHrP antibodies to label sections of psoriatic and unaffected skin. This antibody exclusively stained the granular layer of the epidermis in unaffected skin samples, but failed to label psoriatic lesions (Julin *et al.*, 1992). Given that the psoriatic epidermis does not express markers of the granular layer, as well as the established non-specificity of PTHrP antibodies, one is tempted to disregard this finding. However, a recent survey using reliable RIA methodologies to measure protein levels in the plasma of psoriasis patients found that PTHrP levels were not different than healthy controls, but PTH levels were significantly elevated (Regana *et al.*, 2005). In light of this data, we speculate that uncoupling of the activation PTHrP form EGFR signaling in the psoriatic keratinocytes might contribute to the pathology of the disease. In this context, the positive impact PTH-1-34 novosome cream on psoriatic lesions in a phase 1 trial does not appear quite as surprising. Clearly, the relationship between amphiregulin-EGFR and PTHrP-PPR signaling in the context of psoriasis and other skin diseases merits further study.

MATERIALS AND METHODS

Antibody Labeling

After equilibrating to room temperature, the frozen tissues on the slides were fixed in 4% paraformaldehyde. Tissues were washed in single strength PBS buffer twice and incubated in 1.5 % H_2O_2 diluted in methanol to inactivate endogenous peroxidase activity. After washing in PBS buffer, 5% rabbit serum was applied for 20 minutes at room temperature in a humidified incubator. Then primary antibody (immunoaffinity purified) antibody that had initially been raised against human PTHrP (dilutions indicated in figure legend 1) were applied at 4°C in a humidified incubator overnight. No primary antibody was applied on the tissues for negative control. After washing as above, secondary antibody (biotinylated seconday antibodies 1: 500 dilution) were applied at room temperature in a humidified incubator for 45 minutes. After washing as above, the tissues were incubated with avidin-biotin complex solution for 30 minutes and then diaminobenzidine for 10 minutes. The avidin-biotin complex and diaminobenzidine were purchased from Vector Laboratories, Burlingame, CA. After washing in distilled water, tissues were counter-stained with methylene green and mounted for microscopic examination.

Mice and Tissue Harvesting

All experiments that used animals were approved by the Indiana University IACUC and were performed in compliance with stipulations of that body. New born fetuses were harvested from less than 1-hour-old litters generated from crosses of PTHrP+/- or PPR+/- mice. PTHrP and PPR knockout pups were visually identified and normal appearing mice were taken as controls. Skins were removed and fixed in 10% buffered formalin, paraffin embedded, sectioned and stained with Hematoxylin and Eosin. PCR was performed on tail biopsies as in Foley et al, 2001 to confirm the identification of knockouts and establish the genotypes of controls.

Grafting

For skin grafts, fetal mice were harvested at E18.5 and viable PTHrP and PPR knockout fetuses were visually identified. The entire dorsal skin was removed from the knockout and control mice as a single pelt within a laminar air flow hood and stitched into an excision on the dorsal surface of athymic nude mice or $Foxn1^{n/n}$ (Harlan, Indianapolis). The graft was covered with a bandage for 3 days and then treated with petrolatum until hair began to emerge. PCR was performed on tails biopsy as in Foley *et al.*, 2001 to confirm the identification of knockouts and establish the genotypes of control grafts. Grafts were maintained on the mice for 10 to 16 weeks. . The hair on some of the grafts was clipped at 4 weeks after its emergence and then observed every few days to monitor hair growth. At the termination of the experiment, the graft and surrounding skin was removed, fixed in Bouis or formalin for various histological and immunohistochemistry assays. Upon microscopic examination of these samples, regions that contained *Foxn1*$^{n/n}$ epidermal cells were clearly distinguishable from the grafted skin due to the uniquely thickened epidermis and unusual hair follicle morphology. Numbers of grafts were as follows: PTHrP knockout N=12, littermate N=10; PPR knockout N=4, and littermates N=4.

In situ Hybridization

Sections of dissected mouse vibrissa were processed as in Cho *et al.*, 2003

Acknowledgements

This work was supported by National Institutes of Health grant R01 AR45585. Parts of this review were contained in a Masters of Science thesis prepared by A. G. Diamond. A special thanks to Sue Childress for her prompt and professional histological

technical support. We thank Dr. Henry Kronenberg (Massachusetts General Hospital) for providing the PPR and PTHrP-KO mice. We are greatly indebted to Dr. Arthur Broadus who has provided the K14-PTHrP mouse, shared unpublished information regarding the PTHrP-β-gal knockin mouse as well as enthusiastically encouraged our scholarship in this area of study.

References

Abdalkhani, A., Sellers, R., Gent, J., Wulitich, H., Childress, S., Stein, B., Boissy, R. E., Wysolmerski, J. J., and Foley, J. (2002). Nipple connective tissue and its development: insights from the K14-PTHrP mouse. *Mech Dev 115*, 63-77.

Aklilu, F., Park, M., Goltzman, D., and Rabbani, S. A. (1997). Induction of parathyroid hormone-related peptide by the Ras oncogene: role of Ras farnesylation inhibitors as potential therapeutic agents for hypercalcemia of malignancy. *Cancer Res 57*, 4517-4522.

Atillasoy, E. J., Burtis, W. J., and Milstone, L. M. (1991). Immunohistochemical localization of parathyroid hormone-related protein (PTHRP) in normal human skin. *J Invest Dermatol 96*, 277-280.

Bakre, M. M., Zhu, Y., Yin, H., Burton, D. W., Terkeltaub, R., Deftos, L. J., and Varner, J. A. (2002). Parathyroid hormone-related peptide is a naturally occurring, protein kinase A-dependent angiogenesis inhibitor. *Nat Med 8*, 995-1003.

Barrandon, Y., and Green, H. (1987). Three clonal types of keratinocyte with different capacities for multiplication. *Proc Natl Acad Sci U S A 84*, 2302-2306.

Beaudoin, G. M., 3rd, Sisk, J. M., Coulombe, P. A., and Thompson, C. C. (2005). Hairless triggers reactivation of hair growth by promoting Wnt signaling. *Proc Natl Acad Sci U S A 102*, 14653-14658.

Bhagavathula, N., Nerusu, K. C., Fisher, G. J., Liu, G., Thakur, A. B., Gemmell, L., Kumar, S., Xu, Z. H., Hinton, P., Tsurushita, N., *et al.* (2005). Amphiregulin and epidermal hyperplasia: amphiregulin is required to maintain the psoriatic phenotype of human skin grafts on severe combined immunodeficient mice. *Am J Pathol 166*, 1009-1016.

Bierie, B., and Moses, H. L. (2006). Tumour microenvironment: TGFbeta: the molecular Jekyll and Hyde of cancer. *Nat Rev Cancer 6*, 506-520.

Blomme, E. A., Zhou, H., Kartsogiannis, V., Capen, C. C., and Rosol, T. J. (1999). Spatial and temporal expression of parathyroid hormone-related protein during wound healing. *J Invest Dermatol 112*, 788-795.

Botchkarev, V. A., Botchkareva, N. V., Roth, W., Nakamura, M., Chen, L. H., Herzog, W., Lindner, G., McMahon, J. A., Peters, C., Lauster, R., *et al.* (1999). Noggin is a mesenchymally derived stimulator of hair-follicle induction. *Nat Cell Biol 1*, 158-164.

Botchkarev, V. A., and Sharov, A. A. (2004). BMP signaling in the control of skin development and hair follicle growth. *Differentiation 72*, 512-526.

Callahan, C. A., and Oro, A. E. (2001). Monstrous attempts at adnexogenesis: regulating hair follicle progenitors through Sonic hedgehog signaling. Curr Opin Genet Dev *11*, 541-546.

Chase, H. B. (1954). Growth of the hair. *Physiol Rev 34*, 113-126.

Chen, X., Macica, C. M., Dreyer, B. E., Hammond, V. E., Hens, J. R., Philbrick, W. M., and Broadus, A. E. (2006). Initial characterization of PTH-related protein gene-driven lacZ expression in the mouse. *J Bone Miner Res 21*, 113-123.

Cho, Y. M., Lewis, D. A., Koltz, P. F., Richard, V., Gocken, T. A., Rosol, T. J., Konger, R. L., Spandau, D. F., and Foley, J. (2004). Regulation of parathyroid hormone-related protein gene expression by epidermal growth factor-family ligands in primary human keratinocytes. *J Endocrinol 181*, 179-190.

Cho, Y. M., Woodard, G. L., Dunbar, M., Gocken, T., Jimenez, J. A., and Foley, J. (2003). Hair-cycle-dependent expression of parathyroid hormone-related protein and its type I receptor: evidence for regulation at the anagen to catagen transition. *J Invest Dermatol 120*, 715-727.

Chu, D. H., Haake, A. R., Holbrook, K., and Loomis, C. A. (2003). The Structure and Development of the Skin, In: *Dermatology in General Medicine*, I. Freedberg, ed. (New York: Mcgraw Hill), pp. 107-118.

Chu, E. Y., Hens, J., Andl, T., Kairo, A., Yamaguchi, T. P., Brisken, C., Glick, A., Wysolmerski, J. J., and Millar, S. E. (2004). Canonical WNT signaling promotes mammary placode development and is essential for initiation of mammary gland morphogenesis. *Development 131*, 4819-4829.

Chuong, C.-M. (1998). *Molecular basis of epithelial appendage morphogenesis* (Austin, Tex.: R.G. Landes).

Cook, P. W., Piepkorn, M., Clegg, C. H., Plowman, G. D., DeMay, J. M., Brown, J. R., and Pittelkow, M. R. (1997). Transgenic expression of the human amphiregulin gene induces a psoriasis-like phenotype. *J Clin Invest 100*, 2286-2294.

Cook, P. W., Pittelkow, M. R., Keeble, W. W., Graves-Deal, R., Coffey, R. J., Jr., and Shipley, G. D. (1992). Amphiregulin messenger RNA is elevated in psoriatic epidermis and gastrointestinal carcinomas. *Cancer Res 52*, 3224-3227.

Cotsarelis, G., Sun, T. T., and Lavker, R. M. (1990). Label-retaining cells reside in the bulge area of pilosebaceous unit: implications for follicular stem cells, hair cycle, and skin carcinogenesis. *Cell 61*, 1329-1337.

Danks, J. A., Ebeling, P. R., Hayman, J., Chou, S. T., Moseley, J. M., Dunlop, J., Kemp, B. E., and Martin, T. J. (1989). Parathyroid hormone-related protein: immunohistochemical localization in cancers and in normal skin. *J Bone Miner Res 4*, 273-278.

Danks, J. A., Martin, T. J., Moseley, J. M., and Hayman, J. A. (1991). Do all epidermal keratinocytes contain parathyroid hormone related protein (PTHrP)? *J Invest Dermatol 97*, 1086-1087.

Diamond, A. G., Gonterman, R. M., Anderson, A. L., Menon, K., Offutt, C. D., Weaver, C. H., Philbrick, W. M., and Foley, J. (2006). Parathyroid hormone hormone-related protein and the PTH receptor regulate angiogenesis of the skin. *J Invest Dermatol 126*, 2127-2134.

Dunbar, M. E., Dann, P. R., Robinson, G. W., Hennighausen, L., Zhang, J. P., and Wysolmerski, J. J. (1999). Parathyroid hormone-related protein signaling is necessary for sexual dimorphism during embryonic mammary development. *Development 126*, 3485-3493.

Dunbar, M. E., Young, P., Zhang, J. P., McCaughern-Carucci, J., Lanske, B., Orloff, J. J., Karaplis, A., Cunha, G., and Wysolmerski, J. J. (1998). Stromal cells are critical targets in the regulation of mammary ductal morphogenesis by parathyroid hormone-related protein. *Dev Biol 203*, 75-89.

Eastwood, J., Offutt, C. D., Mennon, K., M., K., Hrncirova, P., Novotny, M. V., Arnold, R. J., and Foley, J. (2006). Identification of markers for nipple epidermis: changes during pregnancy and lactation. *differentiation 74*, 1-9.

Elias, P., Feingold, K., and Fluhr, J. (2003). Overview of the protective functions of the skin, In: *Dermatology in General Medicine I*. Freedberg, ed. (McGraw Hill), pp. 107-118.

Errazahi, A., Bouizar, Z., Lieberherr, M., Souil, E., and Rizk-Rabin, M. (2003). Functional type I PTH/PTHrP receptor in freshly isolated newborn rat keratinocytes: identification by RT-PCR and immunohistochemistry. *J Bone Miner Res 18*, 737-750.

Foley, J., Dann, P., Hong, J , Cosgrove, J., Dreyer, B., Rimm, D., Dunbar, M., Philbrick, W., and Wysolmerski, J. (2001). Parathyroid hormone-related protein maintains mammary epithelial fate and triggers nipple skin differentiation during embryonic breast development. *Development 128*, 513-525.

Foley, J., Longely, B. J., Wysolmerski, J. J., Dreyer, B. E., Broadus, A. E., and Philbrick, W. M. (1998). PTHrP regulates epidermal differentiation in adult mice. *J Invest Dermatol 111*, 1122-1128.

Freedberg, I. M., Tomic-Canic, M., Komine, M., and Blumenberg, M. (2001). Keratins and the keratinocyte activation cycle. *J Invest Dermatol 116*, 633-640.

Gaich, G., Orloff, J. J., Atillasoy, E. J., Burtis, W. J., Ganz, M. B., and Stewart, A. F. (1993). Amino-terminal parathyroid hormone-related protein: specific binding and cytosolic calcium responses in rat insulinoma cells. *Endocrinology 132*, 1402-1409.

Grachtchouk, M., Liu, J., Hutchin, M. E., Wang, A., Glick, A., and Dlugosz, A. A. (2005). Hedgehog signaling and sebocyte development. *Journal of Investigative Dermatology 125*, A648.

Hanafin, N. M., Chen, T. C., Heinrich, G., Segre, G. V., and Holick, M. F. (1995). Cultured human fibroblasts and not cultured human keratinocytes express a PTH/PTHrP receptor mRNA. *J Invest Dermatol 105*, 133-137.

Hardy, M. H. (1992). The secret life of the hair follicle. *Trends Genet 8*, 55-61.

Hatsell, S. J., and Cowin, P. (2006). Gli3-mediated repression of Hedgehog targets is required for normal mammary development. *Development 133*, 3661-3670.

Hayman, J. A., Danks, J. A., Ebeling, P. R., Moseley, J. M., Kemp, B. E., and Martin, T. J. (1989). Expression of parathyroid hormone related protein in normal skin and in tumours of skin and skin appendages. *J Pathol 158*, 293-296.

He, B., Deckelbaum, R. A., Miao, D., Lipman, M. L., Pollak, M., Goltzman, D., and Karaplis, A. C. (2001). Tissue-specific targeting of the pthrp gene: the generation of mice with floxed alleles. *Endocrinology 142*, 2070-2077.

Heath, J. K., Southby, J., Fukumoto, S., O'Keeffe, L. M., Martin, T. J., and Gillespie, M. T. (1995). Epidermal growth factor-stimulated parathyroid hormone-related protein expression involves increased gene transcription and mRNA stability. *Biochem J 307 (Pt 1)*, 159-167.

Hens, J. R., Dann, P., Zhang, J. P., Harris, S., Robinson, G. W., and Wysolmerski, J. (2007). BMP4 and PTHrP interact to stimulate ductal outgrowth during embryonic mammary development and to inhibit hair follicle induction. *Development 134*, 1221-1230.

Holick, M. F., Chimeh, F. N., and Ray, S. (2003). Topical PTH (1-34) is a novel, safe and effective treatment for psoriasis: a randomized self-controlled trial and an open trial. *Br J Dermatol 149*, 370-376.

Holick, M. F., Ray, S., Chen, T. C., Tian, X., and Persons, K. S. (1994). A parathyroid hormone antagonist stimulates epidermal proliferation and hair growth in mice. *Proc Natl Acad Sci U S A 91*, 8014-8016.

Ikeda, K., Arnold, A., Mangin, M., Kinder, B., Vydelingum, N. A., Brennan, M. F., and Broadus, A. E. (1989). Expression of transcripts encoding a parathyroid hormone-related peptide in abnormal human parathyroid tissues. *J Clin Endocrinol Metab 69*, 1240-1248.

Insogna, K. L., Stewart, A. F., Ikeda, K., Centrella, M., and Milstone, L. M. (1988). Characterization of a parathyroid hormonelike peptide secreted by human keratinocytes. *Ann N Y Acad Sci 548*, 146-159.

Isales, C. M., Sumpio, B., Bollag, R. J., Zhong, Q., Ding, K. H., Du, W., Rodriguez-Commes, J., Lopez, R., Rosales, O. R., Gasalla-Herraiz, J., *et al.* (2000). Functional parathyroid hormone receptors are present in an umbilical vein endothelial cell line. *Am J Physiol Endocrinol Metab 279*, E654-662.

Jiang, C. K., Magnaldo, T., Ohtsuki, M., Freedberg, I. M., Bernerd, F., and Blumenberg, M. (1993). Epidermal growth factor and transforming growth factor alpha specifically induce the activation- and hyperproliferation-associated keratins 6 and 16. *Proc Natl Acad Sci USA 90*, 6786-6790.

Jones, P. H., Harper, S., and Watt, F. M. (1995). Stem cell patterning and fate in human epidermis. *Cell 80*, 83-93.

Juhlin, L., Hagforsen, E., and Juhlin, C. (1992). Parathyroid hormone related protein is localized in the granular layer of normal skin and in the dermal infiltrates of mycosis fungoides but is absent in psoriatic lesions. *Acta Derm Venereol 72*, 81-83.

Kaiser, S. M., Laneuville, P., Bernier, S. M., Rhim, J. S., Kremer, R., and Goltzman, D. (1992). Enhanced growth of a human keratinocyte cell line induced by antisense RNA for parathyroid hormone-related peptide. *J Biol Chem 267*, 13623-13628.

Kaiser, S. M., Sebag, M., Rhim, J. S., Kremer, R., and Goltzman, D. (1994). Antisense-mediated inhibition of parathyroid hormone-related peptide production in a keratinocyte cell line impedes differentiation. *Mol Endocrinol 8*, 139-147.

Karaplis, A. C., Luz, A., Glowacki, J., Bronson, R. T., Tybulewicz, V. L., Kronenberg, H. M., and Mulligan, R. C (1994). Lethal skeletal dysplasia from targeted disruption of the parathyroid hormone-related peptide gene. *Genes Dev 8*, 277-289.

Kishimoto, J., Burgeson, R. E., and Morgan, B. A. (2000). Wnt signaling maintains the hair-inducing activity of the dermal papilla. *Genes Dev 14*, 1181-1185.

Kitazawa, S., Fukase, M., Kitazawa, R., Takenaka, A., Gotoh, A., Fujita, T., and Maeda, S. (1991). Immunohistologic evaluation of parathyroid hormone-related protein in human lung cancer and normal tissue with newly developed monoclonal antibody. *Cancer 67*, 984-989.

Kratochwil, K., Dull, M., Farinas, I., Galceran, J., and Grosschedl, R. (1996). Lefl expression is activated by BMP-4 and regulates inductive tissue interactions in tooth and hair development. *Genes Dev 10*, 1382-1394.

Kremer, R., Karaplis, A. C., Henderson, J., Gulliver, W., Banville, D., Hendy, G. N., and Goltzman, D. (1991). Regulation of parathyroid hormone-like peptide in cultured normal human keratinocytes. Effect of growth factors and 1,25 dihydroxyvitamin D3 on gene expression and secretion. *J Clin Invest 87*, 884-893.

Kremer, R., Sebag, M., Champigny, C., Meerovitch, K., Hendy, G. N., White, J., and Goltzman, D. (1996). Identification and characterization of 1,25-dihydroxyvitamin D3-responsive repressor sequences in the rat parathyroid hormone-related peptide gene. *J Biol Chem 271*, 16310-16316.

Langbein, L., Rogers, M. A., Winter, H., Praetzel, S., and Schweizer, J. (2001). The catalog of human hair keratins. II. Expression of the six type II members in the hair follicle and the combined catalog of human type I and II keratins. *J Biol Chem 276*, 35123-35132.

Lanske, B., Karaplis, A. C., Lee, K., Luz, A., Vortkamp, A., Pirro, A., Karperien, M., Defize, L. H., Ho, C., Mulligan, R. C., *et al.* (1996). PTH/PTHrP receptor in early development and Indian hedgehog-regulated bone growth. *Science 273*, 663-666.

Lee, K., Deeds, J. D., and Segre, G. V. (1995). Expression of parathyroid hormone-related peptide and its receptor messenger ribonucleic acids during fetal development of rats. *Endocrinology 136*, 453-463.

Mahler, B., Gocken, T., Brojan, M., Childress, S., Spandau, D. F., and Foley, J. (2004). Keratin 2e: a marker for murine nipple epidermis. *Cells Tissues Organs 176*, 169-177.

Maioli, E., Fortino, V., Torricelli, C., Arezzini, B., and Gardi, C. (2002). Effect of parathyroid hormone-related protein on fibroblast proliferation and collagen metabolism in human skin. *Exp Dermatol 11*, 302-310.

Mangin, M., Webb, A., Dreyer, B., Posillico, J., Ikeda, K., Weir, E., Stewart, A., Bander, N., Milstone, L., Barton, D., and Broadus, A. E. (1988). Identification of a cDNA encoding a parathyroid hormone-like peptide from a human tumor associated with humoral hypercalcemia of malignancy. *Proceedings of the National Academy of Sciences of the United States of America 85*, 597-601.

Marques, M. M., Martinez, N., Rodriguez-Garcia, I., and Alonso, A. (1999). EGFR family-mediated signal transduction in the human keratinocyte cell line HaCaT. *Exp Cell Res 252*, 432-438.

Mathur, M., and Doe, M. G. (1976). Kinetics of proliferation and differentiation in the hair follicle and epidermis in neonatally undernourished rats. *Am J Pathol 82*, 9-24.

McCauley, L. K., Rosol, T. J., Merryman, J. I., and Capen, C. C. (1992). Parathyroid hormone-related protein binding to human T-cell lymphotropic virus type I-infected lymphocytes. *Endocrinology 130*, 300-306.

McElwee, K., and Hoffmann, R. (2000). Growth factors in early hair follicle morphogenesis. *Eur J Dermatol 10*, 341-350.

Mecklenburg, L., Tobin, D. J., Muller-Rover, S., Handjiski, B., Wendt, G., Peters, E. M., Pohl, S., Moll, I., and Paus, R. (2000). Active hair growth (anagen) is associated with angiogenesis. *J Invest Dermatol 114*, 909-916.

Merendino, J. J., Jr., Insogna, K. L., Milstone, L. M., Broadus, A. E., and Stewart, A. F. (1986). A parathyroid hormone-like protein from cultured human keratinocytes. *Science 231*, 388-390.

Millar, S. E. (2002). Molecular mechanisms regulating hair follicle development. *J Invest Dermatol 118*, 216-225.

Moniz, C., Burton, P. B., Malik, A. N., Dixit, M., Banga, J. P., Nicolaides, K., Quirke, P., Knight, D. E., and McGregor, A. M. (1990). Parathyroid hormone-related peptide in normal human fetal development. *J Mol Endocrinol 5*, 259-266.

Nickoloff, B. J., Bonish, B. K., Marble, D. J., Schriedel, K. A., Dipietro, L. A., Gordon, K. B., and Lingen, M. W. (2006). Lessons learned from psoriatic plaques concerning mechanisms of tissue repair, remodeling, and inflammation. *J Invest Dermatol 126 Suppl*, 16-29.

Niemann, C., Unden, A. B., Lyle, S., Zouboulis Ch, C., Toftgard, R., and Watt, F. M. (2003). Indian hedgehog and beta-catenin signaling: role in the sebaceous lineage of normal and neoplastic mammalian epidermis. *Proc Natl Acad Sci U S A 100 Suppl 1*, 11873-11880.

Okano, K., Wu, S., Huang, X., Pirola, C. J., Juppner, H., Abou-Samra, A. B., Segre, G. V., Iwasaki, K., Fagin, J. A., and Clemens, T. L. (1994). Parathyroid hormone (PTH)/PTH-related protein (PTHrP) receptor and its messenger ribonucleic acid in rat aortic vascular smooth muscle cells and UMR osteoblast-like cells: cell-specific regulation by angiotensin-II and PTHrP. *Endocrinology 135*, 1093-1099.

Olivera-Martinez, I., Thelu, J., Teillet, M. A., and Dhouailly, D. (2001). Dorsal dermis development depends on a signal from the dorsal neural tube, which can be substituted by Wnt-1. *Mech Dev 100*, 233-244.

Orloff, J. J., Ganz, M. B., Nathanson, M. H., Moyer, M. S., Kats, Y., Mitnick, M., Behal, A., Gasalla-Herraiz, J., and Isales, C. M. (1996). A midregion parathyroid hormone-related peptide mobilizes cytosolic calcium and stimulates formation of inositol trisphosphate in a squamous carcinoma cell line. *Endocrinology 137*, 5376-5385.

Orloff, J. J., Ganz, M. B., Ribaudo, A. E., Burtis, W. J., Reiss, M., Milstone, L. M., and Stewart, A. F. (1992). Analysis of PTHRP binding and signal transduction mechanisms in benign and malignant squamous cells. *Am J Physiol 262*, E599-607.

Orloff, J. J., Kats, Y., Urena, P., Schipani, E., Vasavada, R. C., Philbrick, W. M., Behal, A., Abou-Samra, A. B., Segre, G. V., and Juppner, H. (1995). Further evidence for a novel receptor for amino-terminal parathyroid hormone-related protein on keratinocytes and squamous carcinoma cell lines. *Endocrinology 136*, 3016-3023.

Oshima, H., Rochat, A., Kedzia, C., Kobayashi, K., and Barrandon, Y. (2001). Morphogenesis and renewal of hair follicles from adult multipotent stem cells. *Cell 104*, 233-245.

Panteleyev, A. A., Botchkareva, N. V., Sundberg, J. P., Christiano, A. M., and Paus, R. (1999). The role of the hairless (hr) gene in the regulation of hair follicle catagen transformation. *Am J Pathol 155*, 159-171.

Paus, R., and Cotsarelis, G. (1999). The biology of hair follicles. N Engl J Med *341*, 491-497.

Paus, R., and Foitzik, K. (2004). In search of the "hair cycle clock": a guided tour. *Differentiation 72*, 489-511.

Paus, R., Muller-Rover, S., and Botchkarev, V. A. (1999). Chronobiology of the hair follicle: hunting the " hair cycle clock". *J Investig Dermatol Symp Proc 4*, 338-345.

Peters, E. M., Foitzik, K., Paus, R., Ray, S., and Holick, M. F. (2001). A new strategy for modulating chemotherapy-induced alopecia, using PTH/PTHrP receptor agonist and antagonist. *J Invest Dermatol 117*, 173-178.

Philbrick, W. M., Dreyer, B. E., Nakchbandi, I. A., and Karaplis, A. C. (1998). Parathyroid hormone-related protein is required for tooth eruption. *Proc Natl Acad Sci U S A 95*, 11846-11851.

Piepkorn, M., Pittelkow, M. R., and Cook, P. W. (1998). Autocrine regulation of keratinocytes: the emerging role of heparin-binding, epidermal growth factor-related growth factors. *J Invest Dermatol 111*, 715-721.

Plikus, M., Wang, W. P., Liu, J., Wang, X., Jiang, T. X., and Chuong, C. M. (2004). Morpho-regulation of ectodermal organs: integument pathology and phenotypic variations in K14-Noggin engineered mice through modulation of bone morphogenic protein pathway. *Am J Pathol 164*, 1099-1114.

Pun, K. K., and Tam, S. M. (1995). Parathyroid hormone-activated phosphoinositide degradation and calcium channels in human dermal fibroblasts. *Biol Signals 4*, 19-23.

Quinn, A. G., and Epstein, E., Jr. (2003). Patched, hedgehog, and skin cancer. *Methods Mol Biol 222*, 85-95.

Regana, M. S., Ezquerra, G. M., and Millet, P. U. (2005). Serum levels of parathyroid hormone and parathyroid-related peptide in psoriasis. *Acta Derm Venereol 85*, 420-423.

Rosol, T. J., Steinmeyer, C. L., McCauley, L. K., Merryman, J. I., Werkmeister, J. R., Grone, A., Weckmann, M. T., Swayne, D. E., and Capen, C. C. (1993). Studies on chicken polyclonal anti-peptide antibodies specific for parathyroid hormone-related protein (1-36). *Vet Immunol Immunopathol 35*, 321-337.

Safer, J. D., Ray, S., and Holick, M. F. (2006). A Topical PTH/PTHrP Receptor Antagonist Stimulates Hair Growth in Mice. *Endocrinology*.

Sakakura, T. (1987). Mammary embryogenesis, In: *The Mammary gland: development, regulation, and function*, M. C. Neville, and C. W. Daniel, eds. (New York: Plenum Press), pp. 37-66.

Schilli, M. B., Ray, S., Paus, R., Obi-Tabot, E., and Holick, M. F. (1997). Control of hair growth with parathyroid hormone (7-34). *J Invest Dermatol 108*, 928-932.

Sengel, P. (1976). Morphogenesis of skin (Cambridge, Eng.; New York: Cambridge University Press).

Sharpe, G. R., Dillon, J. P., Durham, B., Gallagher, J. A., and Fraser, W. D. (1998). Human keratinocytes express transcripts for three isoforms of parathyroid hormone-related protein (PTHrP), but not for the parathyroid hormone/PTHrP receptor: effects of 1,25(OH)2 vitamin D3. *Br J Dermatol 138*, 944-951.

Shin, J. H., Ji, C., Casinghino, S., McCarthy, T. L., and Centrella, M. (1997). Parathyroid hormone-related protein enhances insulin-like growth factor-I expression by fetal rat dermal fibroblasts. *J Biol Chem 272*, 23498-23502.

Sorrell, J. M., and Caplan, A. I. (2004). Fibroblast heterogeneity: more than skin deep. J Cell Sci *117*, 667-675.

Suva, L. J., Winslow, G., A., Wettenhall, R. E., Hammonds, R. G., Moseley, J. M., Diefenbach-Jagger, H., Rodda, C. P., Kemp, B. E., Rodriguez, H., Chen, E. Y., and *et al.* (1987). A parathyroid hormone-related protein implicated in malignant hypercalcemia: cloning and expression. *Science 237*, 893-896.

Thiboutot, D. (2004). Regulation of human sebaceous glands. *J Invest Dermatol 123*, 1-12.

Thomson, M., McCarroll, J., Bond, J., Gordon-Thomson, C., E, D. W., and Moore, G. P. (2003). Parathyroid hormone-related peptide modulates signal pathways in skin and hair follicle cells. *Exp Dermatol 12*, 389-395.

Urena, P., Kong, X. F., Abou-Samra, A. B., Juppner, H., Kronenberg, H. M., Potts, J. T., Jr., and Segre, G. V. (1993). Parathyroid hormone (PTH)/PTH-related peptide receptor messenger ribonucleic acids are widely distributed in rat tissues. *Endocrinology 133*, 617-623.

Vortkamp, A., Lee, K., Lanske, B., Segre, G. V., Kronenberg, H. M., and Tabin, C. J. (1996). Regulation of rate of cartilage differentiation by Indian hedgehog and PTH-related protein. *Science 273*, 613-622.

Whitfield, J. F., Isaacs, R. J., Jouishomme, H., MacLean, S., Chakravarthy, B. R., Morley, P., Barisoni, D., Regalia, E., and Armato, U. (1996). C-terminal fragment of parathyroid hormone-related protein, PTHrP-(107-111), stimulates membrane-associated protein kinase C activity and modulates the proliferation of human and murine skin keratinocytes. *J Cell Physiol 166*, 1-11.

Widelitz, R., Veltmaat, J. M., Mayer, J. A., Foley, J., and Chuong, C. M. (2007). Mammary glands and feathers: Comparing two skin appendages which help define novel classes during vertebrate evolution Seminars in Cell and Developmental Biology *in press*.

Wu, T. L., Insogna, K. L., Hough, L. M., Milstone, L., and Stewart, A. F. (1987). Skin-derived fibroblasts respond to human parathyroid hormone-like adenylate cyclase-stimulating proteins. *J Clin Endocrinol Metab 65*, 105-109.

Wysolmerski, J. J., Broadus, A. E., Zhou, J., Fuchs, E., Milstone, L. M., and Philbrick, W. M. (1994). Overexpression of parathyroid hormone-related protein in the skin of transgenic mice interferes with hair follicle development. *Proc Natl Acad Sci U S A 91*, 1133-1137.

Wysolmerski, J. J., Philbrick, W. M., Dunbar, M. E., Lanske, B., Kronenberg, H., and Broadus, A. E. (1998). Rescue of the parathyroid hormone-related protein knockout mouse demonstrates that parathyroid hormone-related protein is essential for mammary gland development. *Development 125*, 1285-1294.

Yano, K., Brown, L. F., and Detmar, M. (2001). Control of hair growth and follicle size by VEGF-mediated angiogenesis. *J Clin Invest 107*, 409-417.

Yuspa, S. H., Hansen, L., Li, L., Joseloff, E., Weinberg, W., and Fernandez-Salas, E. (2000). Interacting signaling pathways in the pathogenesis of squamous cell carcinoma. *Medicina (B Aires) 60*, 689-692.

Zabel, M., Murawski, M., Surdyk-Zasada, J., Salwa-Zurawska, W., and Radziemski, A. (1999). Immunocytochemical localisation of PTHrP (parathormone-related peptide) in myoepithelial cells of human sweat and parotid glands. *Folia Histochem Cytobiol 37*, 167-172.

In: Novel Aspects of PTHrP Physiopathology
Editor: Claudio Luparello, pp. 73-93
ISBN: 978-1-60021-857-6

Chapter IV

NOVEL ASPECTS OF PTHRP IN LUNG BIOLOGY AND PATHOBIOLOGY

John S. Torday* and Virender K. Rehan

Departments of Pediatrics and Obstetrics and Gynecology, The Los Angeles Biomedical Research Institute at Harbor-UCLA Medical Center, Torrance, CA, USA.

ABSTRACT

Evolutionary Developmental Biology allows comparison of Gene Regulatory Networks (GRNs) during development across phyla. For lung evolution, the Parathyroid Hormone-related Protein (PTHrP) GRN exemplifies a continuum from ontogeny to phylogeny, homeostasis and repair. PTHrP signaling between lung endoderm and mesoderm stimulates lipofibroblast differentiation by down-regulating the myofibroblast Wnt signaling pathway, and up-regulating the Protein Kinase A-dependent cAMP signaling pathway, inducing the lipofibroblast phenotype. We speculate that recapitulation of the myofibroblast phenotype during transdifferentiation is consistent with lung injury as lung evolution in reverse. Repair recapitulates ontogeny because it is programmed to express the cross-talk between epithelium and mesoderm through evolution.

A number of biologic characteristics of Parathyroid Hormone-related Protein (PTHrP) are central to its roles in lung alveolar homeostasis and chronic parenchymal lung disease. PTHrP is necessary for the formation of alveoli during normal lung development; it is expressed in the alveolar type II cell, and its receptor is expressed in the adepithelial mesodermal fibroblast, forming a paracrine loop for epithelial-mesodermal interactions during development, homeostasis and repair; both PTHrP and the PTHrP receptor are stretch-regulated, integrating alveolar inflation with PTHrP signaling. PTHrP signaling causes increased production of pulmonary surfactant through a paracrine loop involving stimulation of the lipofibroblast phenotype, consisting of

* Correspondence concerning this article should be addressed to: John S. Torday, Departments of Pediatrics and Obstetrics and Gynecology, The Los Angeles Biomedical Research Institute at Harbor-UCLA Medical Center, Torrance, CA, USA. e-mail: jtorday@labiomed.org.

Adipocyte Differentiation Related Protein, Peroxisome Proliferator Activated Receptor gamma and leptin, which is secreted by the fibroblast and specifically binds to the type II cell leptin receptor, stimulating surfactant phospholipid and protein synthesis. Because of the central role of PTHrP signaling in alveolar homeostasis, it is also a key to understanding the etiology of parenchymal lung disease. Barotrauma, hyperoxia, lipopolysaccharide and nicotine all cause down-regulation of the PTHrP signaling pathway and up-regulation of Wnt signaling, the default pathway for the mesodermal fibroblast. The net effect of these molecular injuries to the epithelial and/or mesodermal cells is myofibroblast transdifferentiation and αSmooth Muscle Actin expression, which are characteristic of lung fibrosis. Genome-wide microarray has established that these injuries cause the decreased lipid synthesis and increased Wnt signaling characteristic of lung fibrosis. Either PTHrP itself or a Peroxisome Proliferator Activated Receptor gamma agonist such as Rosiglitazone or Prostaglandin J_2 can experimentally prevent the molecular injuries to the PTHrP signaling pathway and the structural changes that result, normalizing the PTHrP signaling pathway and lung cytoarchitecture.

This integrated model of lung evolution and repair demonstrates how epithelial-mesenchymal cross-talk, when seen as a recapitulation of ontogeny and phylogeny, predicts novel, effective diagnostic and therapeutic targets.

INTRODUCTION

Evolution is All of Lung Biology

Prior to the publication of the Human Genome biomedical investigation of mechanisms of disease was largely dependent on the pathophysiologic approach devised by Sir William Osler at the turn of the 20th century [1]. However, in the post-Genomic era we must permute and cross-reference phenotypes relevant to biologic processes of interest in order to identify the causal gene regulatory networks (GRNs). For example, the GRNs that determine development, homeostasis and repair can be viewed as a family of parallel lines [2], or simultaneous equations. This integrated phenotypic analysis can be expanded to include other vertebrate phyla (phylogeny), since the interrelationship between ontogeny and phylogeny has reemerged as Evo-Devo [3]. We have taken this systematic approach to deconvolute chronic lung disease by exploiting the Parathyroid Hormone-related Protein (PTHrP) GRN that vertically integrates the cell-molecular mechanisms of development, homeostasis and repair [2].

There are a number of reasons to think that PTHrP has played a pivotal role in vertebrate lung evolution: 1) PTHrP is expressed throughout vertebrate phylogeny, beginning with its expression in the fish swim bladder as an adaptation to gravity; microgravity down-regulates the expression of PTHrP by alveolar type II cells, and by the bones of rats exposed to 0 x g [4], suggesting that PTHrP signaling has evolved in adaptation to 1 x g. PTHrP signaling is up-regulated by stretching alveolar type II cells and interstitial fibroblasts [5], whereas over-distension down-regulates PTHrP and PTHrP receptor expression [6], suggesting an evolutionary adaptation; 2) PTHrP is necessary for the formation of alveoli [7], and alveolarization has 'driven' vertebrate lung evolution [8]; 3) Both surfactant homeostasis and alveolar capillary perfusion are under PTHrP control, indicating that alveolarization and ventilation/perfusion matching may have evolved under selection pressure for PTHrP signaling; 4) Down-regulation of PTHrP signaling causes fibroblast transdifferentiation [6,9], resulting in reversion to primordial mesenchyme characterized by Drosophila genes [10]; conversely, PTHrP treatment down-regulates the Drosophila genes [10] and restores homeostasis, recapitulating lung evolution [11].

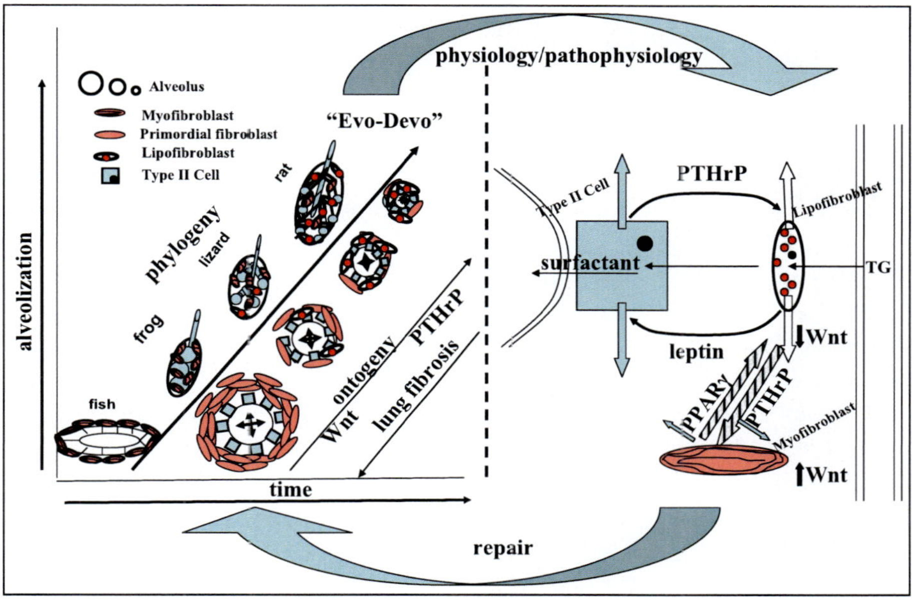

Schematic 1. The Evolutionary Continuum from Lung Development to Physiology/pathophysiology and Repair. On the left-hand side, we compare the progressive phylogenetic and ontogenetic changes in alveolization, or Evo-Devo, over evolutionary (phylogeny) and developmental (ontogeny) time, as alveoli become progressively smaller (see Legend), the alveolar septa become thinner, and the number of interstitial lipofibroblasts increase in proportion to myofibroblasts (phylogeny) or mesenchymal cells (ontogeny). Note that these cellular changes are characterized by a shift from the Wnt signaling pathway to the PTHrP signaling pathway, which is indicative of lung fibrosis. An arching arrow links Evo-Devo to alveolar Homeostasis (right panel), characterized by (1) stretch-enhanced Type II Cell PTHrP expression, (2) PTHrP binding to the stretch-sensitive lipofibroblast PTHrP receptor, down-regulating the Wnt signaling pathway (↓ Wnt), (3) stimulating triglyceride uptake (TG), (4) and up-regulating leptin, (5) which binds to the Type II Cell leptin receptor, (6) stimulating surfactant synthesis. In the absence of PTHrP, lipofibroblasts lose their ability to express PPARγ, becoming Myofibroblasts, which re-express the Wnt signaling pathway (↑Wnt), recapitulating phylogeny and ontogeny ("repair" arrow from the Myofibroblast back to Evo-Devo), a mechanism that can be prevented by PPARγ agonists.

PTHrP is a highly evolutionarily conserved, stretch-regulated gene that is unusual among the paracrine growth factors that have been identified to mediate lung development because 1) the PTHrP knock-out is stage specific and results in failed alveolarization [7], 2) unlike other such growth factors, PTHrP is expressed in the endoderm, and binds to the mesoderm [5], 3) and only PTHrP has been shown to act pleiotropically to integrate surfactant synthesis [5] and alveolar capillary perfusion [12], i.e. alveolar homeostasis. In contrast to this, others have focused on the importance of the epithelial-mesenchymal trophic unit [65] and on the importance of the fibroblasts of the 'scaffold' that act as 'sentinels' to regulate local inflammatory responses [14]. These structural entities are underpinned by PTHrP signaling from the epithelium to the mesoderm, which is highly significant because the earliest developmental signals emanate from the endoderm [15], and we have demonstrated the dependence of the fibroblast phenotype on epithelially-derived PTHrP for development [7], homeostasis [5] and repair [9]. All of these features of PTHrP biology justify its use as an archetype for our proposed model of lung evolution. We have schematized this integrated approach for lung developmental and comparative biology, homeostasis and repair (see Schematic 1).

Ontogeny and Homeostasis

Stimulation of PTHrP and its receptor by alveolar wall distension coordinately increases surfactant production [5] and alveolar capillary blood flow [12]- referred to physiologically as ventilation/perfusion (V/Q) matching. V/Q matching is the net result of the evolutionary integration of cell/molecular interactions by which the lung and pulmonary vasculature have functionally adapted to the progressive increase in metabolic demand for oxygen [16-18]. The structural adaptation for gas exchange is 3-fold: (i), the decrease in alveolar diameter [19]; (ii) the thinning of the alveolar wall [20]; (iii) the maximal increase in total surface area [21,22]. These structural adaptations could have resulted from the phylogenetic amplification of the PTHrP signaling pathway. PTHrP signaling through its receptor is coordinately stimulated by stretching the alveolar parenchyma [5]. Binding of PTHrP to its receptor activates the cyclic AMP-dependent Protein Kinase A (PKA) signaling pathway [23]. Stimulation of this signaling pathway results in the differentiation of the alveolar interstitial lipofibroblast, characterized by increased expression of Adipose Differentiation Related Protein (ADRP) and leptin [5]. ADRP is necessary for the trafficking of substrate from the circulation to the alveolar type II cell, the site of pulmonary surfactant production [24], and leptin stimulates the differentiation of the alveolar type II cell [25]. PTHrP affects the cellular composition of the alveolar interstitium in at least three ways: (i) it inhibits fibroblast growth [26], and stimulates apoptosis [27] causing septal thinning; (ii) stimulation of epithelial type II cell differentiation by leptin [25] can inhibit epithelia cell growth [27]; (iii) leptin may up-regulate type IV collagen synthesis [28], reinforcing the alveolar wall [29].

Ontogeny and Phylogeny

Primordial lung endoderm and mesoderm differentiate into over 40 different cell-types. We know a great deal about growth factor signaling that determines these processes, and the down-stream signals that alter nuclear read-out. And because a great deal of effort has been put into understanding the physiologic and pathophysiologic consequences of preterm birth, we also know how these mechanisms lead to homeostasis, or fail to do so, in which case the phenotype for chronic lung disease informs us of the mechanism of lung fibrosis.

Embryonic lung development is subdivided into branching morphogenesis and alveolarization, the latter being "plastic" [29]. Deleting the PTHrP gene results in failed alveolarization [7], inferring the relevance of PTHrP to lung evolution, since alveolarization is the mechanism for vertebrate lung evolution [30,31]. Because PTHrP and its receptor are highly conserved and coordinately stretch-regulated, functionally linking the endoderm and mesoderm to the vasculature [32], we are compelled to investigate its overall role in lung phylogeny and evolution.

The combined effects of i-iii in the previous section would lead to natural selection for progressive, concomitant decreases in both alveolar diameter and alveolar wall thickness through ontogeny [33] and phylogeny [34-36], exponentially increasing the surface area-to-volume ratio of the lung due to receptor-mediated second messaging. PTHrP turns off myofibroblast differentiation by inhibiting Gli [37], the first molecular step in the mesodermal Wingless/int (Wnt) pathway, and by inactivating βcatenin [38], followed by the sequential activation of LEF-1/TCP, C/EBPα and PPARγ. The down-stream targets for PPARγ are adipogenic regulatory genes such as ADRP and leptin. PTHrP induces the lipofibroblast phenotype, first described by Vaccaro and Brody [39]. This cell-type is expressed in the lungs of a wide variety of species [40], including both newborn and adult humans [41]. Lipofibroblasts are found next to type II cells in the interstitium [42], and are characterized by neutral lipid inclusions wrapped in ADRP, which mediates the uptake and trafficking of lipid from the lipofibroblast to the type II cell for surfactant phospholipid synthesis [43], and protects the alveolar acinus against oxidant injury [44]. The concomitant inhibitory effects of PTHrP on both fibroblast and type II cell growth, in combination with PTHrP augmentation of surfactant production, would have the net effect of distending and "stenting" the thinning alveolar wall, synergizing with the up-regulation of PTHrP, and physiologically stabilizing what otherwise would result in an unstable structure that would collapse [45].

Myofibroblast Transdifferentiation as Evolution in Reverse

Lung development prepares the fetus for birth and physiologic homeostasis [46]. Surfactant production, in particular, is crucial for effective gas exchange [47]. Based on this functional linkage between lung development and homeostasis, we have generated data demonstrating that the underlying mechanisms of repair may recapitulate ontogeny. If lung fibroblasts are deprived of PTHrP, their structure and function change [6,48]: first, the PTHrP receptor is down-regulated, as are its down-stream targets ADRP and leptin: the decline in the lipofibroblast phenotype is mirrored by the gain of the myofibroblast phenotype, characteristic of fibrosis.

During the process of fetal lung development the mesodermal fibroblasts are characterized by Wnt/beta catenin signaling that determines the splanchnic mesodermal fibroblast [49]. We have shown that during alveolarization, the physiologic distension of the lung by lung liquid up-regulates the PTHrP signaling pathway in the endoderm, causing the down-regulation of the Wnt/beta-catenin pathway [10], leading to the differentiation of the lipofibroblast. These cells dominate the alveolar acinus during fetal lung development, but are highly apoptotic in the post-natal lung [50,51], giving rise to the alveolar septa [52]. Central to this paracrine determination of the mesodermal cell-types is the failure of the fibroblast to terminally differentiate [53].

Phylogenetically, the swim bladder and frog lung interstitium are characterized by myofibroblasts- lipofibroblasts don't appear in the lung until reptiles and mammals [16-18, 35]. The recapitulation of myofibroblasts during lung injury is consistent with the similarities between lung ontogeny and phylogeny, and with the molecular mechanisms of fibroblast transdifferentiation described above, and may, therefore, represent lung evolution in reverse.

A wide variety of factors can inhibit the normal paracrine induction of the lipofibroblast, and promote myofibroblast proliferation and fibrosis, including prematurity, barotrauma, oxotrauma, nicotine and infection. In all of these instances, injury of the epithelial type II cell can cause down-regulation of PTHrP [28], causing the mesodermal fibroblasts to default to the myofibroblast phenotype [6]. Importantly, myofibroblasts cannot promote the growth and differentiation of the alveolar type II cell for alveolarization [6], and produce angiotensin II, which further damages the type II cell population [54-58].

The PTHrP receptor is present on the adepithelial fibroblasts [5]. Stretching of the alveolus by fluid or air up-regulates both PTHrP ligand (59) and PTHrP receptor activity [5], promoting surfactant production by the type II cell, and lipofibroblast neutral lipid uptake, protecting them against oxidant injury [44]. PTHrP receptor binding stimulates cAMP-dependent PKA expression, which determines the lipofibroblast phenotype. Treatment of the transdifferentiating myofibroblast either in vitro [6] or in vivo [60] with PPARγ agonists blocks the transdifferentiation of the myofibroblast, preventing fibrotic injury [61].

The Role of PPAR Gamma in Ontogeny and Repair

PTHrP induces lipofibroblast differentiation via the PKA pathway, blocking Wnt signaling by inhibiting both Gli and GSK 3beta, consequently up-regulating the lipofibroblast phenotype, characterized by PTHrP receptor, ADRP, leptin, triglyceride uptake, by stimulating PPAR gamma expression [10,60].

Based on the minimalist idea that development culminates in homeostasis, disruption of homeostasis may atavistically lead back to primordial developmental cell/molecular motifs [11]. This occurs in various lung diseases [61,62], and by focusing on the continuum from development to homeostasis we can select treatments that are more consistent with promoting cellular reintegration than stopping inflammation. For example, Bronchopulmonary Dysplasia (BPD), the chronic lung disease of the newborn, can be induced by overdistending an otherwise healthy, but immature newborn baboon lung [63]. Changing the homeostatic balance of the alveolus by knocking out surfactant protein genes B, C, or D leads to alveolar remodeling that is either grossly flawed (B) or less than optimal (C, D) physiologically. Interfering with cell-cell signaling blocks lung development [6], usually resulting in parenchymal simplification. Conversely, replacing missing developmental molecular elements can re-establish lung development [6], homeostasis [60] and structure [60].

Repair recapitulates ontogeny because it is programmed to express the cross-talk between epithelium and mesoderm through evolution [11]. This model is based on three key principles: (i) the cross-talk between the epithelium and mesoderm is necessary for homeostasis; (ii) damage to the epithelium impairs the cross-talk, leading to loss of homeostasis and re-adaptation through myofibroblast proliferation; and (iii) normal physiology will either be re-established, or cell/tissue remodeling//altered lung function may occur, and/or fibrosis will persist, leading to chronic lung disease. The cell-molecular injury affecting epithelial-mesenchymal cross-talk recapitulates ontogeny (in reverse), providing effective diagnostic and therapeutic targets.

From Lung Evolution to Disease: Chronic Lung Disease as Maladaptation

The Mechanistic Relationship Between Lung Development and Repair

Lung morphogenesis and repair are characterized by a complex sequence of cell-cell interactions of endodermal and mesodermal origins, which has evolved an alveolar structure that can effectively exchange gases between the circulation and the alveolar space [11]. By determining the spatio-temporal nature of this process, we gain insights into the pathophysiology of a broad spectrum of chronic lung diseases caused by both intrinsic and extrinsic factors, bearing in mind that they phenotypically funnel into only a few pathologies-epithelial, interstitial, and/or vascular.

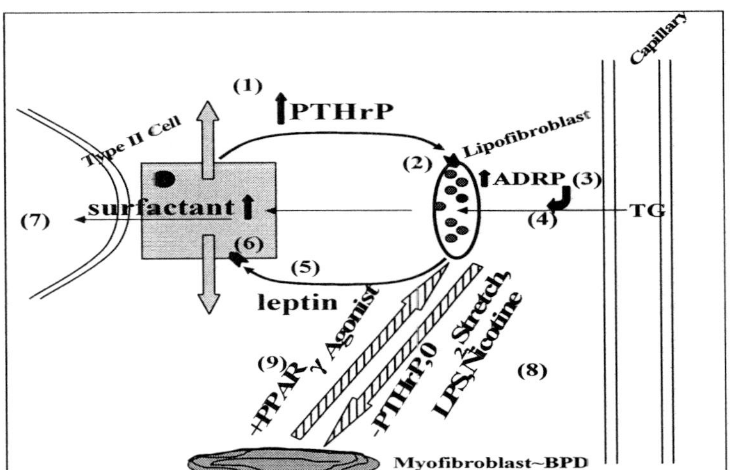

Schematic 2. Determinants of Alveolar Homeostasis and Chronic Lung Disease. Stretch coordinates alveolar type II cell expression of PTHrP (*step 1*), with up-regulation of the lipofibroblast PTHrP receptor (*step 2*), its downstream effect on lipofibroblast ADRP expression (*step 3*) and triglyceride uptake (*step 4*), and on the interaction between lipofibroblast-produced leptin (*step 5*) and the alveolar type II cell leptin receptor (*step 6*), stimulating de novo surfactant synthesis by alveolar type II cells (*step 7*). The schematic depicts lipofibroblast-to-myofibroblast transdifferentiation (*step 8*) due to decreased PTHrP (-PTHrP) in response to hyperoxia (O_2), barotrauma/volutrauma (stretch), infection (LPS) or maternal smoking (nicotine). All of these effects are prevented or rescued by PPARγ agonists (*step 9*).

The global mechanisms that mediate mesenchymal-epithelial interactions and the plasticity of mesenchymal cells in normal lung development and remodeling provide a functional genomic model that offers insights to the cell/molecular basis for lung homeostasis [11], as depicted in Schematic 2. Since we can effectively recapitulate the natural processes of development that determine normal lung structure, function and homeostasis using this approach, we should be able to exploit this knowledge to understand the cell/molecular basis for lung pathophysiology, and therefore treat it effectively.

The pathophysiology of BPD involves interactions between multiple extrinsic and intrinsic factors, including oxygen free radicals, ventilator-induced lung injury, and release of inflammatory cytokines and cytotoxic enzymes such as proteases and elastases. Injury at early developmental stages leads to an arrest of both alveolar and vascular growth, which has been attributed to perturbations in key cellular factors associated with normal alveolarization such as Retinoic Acid [66], Vascular Endothelial Growth Factor [67], and PTHrP [68]. Of these, perturbation in PTHrP signaling is compelling, as alluded to above, since 1) PTHrP is stretch-regulated; 2) its deletion results in failed alveolarization; 3) PTHrP has been shown to act pleiotropically to integrate ventilation (surfactant synthesis) and perfusion (alveolar capillary dilatation), i.e. alveolar homeostasis; and 4) the lungs of infants with BPD are PTHrP deficient [68]. We will review the role of PTHrP in lung development, homeostasis and repair.

Epithelial-Mesenchymal Interactions Determine Alveolar Lung Development

Our laboratory has used a developmental biologic approach to understand the etiology of CLD in newborns. We began with a paracrine growth factor model for the maturation of the pulmonary surfactant system based on classic mesenchymal-epithelial interactions (see Schematic, steps 2-7). These studies were originally fostered by Barry Smith's seminal observation [69] that glucocorticoids accelerate alveolar type II cell surfactant synthesis by stimulating fibroblast synthesis of an oligopeptide he termed Fibroblast-Pneumonocyte Factor (FPF). It was known at that time that lung, prostate and mammary mesodermal development were under endocrine control, and importantly, it had clearly been shown that early signals emanated from the epithelium to differentiate the immature mesenchyme in the neighboring epithelium [70]. Moreover, Brody's laboratory had shown that the developing lung fibroblast acquired an adipocyte-like phenotype [71], termed the lipid-laden fibroblast, leaving open the question as to whether these cells might be a source of lipid substrate for surfactant synthesis by the alveolar type II cell. We discovered that co-culture of the lipid-laden fibroblasts with type II cells resulted in the trafficking of the lipid from the fibroblast to the type II cell and its highly enriched incorporation into surfactant phospholipids, particularly when treated with glucocorticoids, suggesting a specific, regulated mechanism for neutral lipid trafficking [72]. Interestingly, the fibroblasts took up the neutral lipid, but did not release it unless they were in the presence of type II cells; conversely, the type II cells were unable to take up neutral lipid. These observations led to the discovery that type II cell secretion of prostaglandin E_2 caused the release of neutral lipid from the fibroblasts [73], but the nature of the lipid uptake mechanism by the type II cells remained unknown. Yet we were aware that the synthesis of pulmonary surfactant was an 'on demand' system [74-76] in which increased respiration resulted in increased surfactant production, suggesting a stretch-sensitive signal from the type II cell. With this in mind, we began studying the role of PTHrP in lung development because a) it was expressed in the embryonic endoderm, b) its receptor was present on the adepithelial mesoderm, c) it had been shown to be stretch-regulated in the urinary bladder [77] and uterus [78], and distension of the lung was known to be of physiologic significance to normal lung development [79], d) knock-out of PTHrP caused stage-specific inhibition of fetal lung alveolarization in the transition from the pseudoglandular to the canalicular stage [10], the stage at which PTHrP and its receptor appear during normal lung development.

Early functional studies of PTHrP had shown that it was a paracrine factor that stimulated surfactant phospholipid synthesis, and that it was stretch-regulated. We subsequently discovered that PTHrP stimulated neutral lipid uptake by the developing lung fibroblast, which we chose to call a lipofibroblast, by up-regulating ADRP, a molecule shown to be necessary for lipid uptake and storage. We subsequently found that ADRP was the factor necessary for the transit of neutral lipid from the lipofibroblast to the alveolar type II cell for surfactant phospholipid synthesis. The missing component for PTHrP regulation of lung surfactant was the lipofibroblast paracrine factor that stimulated surfactant synthesis. Reasoning that lipofibroblasts were similar to adipocytes, we hypothesized that lipofibroblasts would, like fat cells, express and secrete leptin, which would bind to the type II cell and stimulate surfactant synthesis- we found that lipofibroblasts do express leptin during rat lung development just prior to the onset of surfactant synthesis by the type II cell [25]. Importantly, type II cells express the leptin receptor [25], thus providing a ligand-receptor signaling pathway between the lipofibroblast and type II cell. Moreover, PTHrP was discovered to stimulate leptin expression by fetal lung fibroblasts [5], thus providing a complete growth factor-mediated paracrine loop for the synthesis of pulmonary surfactant, as predicted by the PTHrP-based model of lung development.

Since the major inducers of BPD- barotrauma [80], oxotrauma [81] and infection [82]- inhibit PTHrP expression by the alveolar type II cell, we investigated the effects of PTHrP deprivation on the lipofibroblast phenotype, only to discover that in the absence of PTHrP, the lipofibroblast transdifferentiates to a myofibroblast, the cell-type that characterizes lung fibrosis. Furthermore, myofibroblasts cannot sustain type II cell growth and differentiation, whereas the lipofibroblast can [6], demonstrating the functional significance of these two fibroblast phenotypes for lung development. Importantly, when myofibroblasts are treated with a PPARγ agonist they revert back to the lipofibroblast phenotype, including their ability to promote type II cell growth and differentiation.

We have exploited these novel observations regarding the regulated development of the alveolus by paracrine growth factors as a model for determining several cell/molecular causes of neonatal lung injury, including barotrauma/volutrauma, oxotrauma, infection and maternal smoke (nicotine) exposure, as follows.

Breakdown in PTHrP Signaling and Chronic Lung Disease

The Effect of Barotrauma/Volutrauma on PTHrP Signaling

The effective distension of the newborn lung has a profound physiologic effect on pulmonary homeostasis [83]. Conversely, overdistension can instantaneously disrupt that homeostatic mechanism (refer to Schematic 2, step 8), resulting in barotrauma/volutrauma/atelectrauma. As indicated above, the stretching of the alveolar type II cell increases the expression and production of PTHrP, potentially explaining why increased lung tidal volume stimulates pulmonary surfactant synthesis. And may explain why Wirtz and Dobbs [84] observed secretion of surfactant by isolated type II cells, but only after one stretching maneuver, without any effect of subsequent stretching, perhaps due to the absence of lipid substrate from the neighboring fibroblast. In contrast to the increased synthesis of surfactant in response to mild stretch (3-5%), overdistension of the type II cell results in down-regulation of PTHrP expression, simulating the consequences of volutrauma or atelectrauma. The effect of barotrauma/volutrauma/atelectrauma could be reversed by treatment with a PPARγ agonist prostaglandin J_2 (PGJ_2), as depicted in Schematic 2, step 9. In other experiments, we found that when the type II cell contracts under the simulated microgravity conditions created by a Rotating Wall Bioreactor, that PTHrP is also down-regulated [4], indicating that the set-point for the effect of stretch on type II cells is finely regulated and has likely evolved to optimally regulate surfactant synthesis [2].

The Effect of Oxotrauma on PTHrP Signaling

In vitro [85]: Since lipofibroblasts play an important role in injury-repair mechanisms in the lung, we studied the effects of hyperoxia on the fibroblast phenotype in immature and relatively mature alveolar interstitial fibroblasts, and found that exposure to hyperoxia down-regulated PTHrP signaling, augmenting the transdifferentiation of pulmonary lipofibroblasts to myofibroblasts (refer to Schematic, step 8). Fetal rat lung fibroblasts (FRLF) from e (embryonic, term = e22) 18 and e21 gestation were studied. After initial culture in Minimum Essential Medium (MEM) and 10% fetal bovine serum (FBS) in 21% O_2 / 5% CO_2 at 37^{0}C, FRLF were maintained in MEM and 10%FBS at 37^{0}C under control (21% O_2 / 5% CO_2) and experimental conditions (24h exposure to 95% O_2 /5% CO_2) at passages (P) 1 and P5. Passage 1 and 5 cells were analyzed for the expression of well-characterized lipogenic and myogenic markers [PTHrP receptor, ADRP, and αSMA] based on semi-quantitative competitive RT-PCR, triglyceride uptake, and leptin assay. Serial passaging and maintenance of cells in 21% O_2 resulted in a significant spontaneous decrease in the expression of the lipogenic markers between P1 and P5. This decrease was greater for immature (e18) than for (near-mature) e21 FRLFs. However, exposing cells to 95% O_2 augmented the loss of the lipogenic markers and gain of the myogenic marker from P1 to P5 in comparison to cells maintained in 21% O_2. This augmentation was also greater for e18 versus e21 lipofibroblasts. The changes in mRNA expression were accompanied by decreased triglyceride uptake and leptin secretion on exposure to hyperoxia. These data suggest that exposure to hyperoxia augments the transdifferentiation of pulmonary lipofibroblasts to myofibroblasts. Further, pretreatment with PGJ_2, at least partially attenuated the hyperoxia-augmented lipo-to-myofibroblast transdifferentiation [see Schematic 2, step 9).

In an accompanying series of experiments [48], using [1,2-$^{13}C_2$]-D-glucose tracer and gas chromatography/mass spectrometry, we metabolically profiled e18 and e21 FRLFs with and without hyperoxia exposure at passages 1, 4, 7, and 10. For this series of studies, glucose carbon redistribution between the nucleic acid ribose, lactate, and palmitate synthetic pathways and ADRP expression by RT-PCR were examined. Exposure to hyperoxia at each passage caused a decrease in ADRP mRNA expression. This passage- dependent transdifferentiation was accompanied by a moderate (9% to 20%) increase in the synthesis of nucleic acid ribose from glucose through the non-oxidative steps of the pentose cycle. E18 fibroblasts showed over an 85% decrease in the de novo synthesis of palmitate from glucose, while e21 fibroblasts showed a less pronounced 32% to 38% decrease in de novo lipid synthesis in hyperoxia-exposed cultures. From these data we conclude that 1) there is a maturation-dependent sensitivity to hyperoxia; 2) transdifferentiation of the lipofibroblast, as demonstrated by changes in ADRP expression, is accompanied by metabolic enzyme changes affecting ribose synthesis from glucose, and 3) hyperoxia specifically inhibits lipogenesis from glucose. These molecular and metabolomic data were further complemented by genome-wide microarray analysis of RNA extracted from P1 and P10 e19 FRLFs with or without exposure to hyperoxia (95% O_2 for 24h) (41). Rat chip RAE230, which has 15,923 RNA transcripts, including most genes of interest, e.g., PTHrP, PPARγ, Adipophilin (moderate homology with ADRP) was used. Genome-wide expression was analyzed using Affymetrix GeneChip Operating Software and Netaffx, Genespring 6.2 (Silicon Genetics), and Gene Microarray Pathway Profiler (Gladstone Institute). Once data files created in GCOS were imported into Genespring, the transcripts were normalized using, "Per Gene: Normalize to Median". Next, transcripts were filtered based on the following criteria: increase or decrease with a p value <0.006 or >0.994; a signal log ratio of <-0.6 or >0.6; a present call; and a minimal signal intensity of 50 in at least one experimental file. Filtered transcripts were then clustered using SOM and K-means clustering. In accord with our molecular and metabolomic data, cluster analysis of the microarray data confirmed the down-regulation of cholesterol and fatty acid synthetic genes and up-regulation of fatty acid degradation and Wnt signaling pathway genes on passaging e19 FRLFs from P1 to P10, and on exposure to hyperoxia at passages 1 and 10, thereby confirming lipo-to-myofibroblast transdifferenation under these conditions. Based on these data, it appears that lipo-to-myofibroblast transdifferentiation may be an important mechanism for hyperoxia-induced lung injury and likely a key element in the pathophysiology of BPD, allowing us to speculate that induction of adipogenic transcription factors may not only prevent, but in fact may revert the myogenic fibroblast phenotype back to the adipogenic fibroblast phenotype.

In vivo [60]:Following our *in vitro* studies, as outlined above, we next determined whether upon exposure to hyperoxia, pulmonary alveolar lipo-to-myofibroblast transdifferentiation occurs *in vivo*, and whether treatment with a potent PPARγ (the key lipogenic fibroblast nuclear transcription factor) agonist, Rosiglitazone (RGZ), would prevent this process (see Schematic, step 9). Newborn Sprague Dawley rat pups were exposed to control (21% O_2), hyperoxia alone (95% O_2 for 24h), or hyperoxia with RGZ (95% O_2 for 24h + RGZ, 3 mg/kg, administered intraperitoneally) conditions. All experiments were conducted as paired exposures, with one exposure chamber receiving 95% O_2 and the other receiving 21% O_2. On the day of delivery, each animal was placed in a 60 x 40 x 35 cm plastic chamber with 12h:12h light:dark cycles. Food and water were provided ad libitum. Chambers were connected to either 95% O_2 or 21% O_2 source before placing animals in the chambers and delivery occurred in the selected gas conditions. Oxygen concentration within the chambers was monitored at the beginning and at the end of experiments using an oxygen analyzer (Nellcor Inc.). Gas flow was adjusted to maintain minimal chamber humidity. The number of pups in each paired litter was adjusted to 8-10 pups at the onset of the exposure period. At the end of 24 hours, pups were sacrificed and lung tissue was analyzed by morphometry, and by RT-PCR, Western hybridization, and immunohistochemistry for the expression of key lipogenic and myogenic markers. We observed a significant decrease in the expression of lipogenic markers, and a significant increase in the expression of myogenic markers in the hyperoxia alone group. Exposure of rat pups to 24 hours of hyperoxia dramatically affected normal postnatal lung development. Histologic examination of lungs obtained from hyperoxic pups revealed a remarkable arrest of alveolarization compared with their normoxic littermate controls. Hyperoxia-exposed lungs demonstrated relatively large air spaces, thinned interstitia, and decreased secondary septal crests compared to air-exposed controls. In lungs from hyperoxic animals, septal thickness was reduced significantly (40%) compared to control lungs. Furthermore, quantitative analysis of alveolar number demonstrated a significant reduction (50%) in average radial alveolar counts in hyperoxic animals compared to controls. Pre-treatment with RGZ virtually prevented the hyperoxia-induced changes in lung morphology, including the effects on septal thickness and radial alveolar counts. The hyperoxia-induced morphologic, molecular, and immunohistochemical changes were virtually prevented by RGZ (see Schematic 2, step 9). This is the first evidence of *in vivo* lipo-to-myofibroblast transdifferentiation and its virtual prevention by RGZ, prompting us to conclude that administration of PPARγ agonists may be a novel, effective strategy to prevent the hyperoxia-induced lung molecular injury that has been implicated in the pathogenesis of BPD.

The Effect of Lipopolysaccharide on PTHrP Signaling

Since lung inflammation is a key factor that predisposes preterm infants to BPD, in a series of studies [86] we determined the effects of Lipopolysaccharide- (LPS) on PTHrP-driven pulmonary epithelial-mesenchymal interactions that have been shown by us to be essential in the maintenance of lung homeostasis (refer to the Schematic). Lung explants derived from e19.5 Sprague Dawley rat pups were treated with LPS (0-50 ng/ml) with or without a PTHrP pathway agonist, PGJ_2, for up to 72 hours. LPS treatment affected the expression of the key markers of the epithelial-mesenchymal paracrine loop in a dose- and time-dependent manner. There were acute (24 hour), significant increases in the expression of PTHrP, PPARγ, ADRP, and Surfactant Protein-B (SP-B), without any significant effects on the expression of αSMA. This was followed (72 hours) by significant decreases in the expression of PTHrP, PPARγ, ADRP, and SP-B, accompanied by a significant increase in the expression of αSMA, the key functional marker for BPD. These changes were completely prevented by concomitant treatment with PGJ_2, providing an integrated mechanism for the acute stimulation of lung maturation, accompanied paradoxically by BPD following intrauterine inflammation. Further, as in our *in vivo* hyperoxia model, treatment with a specific agonist of epithelial-mesenchymal interactions prevented the inflammation-induced molecular lung injury that is known to result in BPD [see Schematic 2, step 9).

The Effect of Nicotine on PTHrP Signaling

Maternal smoking during pregnancy adversely affects fetal lung growth that may result in adverse long-term consequences such as increased occurrence of lower respiratory tract illnesses and altered pulmonary mechanics on pulmonary function testing [87]. The mechanisms underlying the general effects of maternal smoking on fetal viability and growth are generally thought to be due to fetal hypoxia, yet the mechanisms underlying the pulmonary outcomes seem more complicated and are poorly understood [88]- on the one hand, there is evidence of increased surfactant production at birth, perhaps explaining why there is a lower incidence of RDS [89]. On the other hand, there is equally strong evidence for deleterious effects on pre- and postnatal lung growth and development following in utero exposure to maternal smoking [90,91]. The mechanisms underlying these seemingly paradoxical effects remain largely unknown. We tested the hypothesis that in vitro nicotine exposure would disrupt specific epithelial-mesenchymal paracrine signaling pathways and result in pulmonary lipo-to-myofibroblast transdifferentiation, resulting in altered pulmonary development and function [92,93; see Schematic, step 8. WI38 cells, a human embryonic pulmonary fibroblast cell line, were treated with nicotine (1×10^{-9}M - 1×10^{-6}M) with or without specific agonists of the alveolar fibroblast lipogenic pathway, namely PTHrP (5×10^{-7}M), dibutyryl cAMP (1×10^{-5}M) or the potent PPARγ stimulant RGZ (1×10^{-5}M), for 7 days. Expression of key lipogenic and myogenic markers was examined by RT-PCR, Western hybridization, and immunohistochemistry. The effects of nicotine on triglyceride uptake by WI38 cells, and PTHrP binding to its receptor were also determined. Finally, the effect of transfecting WI38 cells with a PPARγ expression vector on nicotine-induced lipo-to-myofibroblast transdifferentiation was determined. Nicotine treatment resulted in significantly decreased expression of lipogenic, and increased expression of myogenic markers in a dose-dependent manner, indicating nicotine-induced lipo-to-myofibroblast transdifferentiation. This was accompanied by decreased PTHrP binding to its receptor. The nicotine-induced lipo-to-myofibroblast transdifferentiation was completely prevented by concomitant treatment with either PTHrP, dibutyryl cAMP, or RGZ, and by overexpressing PPARγ (see Schematic, step 9). Our data suggest that nicotine induces alveolar lipo-to-myofibroblast transdifferentiation through a mechanism involving down-regulation of the lipogenic, PTHrP-mediated, cAMP-dependent PKA signaling pathway, which can be prevented by focusing on specific molecular targets.

PTHrP Signaling in BPD

Since PTHrP secreted by pulmonary alveolar type II cells is a key physiologic paracrine factor in maintaining alveolar homeostasis (see Schematic 2, steps 1-8), we hypothesized that its levels in the tracheal aspirates (TA) of ventilated Very Low Birth Weight Infants (VLBWI) would predict the development of BPD [68]. We examined whether TA PTHrP content during the first week of life correlated with the later development of BPD. Forty VLBWIs (birth weight 943 ± 302 grams (mean ± SD); gestational age 27 ± 2 weeks; 21 males and 19 females), who were ventilated for Respiratory Distress Syndrome, were studied. The TAs were collected once daily until the infants were extubated, and were assayed for PTHrP. The levels of TA PTHrP were compared with the later development of BPD. PTHrP in the TA during the first week of life was significantly lower in those infants who developed BPD (12/40) than among those who did not (28/40). The PTHrP levels also correlated with the duration of mechanical ventilation needed in these infants. A PTHrP level of ≤1.32 pg/mg protein predicts the later development of BPD maximally [84.6% correct classifications (true positives + true negatives)], with a sensitivity = 76.9% and specificity = 88.5%. Using a TA PTHrP level of 1.32 pg/mg protein as the cutoff, we constructed Kaplan-Meier curves to compare the duration of ventilation needed between the two groups, i.e., ≤ and > than 1.32 pg/mg protein TA PTHrP level. Infants with TA PTHrP levels greater than 1.32 pg/mg protein were off ventilatory support significantly earlier. To determine how PTHrP levels compared with the other known predictors of BPD, such as birth weight (< 1000 g), GA (< 28 wk), and male gender, we performed multivariate logistic regression analysis for these 4 variables in predicting the development of BPD. Of these variables, a PTHrP level of ≤1.32 pg/mg protein was the strongest predictor of BPD, and remained so after adjusting for the other 3 variables, i.e., birth weight of < 1000 g, GA of < 28 wk, and male gender. From these data, we concluded that lower TA PTHrP content during the first week of life in ventilated VLBWI inversely correlates with prolonged ventilation and the later development of BPD.

Prevention of Molecular Lung Injuries Leading to BPD with PPARγ Agonists

It is clear from the work outlined above that we have systematically demonstrated the central role of epithelial-mesenchymal interactions in maintaining alveolar homeostasis in barotrauma, oxotrauma, infection and nicotine injury. The lipofibroblast expresses both ADRP and leptin in response to PTHrP signaling from the alveolar type II cell, resulting in direct protection of the mesoderm against oxidant injury [44], and protection against atelectasis by augmenting surfactant phospholipid [25] and protein [5] synthesis. Molecular injury to either the alveolar type II cell or the lipofibroblast down-regulates this molecular signaling pathway, causing myofibroblast transdifferentiation (see Schematic, step 8). Unlike lipofibroblasts, myofibroblasts cannot promote alveolar type II cell growth and differentiation, leading to the failed alveolarization characteristic of BPD [6]. PPARγ is the key nuclear transcription factor that determines the lipofibroblastic phenotype, which supports alveolar type II cell growth and differentiation under the influence of factors implicated in the pathogenesis of BPD. We have shown that a wide variety of factors associated with failed alveolarization- barotrauma (6), oxotrauma [48,85], infection [86] and nicotine [92,93]- all cause myofibroblast transdifferentiation in vitro [6,48,85,86,92,93] and in vivo [62]. More importantly, we have shown that PPARγ agonists such as PGJ_2 and RGZ can prevent or rescue myofibroblast transdifferentiation (see Schematic 2, step 9), potentially preventing the inhibition of alveolarization in the developing lung [6,48,85,86,92,93].

Conclusion

Dobzhansky proclaimed that Evolution encompasses all of biology [94]. With this global concept in mind, in the post-genomic era we must make maximal use of all the phenotypes in lung biology, both in health and disease, in order to deconvolute the underlying genomic bases for physiology and pathophysiology. In the first half of this review we have traced the fundamental interrelationships between lung ontogeny and phylogeny, and their cell-molecular linkages to health and disease based on PTHrP signaling. In the second half of the review, we have shown how this basic biologic approach has been leveraged to elucidate the pathophysiology of Bronchopulmonary Dysplasia. We have determined the paracrine cell/molecular mechanism by which stretch coordinates PTHrP signaling between the alveolar type II cell and the mesoderm to up-regulate key genes for the homeostatic fibroblast phenotype- including PPARγ, ADRP and leptin- and the retrograde stimulation of alveolar type II cell surfactant phospholipid and protein synthesis by leptin. Each of these paracrine interactions requires cell-specific receptors on adjacent cells derived from the endoderm or mesoderm, respectively, i.e. PTHrP receptors on the mesoderm, and leptin receptors on the endoderm, to mediate the signaling pathways within each cell-type. It is this functional compartmentalization that is the key to understanding how specific agonists and antagonists predictably affect this mechanism of alveolar homeostasis. More importantly, it is the cell-specific molecular nature of this mechanism that we have exploited in order to effectively prevent and treat lung injuries that affect this signaling pathway.

References

[1] Bryan CS. What is the Oslerian Tradition? *Annals of Medicine*. 1994 120: 682-687.

[2] Torday JS, Rehan VK. Deconvoluting lung evolution using functional/comparative genomics. *Am J Respir Cell Mol Biol*. 2004 31:8-12.

[3] Gilbert SF. The morphogenesis of evolutionary developmental biology. *Int J Dev Biol*. 2003 47:467-477.

[4] Torday, JS. Parathyroid Hormone-related Protein is a Gravisensor in Lung and Bone Cell Biology. *Advances in Space Research*. 2003 32: 1569-1576.

[5] Torday JS, Rehan VK. Stretch-stimulated surfactant synthesis is coordinated by the paracrine actions of PTHrP and leptin. *Am J Physiol Lung Cell Mol Physiol*. 2002 283:L130-L135.

[6] Torday JS, Torres E, Rehan VK. The role of fibroblast transdifferentiation in lung epithelial cell proliferation, differentiation, and repair in vitro. *Pediatr Pathol Mol Med.* 2003 22:189-207.

[7] Rubin LP, Kovacs CS, De Paepe ME, Tsai SW, Torday JS, Kronenberg HM. Arrested pulmonary alveolar cytodifferentiation and defective surfactant synthesis in mice missing the gene for parathyroid hormone-related protein. *Dev Dyn.* 2004 230:278-289.

[8] Maina JN. Structure, function and evolution of the gas exchangers: comparative perspectives. *J Anat.* 2002 201:281-304.

[9] Demayo F, Minoo P, Plopper CG, Schuger L, Shannon J, Torday JS. Mesenchymal-epithelial interactions in lung development and repair: are modeling and remodeling the same process? *Am J Physiol Lung Cell Mol Physiol.* 2002 283:L510-517.

[10] Torday JS, Rehan VK. Up-Regulation of Fetal Rat Lung Parathyroid Hormone-Related Protein Gene Regulatory Network Down-Regulates the Sonic Hedgehog/Wnt/{beta}catenin Gene Regulatory Network. *Pediatr Res.* 2006 60:382-388.

[11] Torday J, Rehan VK. The Evolutionary Continuum from Lung Development to Homeostasis and Repair. *Am J Physiol Lung Cell Mol Physiol. 2006 (in press)*

[12] Gao Y, Raj JU. Parathyroid hormone-related protein-mediated responses in pulmonary arteries and veins of newborn lambs. *Am J Physiol Lung Cell Mol Physiol.* 2005 289:L60-L66.

[13] Torday J. A Periodic Table for Biology. *The Scientist.* 2004 18:32-33.

[14] Cool CD, Groshong SD, Rai PR, Henson PM, Stewart JS, Brown KK. Fibroblast foci are not discrete sites of lung injury or repair: the fibroblast reticulum. *Am J Respir Crit Care Med.* 2006 174:654-658.

[15] Heuberger B, Fitzka I, Wasner G, Kratochwil K. Induction of androgen receptor formation by epithelium-mesenchyme interaction in embryonic mouse mammary gland. *Proc Natl Acad Sci U S A.* 1982 79:2957-2961.

[16] Maina JN. Comparative respiratory morphology: themes and principles in the design and construction of the gas exchangers. *Anat Rec.* 2000 261:25-44.

[17] Maina JN. Fundamental structural aspects and features in the bioengineering of the gas exchangers: comparative perspectives. *Adv Anat Embryol.* 2002 Cell Biol 163:III-XII, 1-108.

[18] Maina JN. Structure, function and evolution of the gas exchangers: comparative perspectives. *J Anat.* 2002 201:281-304.

[19] Daniels CB, Orgeig S. Pulmonary surfactant: the key to the evolution of air breathing. *News Physiol Sci.* 2003 18:151-157.

[20] Massaro D, Massaro GD. Retinoids, alveolus formation, and alveolar deficiency: clinical implications. *Am J Respir Cell Mol Biol.* 2003 28:271-274.

[21] Clements JA, Nellenbogen J, Trahan HJ. Pulmonary surfactant and evolution of the lungs. *Science.* 1970 169:603-604.

[22] Weibel ER, Taylor CR, Hoppeler H. Variations in function and design: testing symmorphosis in the respiratory system. *Respir Physiol.* 1992 87:325-348.

[23] Rubin LP, Kifor O, Hua J, Brown EM, Torday JS. Parathyroid hormone (PTH) and PTH-related protein stimulate surfactant phospholipid synthesis in rat fetal lung,

apparently by a mesenchymal-epithelial mechanism. *Biochim Biophys Acta.* 1994 1223:91-100.

[24] Schultz CJ, Torres E, Londos C, Torday JS. Role of adipocyte differentiation-related protein in surfactant phospholipids synthesis by type II cells. *Am J Physiol Lung Cell Mol Physiol.* 2002 283:L288-L296.

[25] Torday JS, Sun H, Wang L, Torres E, Sunday ME, Rubin LP. Leptin mediates the parathyroid hormone-related protein paracrine stimulation of fetal lung maturation. *Am J Physiol Lung Cell Mol Physiol.* 2002 282:L405-L410.

[26] Ortega A, Ramila D, Ardura JA, Esteban V, Ruiz-Ortega M, Barat A, Gazapo R, Bosch RJ, Esbrit P. Role of parathyroid hormone-related protein in tubulointerstitial apoptosis and fibrosis after folic acid-induced nephrotoxicity. *J Am Soc Nephrol.* 2006 17:1594-1603.

[27] Wolf G, Ziyadeh FN. Leptin and renal fibrosis. *Contrib Nephrol.* 2006 151:175-183.

[28] Mason RJ. Biology of alveolar type II cells. *Respirology.* 2006 11:S12-S15.

[29] Warburton D, Schwarz M, Tefft D, Flores-Delgado G, Anderson KD, Cardoso WV. The molecular basis of lung morphogenesis. *Mech Dev.* 2000 92:55-81.

[30] Liem KF. Form and Function of Lungs: The Evolution of Air Breathing Mechanisms. *American Zoologist.* 1988 28:739-759.

[31] Perry SF, Sander M. Reconstructing the evolution of the respiratory apparatus in tetrapods. *Respir Physiol Neurobiol.* 2004 144:125-39.

[32] Jiang B, Morimoto S, Yang J, Niinoabu T, Fukuo K, Ogihara T. Expression of parathyroid hormone/parathyroid hormone-related protein receptor in vascular endothelial cells. *J Cardiovasc Pharmacol.* 1998 1:S142-S144.

[33] Meyrick B, Reid L. Ultrastructure of alveolar lining and its development. In: *Development of the Lung.* 1977 New York: Marcel Dekker, p. 135-214.

[34] Maina JN, West JB. Thin and strong! The bioengineering dilemma in the structural and functional design of the blood-gas barrier. *Physiol Rev* 2005 85:811-844.

[35] Piiper J. Alveolar-capillary gas transfer in lungs: development of concepts and current state. *Adv Exp Med Biol.* 1994 345:7-14.

[36] Massaro D, Massaro GD. Retinoids, alveolus formation, and alveolar deficiency: clinical implications. *Am J Respir Cell Mol Biol.* 2003 28:271-274.

[37] Kaesler S, Luscher B, Ruther U. Transcriptional activity of GLI1 is negatively regulated by protein kinase A. *Biol Chem.* 2000 381:545-551.

[38] Hino S, Tanji C, Nakayama KI, Kikuchi A. Phosphorylation of beta-catenin by cyclic AMP-dependent protein kinase stabilizes beta-catenin through inhibition of its ubiquitination. *Mol Cell Biol.* 2005 25:9063-9072.

[39] Vaccaro C, Brody JS. Ultrastructure of developing alveoli. I. The role of the interstitial fibroblast. *Anat Rec.* 1978 192: 467-479.

[40] McGowan SE, Torday JS. The pulmonary lipofibroblast (lipid interstitial cell) and its contributions to alveolar development. *Annu Rev Physiol.* 1997 59:43-62.

[41] Rehan VK, Sugano S, Wang Y, Santos J, Romero S, Dasgupta C, Keane MP, Stahlman MT, Torday JS. Evidence for the presence of lipofibroblasts in human lung. *Exp Lung Res.* 2006 32:379-93.

[42] Gewolb IH, Torday JS. High glucose inhibits maturation of the fetal lung in vitro. Morphometric analysis of lamellar bodies and fibroblast lipid inclusions. *Lab Invest* 1995 73:59-63.

[43] Schultz CJ, Torres E, Londos C, Torday JS. Role of adipocyte differentiation-related protein in surfactant phospholipids synthesis by type II cells. *Am J Physiol Lung Cell Mol Physiol*. 2002 283:L288-L296.

[44] Torday JS, Torday DP, Gutnick J, Qin J, Rehan V. Biologic role of fetal lung fibroblast triglycerides as antioxidants. *Pediatr Res*. 2001 49:843-849.

[45] Miskovitz P. The Law of Laplace and additional applications. *Arch Phys Med Rehabil*. 2003 84:303-4.

[46] Kallapur SG, Ikegami M. Physiological consequences of intrauterine insults. *Paediatr Respir Rev*. 2006 7:110-116.

[47] Bourbon J. In: *Pulmonary Surfactant: Biochemical, Functional, Regulatory, and Clinical Concepts*. 1991 London: CRC Press.

[48] Boros LG, Torday JS, Paul Lee WN, Rehan VK. Oxygen-induced metabolic changes and transdifferentiation in immature fetal rat lung lipofibroblasts. *Mol Genet Metab*. 2002 77:230-236.

[49] Shannon JM, Hyatt BA. Epithelial-mesenchymal interactions in the developing lung. *Annu Rev Physiol*. 2004 66:625-645.

[50] Awonusonu F, Srinivasan S, Strange J, Al-Jumaily W, Bruce MC. Developmental shift in the relative percentages of lung fibroblast subsets: role of apoptosis postseptation. *Am J Physiol*. 1999 277:L848-L859.

[51] Bruce MC, Honaker CE, Cross RJ. Lung fibroblasts undergo apoptosis following alveolarization. *Am J Respir Cell Mol Biol*. 1999 20:228-236.

[52] Bostrom H, Willetts K, Pekny M, Leveen P, Lindahl P, Hedstrand H, Pekna M, Hellstrom M, Gebre-Medhin S, Schalling M, Nilsson M, Kurland S, Tornell J, Heath JK, Betsholtz C. PDGF-A signaling is a critical event in lung alveolar myofibroblast development and alveogenesis. *Cell*. 1996 85:863-873.

[53] Hu E, Tontonoz P, Spiegelman BM. Transdifferentiation of myoblasts by the adipogenic transcription factors PPAR gamma and C/EBP alpha. *Proc Natl Acad Sci U S A*. 1995 92:9856-9860.

[54] Wang R, Ramos C, Joshi I, Zagariya A, Pardo A, Selman M, Uhal BD. Human lung myofibroblast-derived inducers of alveolar epithelial apoptosis identified as angiotensin peptides. *Am J Physiol*. 1999 277:L1158-L1164.

[55] Wang R, Alam G, Zagariya A, Gidea C, Pinillos H, Lalude O, Choudhary G, Oezatalay D, Uhal BD. Apoptosis of lung epithelial cells in response to TNF-alpha requires angiotensin II generation de novo. *J Cell Physiol*. 2000 185:253-259.

[56] Dincer HE, Gangopadhyay N, Wang R, Uhal BD. Norepinephrine induces alveolar epithelial apoptosis mediated by alpha-, beta-, and angiotensin receptor activation. *Am J Physiol Lung Cell Mol Physiol*. 2001 281:L624-L630.

[57] Filippatos GS, Gangopadhyay N, Lalude O, Parameswaran N, Said SI, Spielman W, Uhal BD. Regulation of apoptosis by vasoactive peptides. *Am J Physiol Lung Cell Mol Physiol*. 2001 281:L749-L761.

[58] Li X, Rayford H, Uhal BD. Essential roles for angiotensin receptor AT1a in bleomycin-induced apoptosis and lung fibrosis in mice. *Am J Pathol.* 2003 163:2523-2530.

[59] Torday JS, Sanchez-Esteban J, Rubin LP. Paracrine mediators of mechanotransduction in lung development. *Am J Med Sci.* 1998 316:205-208.

[60] Rehan VK, Wang Y, Patel S, Santos J, Torday JS. Rosiglitazone, a peroxisome proliferator-activated receptor-gamma agonist, prevents hyperoxia-induced neonatal rat lung injury in vivo. *Pediatr Pulmonol.* 2006 41:558-569.

[61] Chilosi M, Zamo A, Doglioni C, Reghellin D, Lestani M, Montagna L, Pedron S, Ennas MG, Cancellieri A, Murer B, Poletti V. Migratory marker expression in fibroblast foci of idiopathic pulmonary fibrosis. *Respir Res.* 2006 7:95.

[62] Holgate ST, Holloway J, Wilson S, Bucchieri F, Puddicombe S, Davies DE. Epithelial-mesenchymal communication in the pathogenesis of chronic asthma. *Proc Am Thorac Soc.* 2004 1:93-98.

[63] deLemos RA, Coalson JJ. The contribution of experimental models to our understanding of the pathogenesis and treatment of bronchopulmonary dysplasia. *Clin Perinatol.* 1992 19:521-539.

[64] Voelkel NF, Vandivier RW, Tuder RM. Vascular endothelial growth factor in the lung. *Am J Physiol Lung Cell Mol Physiol.* 290:L209-L221, 2006.

[65] Ingram JL, Bonner JC. EGF and PDGF receptor tyrosine kinases as therapeutic targets for chronic lung diseases. *Curr Mol Med.* 6:409-421, 2006.

[66] Zachman RD. Role of vitamin A in lung development. *J Nutr.* 1995 125:1634S-1638S.

[67] Thebaud B, Ladha F, Michelakis ED, Sawicka M, Thurston G, Eaton F, Hashimoto K, Harry G, Haromy A, Korbutt G, Archer SL. Vascular endothelial growth factor gene therapy increases survival, promotes lung angiogenesis, and prevents alveolar damage in hyperoxia-induced lung injury: evidence that angiogenesis participates in alveolarization. *Circulation.* 2005 112:2477-2486.

[68] Rehan VK, Torday JS. Lower parathyroid hormone-related protein content of tracheal aspirates in very low birth weight infants who develop bronchopulmonary dysplasia. *Pediatr Res.* 2006 60:216-220.

[69] Smith BT. Lung maturation in the fetal rat: acceleration by injection of fibroblast-pneumonocyte factor. *Science.* 1979 204:1094-1095.

[70] Durnberger H, Heuberger B, Schwartz P, Wasner G, Kratochwil K. Mesenchyme-mediated effect of testosterone on embryonic mammary epithelium. *Cancer Res.* 1978 38:4066-4070.

[71] Brody JS, Vaccaro C Postnatal formation of alveoli: interstitial events and physiologic consequences. *Fed Proc.* 1979 38:215-223.

[72] Torday J, Hua J, Slavin R. Metabolism and fate of neutral lipids of fetal lung fibroblast origin. *Biochim Biophys Acta.* 1995 1254:198-206.

[73] Torday JS, Sun H, Qin J. Prostaglandin E2 integrates the effects of fluid distension and glucocorticoid on lung maturation. *Am J Physiol.* 1998 274:L106-L111.

[74] Faridy EE, Permutt S, Riley RL. Effect of ventilation on surface forces in excised dogs' lungs. *J Appl Physiol.* 1966 21:1453-1462.

[75] Wyszogrodski I, Kyei-Aboagye K, Taeusch HW Jr, Avery ME. Surfactant inactivation by hyperventilation: conservation by end-expiratory pressure. *J Appl Physiol.* 1975 38:461-466.

[76] Oyarzun MJ, Clements JA, Baritussio A. Ventilation enhances pulmonary alveolar clearance of radioactive dipalmitoyl phosphatidylcholine in liposomes. *Am Rev Respir Dis.* 1980 121:709-721.

[77] Yamamoto M, Harm SC, Grasser WA, Thiede MA. Parathyroid hormone-related protein in the rat urinary bladder: a smooth muscle relaxant produced locally in response to mechanical stretch. *Proc Natl Acad Sci U S A.* 1992 89:5326-5330.

[78] Daifotis AG, Weir EC, Dreyer BE, Broadus AE. Stretch-induced parathyroid hormone-related peptide gene expression in the rat uterus. *J Biol Chem.* 1992 267:23455-23458.

[79] Alcorn D, Adamson TM, Lambert TF, Maloney JE, Ritchie BC, Robinson PM. Morphological effects of chronic tracheal ligation and drainage in the fetal lamb lung. *J Anat.* 1977 123:649-660.

[80] Coalson JJ. Experimental models of bronchopulmonary dysplasia. *Biol Neonate.* 1997 71:35-38.

[81] Davis JM. Role of oxidant injury in the pathogenesis of neonatal lung disease. *Acta Paediatr.* 2002 91:23-25.

[82] Jobe AH. Antenatal associations with lung maturation and infection. *J Perinatol.* 2005 25:S31-S35.

[83] Scarpelli EM. Perinatal lung mechanics and the first breath. *Lung.* 1984 162:61-71.

[84] Wirtz HR, Dobbs LG. Calcium mobilization and exocytosis after one mechanical stretch of lung epithelial cells. *Science.* 1990 250:1266-1269.

[85] Rehan V, Torday J. Hyperoxia augments pulmonary lipofibroblast-to-myofibroblast transdifferentiation. *Cell Biochem Biophys.* 2003 38:239-250.

[86] Soina Dargan-Batra, Sonia Romero, Sharon Sugano, Jamie Santos, Ying Wang, John S. Torday, and Virender K. Rehan. Prenatal Lung Inflammation: The Mechanism for the Decrease in Respiratory Distress Syndrome and the Increase in Bronchopulmonary Dysplasia. *Peds Res. (In Press)*

[87] Hanrahan JP, Tager IB, Segal MR, Tosteson TD, Castile RG, Van Vunakis H, Weiss ST, and Speizer FE. The effect of maternal smoking during pregnancy on early infant lung function. *Am Rev Respir Dis.* 1992 145: 1129-1135.

[88] Pierce RA, Nguyen NM. Prenatal nicotine exposure and abnormal lung function. *Am J Respir Cell Mol Biol.* 2002 26: 10-13.

[89] Lieberman E, Torday J, Barbieri R, Cohen A, Van Vunakin H,Weiss ST. Association of intrauterine cigarette smoke exposure with indices of fetal lung maturation. *Obstet Gynecol.* 1992 79: 564-570.

[90] Collins MH, Moessinger AC, Kleinerman J, Bassi J, Rosso P, Collins AM, James LS,Blanc WA. Fetal lung hypoplasia associated with maternal smoking: A morphometric analysis. *Pediatr Res.* 1985 19: 408-412.

[91] Sekhon HS, Keller JA, Benowitz NL, Spindel ER. Prenatal nicotine exposure alters pulmonary function in newborn rhesus monkeys. *Am J Respir Crit Care Med.* 2001 164:989-994.

[92] Rehan VK, Wang Y, Sugano S, Romero S, Chen X, Santos J, Khazanchi A, Torday JS. Mechanism of nicotine-induced pulmonary fibroblast transdifferentiation. *Am J Physiol Lung Cell Mol Physiol* 2005 289:L667-L676.

[93] Rehan VK, Sakurai R,Wang Y,Santos J,Huynh K, Torday JS. Reversal of Nicotine-Induced Alveolar Lipofibroblast-to-Myofibroblast Transdifferentiation by Stimulants of Parathyroid Hormone-related Protein Signaling. *Exptl Lung Res. (in Press).*

[94] Jobe AJ. The new BPD: an arrest of lung development. *Pediatr Res*. 1999 46:641-643.

[95] Dobzhansky T. Nothing in Biology Makes Sense Except in the Light of Evolution. *American Biology Teacher*. 1973 35:125-129.

In: Novel Aspects of PTHrP Physiopathology
Editor: Claudio Luparello, pp. 95-113
ISBN: 978-1-60021-857-6

Chapter V

ROLE OF PTHRP IN RENAL PATHOPHYSIOLOGY

Pedro Esbrit[1,*], ***David Ramila***[1], ***Juan Antonio Ardura***[1],
Arantxa Ortega[2], ***Montserrat Romero***[2], ***Ricardo J. Bosch***[2]
[1]Bone and Mineral Metabolism Laboratory, Fundación Jiménez Díaz (Capio Group), Madrid, Spain;
[2]Laboratory of Renal Physiology and Experimental Nephrology, Department of Physiology, Alcalá University, Alcalá de Henares, Spain.

ABSTRACT

Parathyroid hormone (PTH)-related protein (PTHrP) was initially isolated from hypercalcemia-associated tumors. However, PTHrP is present in many normal tissues where it exerts a variety of actions, including regulation of cell proliferation and/or differentiation. This lends support to the notion that PTHrP is a developmental and/or growth-regulating factor, more related to other cytokines and growth factors than to PTH. In the kidney, PTHrP and its receptor, the PTH1 receptor, are abundant throughout the nephron and in the renal vessels. Besides its renal PTH-like effects, PTHrP appears to act as a local regulating agent for renal vessels, glomeruli and the tubular epithelium. Several groups including our own group have provided data supporting that PTHrP upregulation is a common event associated with renal injury and/or repair, but its pathophysiological significance is only recently beginning to be unraveled. To help define the true role of PTHrP in the damaged kidney, several models of experimental nephropathies have been used. In addition, the functional consequences of chronic PTHrP overexpression in the proximal tubule have recently been evaluated in some of these models. Using rats with nephrotoxic acute renal failure (ARF), we demonstrated that angiotensin II (Ang II) blockade prevents PTHrP upregulation related to the improvement in both tubular damage and renal function. Moreover, we have disclosed an intracellular mechanism whereby a nephrotoxic dose of folic acid activates the Ang

* Correspondence concerning this article should be addressed to: Pedro Esbrit, Ph.D. Laboratorio de Metabolismo Mineral y Óseo, Unidad de Investigación Fundación Jiménez Díaz (Capio Group), Avda. Reyes Católicos, 2 28040 Madrid (Spain). Phone: 34-91-550-4894; Fax: 34-91-549-8075; e-mail: pesbrit@fjd.es.

II/Ang II type 1 receptor system leading to increased PTHrP expression in tubuloepithelial cells. In fact, current hypothesis suggests that PTHrP might exert a reciprocal control on, or recapitulate, at least some Ang II effects in the damaged kidney. Recent studies also show that PTHrP, in spite of its prosurvival effect on tubulointerstitial cells, was inefficient to prevent renal damage in experimental ARF. The former effect was instead associated with proinflammatory and profibrogenic features in this setting. Related to these findings, PTHrP seems to be involved in the mechanisms of diabetic nephropathy. Thus, the higher PTHrP and PTH1R levels in the kidney of diabetic mice were found to be associated with a significant increase in proteinuria. Collectively, current findings strongly support the implication of PTHrP as a pathogenic factor in tubular and glomerular diseases. PTHrP might contribute to the progression of renal damage by complex mechanisms: increasing tubulointerstitial cell survival, interstitial cell infiltration and fibroblastic activation, and/or affecting glomerular cell function.

Introduction

Parathyroid hormone-related protein (PTHrP) was discovered at the end of the 1980s as the factor responsible for humoral hypercalcemia of malignancy [1]. Overproduction of PTHrP by tumor cells and its release into the circulation allowed this protein to exert PTH-like actions, such as increasing both renal calcium reabsorption and bone resorption, by interaction with the common PTH/PTHrP type 1 receptor (PTH1R) [2]. Partial sequence and conformational homologies within the N-terminal domain of both PTH and PTHrP account for their similar binding affinity to the PTH1R [3]. However, while PTH is a well characterized endocrine regulator of mineral homeostasis, PTHrP is widely expressed in nonmalignant fetal and adult tissues [4]. Indeed, PTH and PTHrP are the products of different genes on distinct chromosomes, differing in their complexity. Thus, some structural features of PTHrP gene (e.g., instability motifs in its 3'-untranslated regions) are reminiscent of those found in many cytokines and growth factors [1,4]. The PTHrP gene contains 9 exons which give rise by alternative splicing to three different transcripts generating three protein isoforms with a different C-terminus of 139, 141 or 173 aminoacids. Furthermore, PTHrP post-translational processing generates various fragments lacking PTH homology, whose biological activity remains to be clarified [5] (Figure 1).

Despite the widespread production of PTHrP in normal tissues, its circulating concentration in healthy subjects is below the detectable limit of the majority of current assays [6]. Thus, in contrast to the situation of humoral hypercalcemia of malignancy in which PTHrP plays the role of a classical hormone, PTHrP exerts paracrine, autocrine and/or even intracrine actions in normal tissues. PTHrP is a key regulator of placental calcium transport in the foetus, and it appears to be a physiological modulator of smooth muscle tone. In addition, a growing body of evidence supports the notion that PTHrP can act as a developmental and growth-regulating factor, much like other known cytokines and growth factors than PTH [1,4,7].

The developmental and physiological aspects of PTHrP in the kidney have received attention and compiled in a recent review [7]. The following paragraphs are thus included here to provide a *physiological framework* in which to fit our present review, focused on the putative roles of PTHrP in kidney injury.

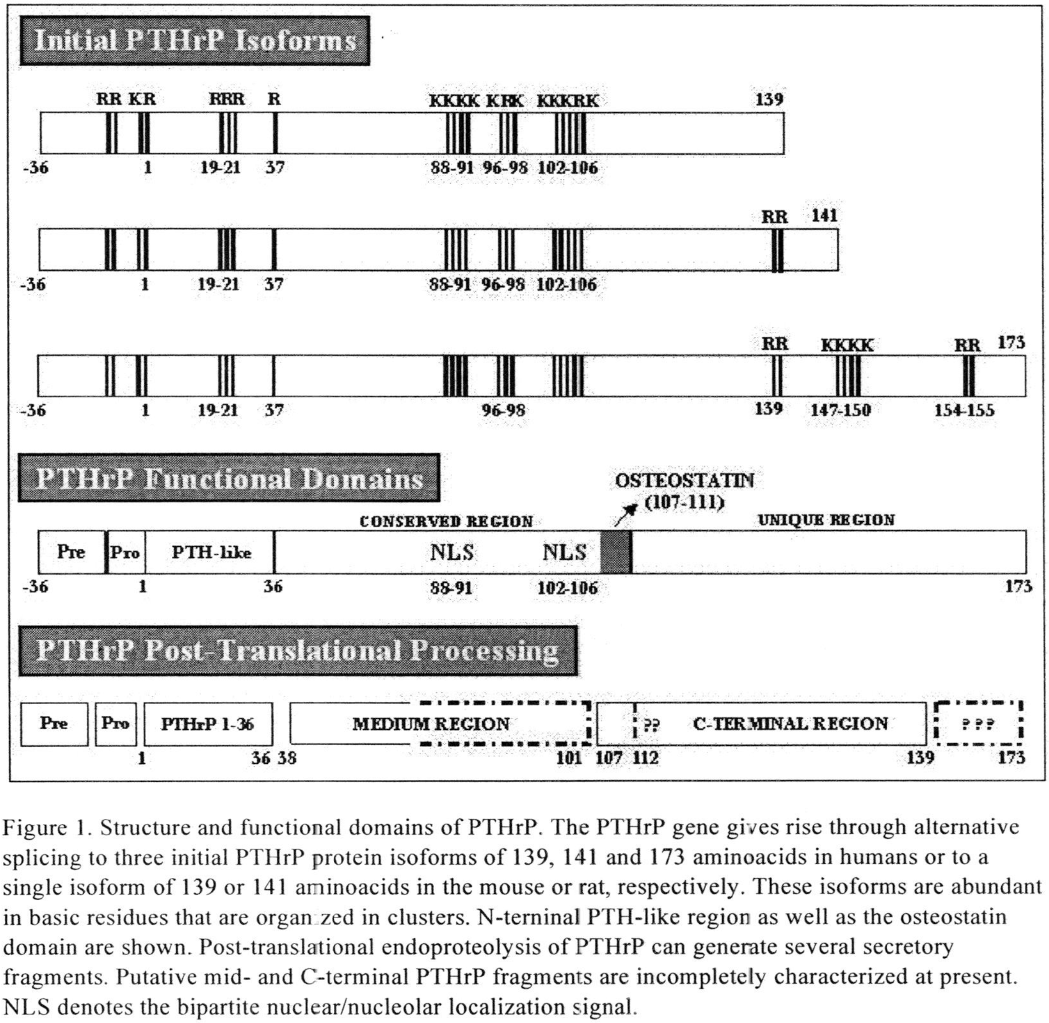

Figure 1. Structure and functional domains of PTHrP. The PTHrP gene gives rise through alternative splicing to three initial PTHrP protein isoforms of 139, 141 and 173 aminoacids in humans or to a single isoform of 139 or 141 aminoacids in the mouse or rat, respectively. These isoforms are abundant in basic residues that are organized in clusters. N-terminal PTH-like region as well as the osteostatin domain are shown. Post-translational endoproteolysis of PTHrP can generate several secretory fragments. Putative mid- and C-terminal PTHrP fragments are incompletely characterized at present. NLS denotes the bipartite nuclear/nucleolar localization signal.

PTHrP and its Receptors in the Kidney

The expression of PTHrP and the PTH1R has been examined in the developing mouse kidney [8]. High PTHrP mRNA levels were found in the collecting duct, urothelium of the pelvis, and immature elements of the glomeruli. In contrast, the PTH1R mRNA was not found in the two former sites, but it increased in the developing tubules and glomeruli associated with the maturation process [8]. These findings suggest a role for PTHrP during mouse renal development. However, this notion is controversial, since mice with targeted disruption of the PTHrP gene show a normal kidney morphology; although a possible altered renal function is unknown as these mice die at birth [9]. More recently, mice overexpressing PTHrP in the renal proximal tubule under the direction of the γ-glutamyl transpeptidase promoter have been generated [10]. PTHrP-overexpressing animals exhibited a normal renal morphology and function, except for a discrete hypophosphatemia, up to at least six months of age [10]. This indicates that PTHrP overexpression in the renal proximal tubule does not appear to interfere in normal nephron development.

In the adult kidney, PTHrP has been identified by immunohistochemistry or *in situ* hybridization in the glomerular podocytes, and proximal, distal, and collecting tubules, as well as in the intrarenal arterial tree, including afferent and efferent arterioles, and in the macula densa [11-15]. In addition, using immunohistochemistry or different mRNA detection techniques, the PTH1R has been detected in both convoluted and straight proximal tubules, in straight ascending limbs, and in distal convoluted tubules, consistent with known sites of PTH action [12-15]. Moreover, the PTH1R is expressed in the glomerulo-vascular system, including podocytes [13,15-18]. Early studies failed to detect the PTH1R mRNA in mesangial cells in both rats and humans by Northern blot, *in situ* hybridization, or RT-PCR [16,19]. However, our recent studies using either the latter technique or RNAse protection assay, have shown that this receptor is expressed in rat mesangial cells [15]. Indeed, this might provide a rationale for the previously reported mitogenic effect of PTHrP in these cells [19,20]. It is possible that some of the aforementioned methods of mRNA analysis might be less efficient to detect putative splice variants of the PTH1R which could be present in mesangial cells [21,22].

Actions of PTHrP in the Glomerulo-Vascular System

In the kidney, as in every tissue examined, PTHrP has shown to be a potent smooth muscle relaxant by acting through the PTH1R [7]. Fritsch *et al* [23] recently demonstrated that induction of PTH1R overexpression in vessels by systemic PTH1R cDNA delivery decreased blood pressure and renal tone in adult rats. In the same way, overexpression of PTHrP or the PTH1R in the arterial wall of transgenic mice resulted in hypotension; an effect which is likely mediated by both NO and cAMP [11,24,25]. Mechanical stretch and a variety of vasoactive factors such as angiotensin II (Ang II), serotonin, and bradykinin rapidly induce PTHrP gene expression in smooth muscle cells [7,26,27]. The effect of Ang II on PTHrP expression is rapid and transient, in a fashion reminiscent of that of immediate response genes in these cells [26]. Thus, at least in certain pathophysiological settings, PTHrP may serve as a counterbalancing modulator of the contractile effects of Ang II, and possibly of other vasoconstrictors. In support of this notion, deregulation of the renal PTHrP system has shown to be associated with an increased renal vascular resistance in a model of genetic hypertension [28]. All these data suggest that the endogenous PTHrP/PTH1R system appears to be a crucial regulator of vascular tone.

Several findings support a local role for PTHrP in the control of glomerular filtration rate in the glomerulus. Using a hydronephrotic rat kidney model, local administration of the N-terminal PTHrP fragment induced vasodilatation of all preglomerular vascular segments, including the afferent arteriole, and an increase in renal blood flow [29]. Furthermore, intrarenal infusion of this fragment into the left renal artery of anaesthetized rats increased renal blood flow, glomerular filtration rate and urine flow in the left kidney [30]. PTHrP (1-

34) has also been found to exert a direct relaxant effect on isolated human mesangial cells [19]; an effect which would promote an increase in both K_f and glomerular filtration rate. Therefore, current data support the notion that locally produced PTHrP might participate in the regulation of renal blood flow and glomerular filtration rate.

Besides its vasoactive effects, PTHrP might also exert other relevant actions in the glomerulus. Soifer *et al* [20] demonstrated an up-regulation of PTHrP expression in the rat glomeruli and tubules during recovery from renal ischemia. Interestingly, these investigators reported a mitogenic effect of PTHrP (1-34) in cultured rat mesangial cells, suggesting its putative role in the recovery of the ischemia-injured kidney [20]. Thus, these authors provided the first evidence for a putative role of PTHrP in the glomerulus in the setting of renal disease. Supporting further this notion, Bosch et al [19] found that PTHrP (1-34) induced a proliferative effect even at <nM doses in human mesangial cells in vitro, which suggests its physiological significance.

Physiology of PTHrP in the Tubular Epithelium

PTHrP interacts with the PTH1R and thus induces PTH-like effects on renal tubular cells: it increases calcium reabsorption in the distal tubule, while inhibits phosphate and bicarbonate reabsorption as well as the Na+/H+ exchange, and stimulates 1α-hydroxylase activity in the renal proximal tubule [2,31]. In fact, some of these PTHrP features allowed its initial characterization and isolation from tumors associated with hypercalcemia [1].

Studies in renal tubuloepithelial cells LLC-PK_1, stably transfected with the PTH1R, show high affinity binding -in the nM range- of the homologous N-terminal domain of PTH and PTHP, associated with cAMP accumulation and intracellular calcium/phospholipase C activation [32,33]. This is in contrast to findings in vascular smooth muscle cells where PTH1R signals exclusively through the cAMP pathway [34]. Current data support the notion that both the PTH1R density and its G protein coupling efficiency provide different mechanisms for regulating the intracellular signaling pathway associated with, and eventually the biological response to, N-terminal PTHrP in renovascular cells [33-35].

In addition, different nephron segments appear to exhibit a distinct pattern of PTH1R signaling. Therefore, in the distal tubule, the mechanism of the PTH1R-dependent increase in transcellular calcium absorption involves a sustained phospholipase D-dependent rise in intracellular calcium not observed in the proximal tubule [36]. In the latter segment, on the other hand, phospholipase C is responsible for intracellular calcium transients and PKC activation through PTH1R [36]. In addition, both PTH and PTHrP similarly inhibit apical Na^+/H^+ exchange, at least in part, by a cAMP-dependent mechanism in the proximal tubule [31,37].

PTHrP has also actions unrelated to those traditionally associated with PTH in renal tissue. Thus, PTHrP is mitogenic for renal tubuloepithelial cells, including proximal and distal tubule cells [38-41]. The proliferative effect of PTHrP in proximal tubule cells appears to occur through PTH1R-associated activation of both cAMP and protein kinase C [40,41]. More recently, PTHrP has been shown to display anti-apoptotic features in renal tubuloepithelial and fibroblastic cells; an effect which seems to occur by interaction with the PTH1R [14,42]. The pathophysiological impact of this recent finding is dealt with below.

PTHrP in Renal Injury

Ischemic and toxic injury to renal tubular epithelial cells can cause both acute and chronic renal failure depending on the intensity and exposure time to the damage [43,44]. Proliferation of injured tubule cells appears to be important for timely tubular recovery after renal injury, and for subsequent functional recovery of the damaged kidney. Several growth factors and cytokines, acting in an autocrine and paracrine manner, appear to participate in the repair process of the tubular epithelium in this setting [10,44-47].

The mitogenic features of PTHrP and its early overexpression after renal injury in experimental models of acute renal failure (ARF) induced by either ischemia or nephrotoxins initially suggested that PTHrP could participate in the regenerative process after ARF [14,20]. However, this putative role of PTHrP in the acutely damaged kidney was intriguing, since the PTH1R gene was found to be rapidly downregulated following ARF [14,20]. This is in sharp contrast to other well characterized renal mitogens, such as epidermal growth factor (EGF) and hepatocyte growth factor, whose receptors are upregulated after ARF [44,46]. Moreover, the PTH1R was also found to decrease in the kidney of protein-overloaded rats with tubulointerstitial damage [13]. Current evidence suggests that factors other than PTHrP or Ang II are likely to account for the PTH1R downregulation associated with kidney damage [10,15]. It is interesting to mention in this context that spliced variants of this receptor showing low expression in the cell surface have shown to be present in the kidney [21]. In addition, the PTH1R can be internalized into the nucleus of renal tubular cells [48]. The pathophysiological relevance of these mechanisms for the PTHrP action in the damaged kidney is presently unknown. The hypothetical beneficial effects of PTHrP as a mitogen in ARF was further questioned when considering that targeted delivery of PTHrP to the proximal tubule in mice failed to provide protection against renal ischemia or folic acid injury [10]. Moreover, experimental data using the latter model in rats showed that pretreatment with Ang II blockers abolished the PTHrP upregulation but not tubular hyperplasia [49]. Thus, current evidence makes it unlikely that PTHrP has a significant role in the regenerative process after acute kidney injury.

Renal PTHrP upregulation was also observed in other experimental nephropathies. Thus, chronic cyclosporin administration, which induces tubular atrophy and interstitial fibrosis, was shown to be associated with an increased PTHrP expression, at both mRNA and protein levels, in the rat renal cortex [50]. Moreover, PTHrP mRNA was found to increase sequentially in the renal cortex during the development of proteinuria in a rat model of tubulointerstitial damage after protein overload [13]. Interestingly, in the latter model, dramatic PTHrP immunostaining was revealed in glomerular mesangial cells, associated with an increased mesangial growth and matrix expansion in those rats with intense proteinuria [13]. These findings suggest that PTHrP could have a role on the mechanisms associated with progression of kidney damage.

Interaction between PTHrP and Angiotensin II in the Damaged Kidney

The renin-angiotensin system is well known to play an important pathogenic role on the mechanisms of renal injury [51,52]. In fact, the main agonist of this system, Ang II, can be envisioned as a growth factor which can promote the progression of kidney damage [53,54]. Activation of components of the renin-angiotensin system, including Ang II, locally in the kidney has shown to occur early in various experimental models of ARF, e.g., folic acid-induced nephrotoxicity or ischemia/reperfusion [14,49,55,56]. Moreover, Ang II antagonists exert beneficial effects on renal function in these models [49,57,58].

Recent data strongly suggest that PTHrP might be involved in the mechanisms related to Ang II-induced renal injury. Exogenously administered Ang II, via its type 1 (AT_1) receptor, increases PTHrP expression in glomerular and tubular cells as well as in vascular smooth muscle cells both *in vivo* and *in vitro* [15,26,27]. Interestingly, a significant correlation between PTHrP overexpression and tubular damage and fibrosis was observed in the rat kidney after systemic Ang II infusion [15]. Furthermore, in nephrotoxic ARF, the improvement of renal function by Ang II antagonists was associated with inhibition of PTHrP overexpression [49].

As mentioned above, Ang II can be synthesized by renal cells where it may act in an autocrine, paracrine or even intracrine manner [55,59,60]. In fact, interaction of intracellular Ang II with Ang II nuclear receptors can increase gene transcription, and occurs associated with disease severity in conditions such as diabetes and hypertension [59-61]. Our recent studies demonstrate that such a mechanism involving the perinuclear relocalization of an Ang II/AT1 receptor complex may account for PTHrP induction by a nephrotoxic dose of folic acid in tubuloepithelial cells [49]. We also disclosed an intracellular pathway whereby Ang II triggers PTHrP gene transcription in these cells. This mechanism requires phosphorylation of extracellular signal-regulated kinases and subsequent activation of cAMP response element-binding protein [49]. Collectively, current data suggest that: 1) Ang II is a likely candidate responsible for PTHrP overexpression; and 2) PTHrP might contribute to the deleterious effects of Ang II, in the damaged kidney. These findings have established a new rationale for further studies focused on the putative contribution of PTHrP to the mechanisms of renal damage.

PTHrP as a Pro-Inflammatory and Pro-Fibrogenic Cytokine in the Damaged Kidney

Inflammation involves complex molecular and cellular mechanisms which are activated against physical, chemical or biological aggressions. This process normally serves a positive biological goal (e.g., to overcome invasion of potentially deleterious agents), but it may have detrimental effects in chronic pathological settings, such as progressive renal disease [62-64]. Tubulointerstitial inflammation is a key event in a variety of nephropathies. Early after renal injury, damaged tubuloepithelial cells begin to overexpress proinflammatory cytokines and chemokines, which promote migration of monocytes/macrophages and T-lymphocytes to the renal interstitium [64,65]. Both infiltrating leukocytes and damaged tubuloepithelial cells activate and induce proliferation of resident fibroblasts in the tubulointerstitial compartment. A severe and prolonged injury will determine a sustained activation of proinflammatory pathways, associated with overexpression of profibrogenic cytokines by tubulointerstitial cells leading to fibrogenesis and renal function loss [66].

Early studies suggested that PTHrP might act as an important mediator of proinflammatory cytokines, namely tumour necrosis factor and interleukin-6, in multi-organ inflammation and rheumatoid arthritis [67]. More recent studies have shown that PTHrP activates nuclear factor (NF)-κB and the expression of NF-κB-dependent cytokines and chemokines [e.g., IL-6 and monocyte chemoattractant protein-1 (MCP-1)] in different cell types [68,69]. PTHrP and MCP-1 were found to colocalize in smooth muscle cells in human atherosclerotic plaques [69-71]. Moreover, our preliminary results in mice with unilateral ureteral obstruction -a well characterized model of renal inflammation- have shown high levels of several cytokines, chemokines and adhesion molecules, and an increased leukocyte infiltration into the interstitium of the obstructed mouse kidney, associated with PTHrP overexpression [72]. Moreover, we recently found a direct induction of various proinflammatory cytokines and chemokines by PTHrP (1-36) in tubulolepithelial cells in culture [42,72]. Since sustained renal inflammation is closeley related to fibrogenesis, these data point to PTHrP as a likely pro-inflammatory and pro-fibrogenic cytokine in the damaged kidney.

Apoptosis is considered to be an important component of the acute response of the tubular epithelium to injury [73,74]. Previous studies showed that PTHrP can inhibit apoptosis in several cell types, like pancreatic β-cells and chondrocytes [75,76]. At least in the latter cells, this antiapoptotic effect appears to involve PTHrP interaction with the PTH1R, and also its internalization into the nucleus [75]. We recently found that PTHrP, interacting with the PTH1R, directly acts as a survival factor for renal tubulointerstitial cells by a dual mechanism involving Bcl-XL upregulation and activation of the phosphatidylinositol-3 kinase/Akt/Bad pathway [42]. Our data, using PTHrP-overexpressing mice with folic acid-induced ARF, suggest that this PTHrP action might have detrimental consequences in the injured kidney. These mice showed a significant delay in renal function recovery and higher focal areas of tubulointerstitial fibrosis than normal mice, associated with a decrease in apoptotic tubulointerstitial cells [42]. The rationale for this association might come from the fact that apoptosis of interstitial fibroblasts appears to be a mechanism to prevent fibrogenesis [43,77].

The process of fibrogenesis involves activation and proliferation of fibroblasts –induced by both tubuloepithelial and infiltrating cells-, as well as secretion of matrix compounds by both activated fibroblasts and tubular cells [78]. In fact, an increased matrix synthesis and deposition, and loss of tubular structural integrity, are paramount events at later stages of fibrogenesis [78]. Our recent studies indicate that the higher number of infiltrating macrophages was associated with increased fibroblast proliferation in the renal interstitium of folic acid-injured kidneys from PTHrP-overexpressing mice [42]. In these mice, an increased immunostaining for α-smooth muscle actin (SMA), a marker of activated fibroblasts or myofibroblasts [79], was also observed in the renal interstitium after folic acid nephrotoxicity [42]. Consistent with the latter *in vivo* finding, PTHrP (1-36) was found to stimulate α-SMA expression in renal fibroblasts *in vitro* [42]. In addition, a higher immunostaining for both types I and IV collagens was observed in the renal interstitium of the obstructed kidneys from PTHrP-overexpressing mice than in their normal littermates [80]. In agreement with this finding, PTHrP (1-36) was found to stimulate the expression of both types of collagens, type-1 procollagen and fibronectin in tubuloepithelial cells and renal fibroblasts *in vitro* [42]. At least part of these effects were abolished by a PTH1R antagonist [42].

Tubuloepithelial cells might also contribute to development of renal fibrosis by directly generating myofibroblasts through a process known as epithelial-mesenchymal transition (EMT) [80,81]. In fact, studies in both human and experimental nephropathies point to EMT as the main source of activated fibroblasts in the renal parenchyma [81]. This process involves disaggregation of epithelia units and epithelium reshaping to facilitate cell movement. Thus, epithelium in transition loses polarity, as well as its tigtht junctions, desmosomes, and intermediate cytokeratin filaments, in order to rearrange their F-actin stress fibers, and begin to form filopodia and lamelipodia. These phenotypic changes require molecular reprogramming of epithelium, with a dramatic proteome change [82-84]. A variety of growth factors, including transforming growth factor (TGF)-β, EGF, insulin growth factor II (IGF-II), and fibroblast growth factor-2 can stimulate EMT [84,85]. Preliminary data from our laboratory also support that PTHrP might interact with some of these factors to promote EMT in tubuloepithelial cells [86]. Collectively, present findings strongly suggest the complex roles of PTHrP as a proinflammatory and profibrogenic factor contributing to progression of kidney injury.

PTHrP and Diabetic Nephropathy

Most studies to assess the actions of PTHrP in the damaged kidney have focused on experimental nephropathies characterized by renal tubuloephitelial damage. Recently, It has been hypothesized that PTHrP might also be involved in the pathogenic mechanisms of glomerular diseases, such as diabetic nephropathy. This condition -the most important cause of chronic renal failure in industrialized societies- is characterized by an initial phase of renal hypertrophy, at both tubular and glomerular level, followed by an increased urinary albumin excretion accompanied by a progressive loss of renal function [87-89]. Izquierdo *et al* [90] have recently evaluated the expression of PTHrP in the kidney of mice with streptozotocin-induced diabetes. This animal model is characterized by development of renal hypertrophy and increased proteinuria early in the course of the disease [91]. Diabetic mice showed a significant increase of both PTHrP and the PTH1R proteins -in the renal tubules and glomeruli- within 2-8 weeks from diabetes onset. In addition, these mice, in contrast to nondiabetic animals, showed a remarkable nuclear immunostaining for PTHrP in the renal tubules [90]. Thus, PTHrP might act in an autocrine, paracrine and/or intracrine fashion in the diabetic mouse kidney. Consistent with these in vivo findings, high glucose medium was found to increase PTHrP and the PTH1R proteins in mouse tubuloepithelial cells, mesangial cells, and podocytes in culture. Interestingly, this increase in PTHrP (but not that of the PTH1R) was inhibited by the AT_1 receptor antagonist losartan in these cell lines [90]. Therefore, Ang II activation might be responsible for PTHrP induction in the diabetic kidney [92,93]. A previous study demonstrated that Ang II increased the PTH1R in the rat kidney *in vivo*, while it failed to affect this receptor expression in either rat mesangial or mouse tubuloepithelial cells *in vitro* [15]. Thus, a putative role of this vasoactive factor on the observed changes in the PTH1R expression in the diabetic kidney cannot be ruled out from current *in vitro* data [15]. Collectively, however, recent findings indicate that hyperglycemia should be added to the increasing list of renal pathophysiological conditions associated with an altered PTHrP/PTH1R system.

The functional consequences of chronic PTHrP overexpression in the mouse diabetic kidney have also recently analyzed in PTHrP-overexpressing mice with streptozotocin-induced diabetes. These animals were found to display a higher degree of renal hypertrophy than their diabetic control littermates [90]. Interestingly, in this regard, our preliminary data have shown that high glucose-induced expression of cell cycle kinase inhibitory protein $p27^{Kip1}$ was inhibited by neutralizing PTHrP antibodies in both mouse podocytes and human mesangial cells in culture [94]. As mentioned above, PTHrP appears to be an important regulatory factor of glomerular haemodynamics [7], and thus it might participate in the pathophysiology of glomerular hyperfiltration. Furthermore, PTHrP might interact with other up-regulated factors in diabetes, namely Ang II and TGF-β, which are known to have important roles in this diabetes-related feature [92]. In fact, this protein may act as a downstream effector of TGF-β at least in some cells [95,96]. As mentioned above in this review, PTHrP has mitogenic features in proximal tubular cells [40]. Interestingly, in this regard, TGF-β can transform a mitogenic stimulus into hypertrophy in tubuloepithelial cells [97,98]. Taken together, these findings suggest that PTHrP might be involved in the mechanisms of diabetic renal hypertrophy.

Diabetic PTHrP-overexpressing mice had increased proteinuria and lower total plasma protein levels than their diabetic control littermates. Indeed, there was a significant increase in the risk of developing proteinuria in those mice with the higher PTHrP and PTH1R levels [90]. The pathophysiological implications of the latter finding come from the fact that the amount of proteinuria is a reliable predictor of diabetic nephropathy [99,100]. It is tempting to speculate that several mechanisms would contribute to the relationship between the PTHrP/PTH1R system and proteinuria in this diabetic model. First, as mentioned above, PTHrP is a potent vasorelaxant which can interact with vasoactive factors affecting glomerular haemodynamics and permeability [7,11,19,30]. Second, due to the pro-inflammatory/pro-fibrogenic properties of PTHrP, which have been dealt with previously in this review, this protein might favour the inflammatory process associated with the development of diabetic nephropathy.

CONCLUSION

The PTHrP/PTH1R system appears to exert several functions in normal renal physiology -including PTH-like actions in the renal tubule and modulation of renal hemodynamics-, and PTHrP upregulation represents a common event in several experimental nephropathies. Current data support the notion that Ang II is a major factor responsible for PTHrP overexpression in both ARF and diabetic nephropathy. In the former condition, PTHrP appears to contribute to the progression of renal damage by increasing tubulointerstitial cell survival, promoting inflammation and fibrogenesis (Figure 2). In diabetic nephropathy, PTHrP can favor renal hypertrophy and proteinuria. Collectively, available data strongly support the implication of PTHrP as a pathogenic factor in kidney disease, and provide novel insights into the protective effects of Ang II antagonists in various nephropathies.

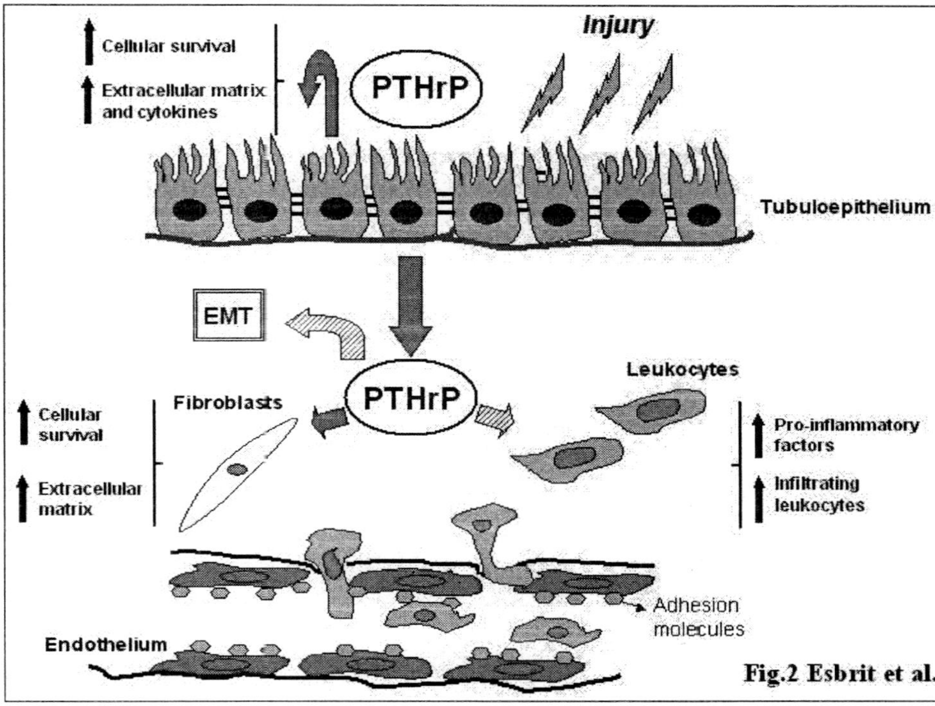

Figure 2. Scheme representing the complex actions whereby PTHrP might promote inflammation and fibrogenesis in the acutely damaged kidney. EMT = Epithelial-mesenchymal transition.

ACKNOWLEDGMENTS

Parts of the studies performed by the authors of this review as described here were supported by grants from the Spanish Ministry of Science and Technology (PB98-0700-C02-01/02 and SAF2002-04356-C03-01/03), the Spanish Ministry of Education and Science (SAF2005-06964), Comunidad Autónoma de Madrid (CAM 08.6/0038/2000-1/2 and GR/SAL/0415/2004), Universidad de Alcalá (CAM-UAH 2005/050), the Spanish Society of Nephrology, and Fundación Renal Íñigo Álvarez de Toledo. A. Ortega and J.A. Ardura were supported by Conchita Rábago Foundation, and D. Rámila from "Ikerketa eta Prestakuntza Programa" from the Basque Government. A. Ortega is currently a recipient of a research contract from "Juan de la Cierva" Program from the Spanish Ministry of Education and Science.

REFERENCES

[1] Martin, T.J., Moseley, J.M., and Williams,E.D. (1997) Parathyroid hormone-related protein: hormone and cytokine. *J Endocrinol, 154* Suppl, S23-S37.

[2] Everhart-Caye, M., Inzucchi, S.E., Guinness-Henry,J., Mitnick,M.A., and Stewart,A.F. (1996) Parathyroid hormone (PTH)-related protein(1-36) is equipotent to PTH(1-34) in humans. *J Clin Endocrinol Metab, 81*, 199-208.

[3] Schipani, E., Karga,H., Karaplis,A.C., Potts,J.T., Jr., Kronenberg,H.M., Segre,G.V., Abou-Samra,A.B., and Juppner,H. (1993) Identical complementary deoxyribonucleic acids encode a human renal and bone parathyroid hormone (PTH)/PTH-related peptide receptor. *Endocrinology, 132*, 2157-2165.

[4] Philbrick,W.M., Wysolmerski,J.J., Galbraith,S., Holt,E., Orloff,J.J., Yang,K.H., Vasavada,R.C., Weir,E.C., Broadus,A.E., and Stewart,A.F. (1996) Defining the roles of parathyroid hormone-related protein in normal physiology. *Physiol Rev., 76*, 127-173.

[5] Yang,K.H., dePapp,A.E., Soifer,N.E., Dreyer,B.E., Wu,T.L., Porter,S.E., Bellantoni,M., Burtis,W.J., Insogna,K.L., Broadus,A.E., and Philbrick, W.M., and Stewart, A.F. (1994) Parathyroid hormone-related protein: evidence for isoform- and tissue-specific posttranslational processing. *Biochemistry, 33*, 7460-7469.

[6] de Miguel,F., Motellón, J.L., Hurtado, J., Jiménez, F.J., and Esbrit, P. (1998) Comparison of two immunoradiometric assays for parathyroid hormone-related protein in the evaluation of cancer patients with and without hypercalcemia. *Clin Chim Acta, 277*, 171-180.

[7] Clemens, T.L., Cormier, S., Eichinger, A., Endlich, K., Fiaschi-Taesch, N., Fischer,E., Friedman, P.A., Karaplis, A.C., Massfelder,T., Rossert, J., Schluter, K.D., Silve,C., Stewart, A.F., Takane, K., and Helwig, J.J. (2001) Parathyroid hormone-related protein and its receptors: nuclear functions and roles in the renal and cardiovascular systems, the placental trophoblasts and the pancreatic islets. *Br J Pharmacol, 134*, 1113-1136.

[8] Aya, K., Tanaka, H., Ichinose, Y., Kobayashi, M., and Seino,Y. (1999) Expression of parathyroid hormone-related peptide messenger ribonucleic acid in developing kidney. *Kidney Int., 55*, 1696-1703.

[9] Karaplis, A.C., Luz, A., Glowacki, J., Bronson, R.T., Tybulewicz, V.L., Kronenberg, H.M., and Mulligan, R.C. (1994) Lethal skeletal dysplasia from targeted disruption of the parathyroid hormone-related peptide gene. *Genes Dev., 8*, 277-289.

[10] Fiaschi-Taesch, N.M., Santos, S., Reddy, V., Van Why, S.K., Philbrick, W.F., Ortega, A., Esbrit, P., Orloff, J.J., and García-Ocaña, A. (2004) Prevention of acute ischemic renal failure by targeted delivery of growth factors to the proximal tubule in transgenic mice: the efficacy of parathyroid hormone-related protein and hepatocyte growth factor. *J Am Soc Nephrol, 15*, 112-125.

[11] Massfelder,T., Stewart, A.F., Endlich, K., Soifer, N., Judes, C., and Helwig, J.J. (1996) Parathyroid hormone-related protein detection and interaction with NO and cyclic AMP in the renovascular system. *Kidney Int., 50*, 1591-1603.

[12] Yang, T., Hassan,S., Huang,Y.G., Smart,A.M., Briggs, J.P., and Schnermann, J.B. (1997) Expression of PTHrP, PTH/PTHrP receptor, and Ca(2+)-sensing receptor mRNAs along the rat nephron. *Am J Physiol, 272*, F751-F758.

[13] Largo, R., Gómez-Garre, D., Santos, S., Peñaranda, C., Blanco, J., Esbrit, P., and Egido, J. (1999) Renal expression of parathyroid hormone-related protein (PTHrP) and PTH/PTHrP receptor in a rat model of tubulointerstitial damage. *Kidney Int., 55*, 82-90.

[14] Santos, S., Bosch, R.J., Ortega, A., Largo, R., Fernández-Agulló, T., Gazapo, R., Egido, J., and Esbrit, P. (2001) Up-regulation of parathyroid hormone-related protein in folic acid-induced acute renal failure. *Kidney Int., 60*, 982-995.

[15] Lorenzo, O., Ruiz-Ortega, M., Esbrit, P., Rupérez, M., Ortega, A., Santos, S., Blanco, J., Ortega, L., and Egido, J. (2002) Angiotensin II increases parathyroid hormone-related protein (PTHrP) and the type 1 PTH/PTHrP receptor in the kidney. *J Am Soc Nephrol., 13*, 1595-1607.

[16] Lee, K., Brown, D., Ureña, P., Ardaillou, N., Ardaillou, R., Deeds, J., and Segre, G.V. (1996) Localization of parathyroid hormone/parathyroid hormone-related peptide receptor mRNA in kidney. *Am J Physiol, 270*, F186-F191.

[17] Endlich,N., Nobiling,R., Kriz,W., and Endlich,K. (2001) Expression and signaling of parathyroid hormone-related protein in cultured podocytes. *Exp Nephrol., 9*, 436-443.

[18] Massfelder,T., Taesch,N., Endlich,N., Eichinger,A., Escande,B., Endlich,K., Barthelmebs,M., and Helwig,J.J. (2001) Paradoxical actions of exogenous and endogenous parathyroid hormone-related protein on renal vascular smooth muscle cell proliferation: reversion in the SHR model of genetic hypertension. *FASEB J., 15*, 707-718.

[19] Bosch, R.J., Rojo-Linares, P., Torrecillas-Casamayor, G., Iglesias-Cruz, M.C., Rodríguez-Puyol, D., and Rodríguez-Puyol, M. (1999) Effects of parathyroid hormone-related protein on human mesangial cells in culture. *Am J Physiol, 277*, E990-E995.

[20] Soifer, N.E., Van Why,S.K., Ganz, M.B., Kashgarian, M., Siegel, N.J., and Stewart, A.F. (1993) Expression of parathyroid hormone-related protein in the rat glomerulus and tubule during recovery from renal ischemia. *J Clin. Invest, 92*, 2850-2857.

[21] Jobert,A.S., Fernandes, I., Turner, G., Coureau, C., Prie, D., Nissenson, R.A., Friedlander,G., and Silve, C. (1996) Expression of alternatively spliced isoforms of the parathyroid hormone (PTH)/PTH-related peptide receptor messenger RNA in human kidney and bone cells. *Mol Endocrinol, 10*, 1066-1076.

[22] Joun, H., Lanske, B., Karperien, M., Qian, F., Defize, L., and Abou-Samra, A. (1997) Tissue-specific transcription start sites and alternative splicing of the parathyroid hormone (PTH)/PTH-related peptide (PTHrP) receptor gene: a new PTH/PTHrP receptor splice variant that lacks the signal peptide. *Endocrinology, 138*, 1742-1749.

[23] Fritsch,S., Lindner,V., Welsch,S., Massfelder,T., Grima,M., Rothhut,S., Barthelmebs,M., and Helwig,J.J. (2004) Intravenous delivery of PTH/PTHrP type 1 receptor cDNA to rats decreases heart rate, blood pressure, renal tone, renin angiotensin system, and stress-induced cardiovascular responses. *J Am Soc Nephrol., 15*, 2588-2600.

[24] Maeda,S., Sutliff,R L., Qian,J., Lorenz,J.N., Wang,J., Tang,H., Nakayama,T., Weber,C., Witte,D., Strauch,A.R., Paul,R.J., Fagin,J.A., and Clemens,T.L. (1999) Targeted overexpression of parathyroid hormone-related protein (PTHrP) to vascular smooth muscle in transgenic mice lowers blood pressure and alters vascular contractility. *Endocrinology, 140*, 1815-1825.

[25] Qian, J., Lorenz, J.N., Maeda, S., Sutliff, R.L., Weber, C., Nakayama,T., Colbert, M.C., Paul, R.J., Fagin, J.A., and Clemens,T.L. (1999) Reduced blood pressure and increased sensitivity of the vasculature to parathyroid hormone-related protein (PTHrP) in transgenic mice overexpressing the PTH/PTHrP receptor in vascular smooth muscle. *Endocrinology, 140*, 1826-1833.

[26] Pirola,C.J., Wang,H.M., Kamyar,A., Wu,S., Enomoto,H., Sharifi,B., Forrester,J.S., Clemens,T.L., and Fagin,J.A. (1993) Angiotensin II regulates parathyroid hormone-related protein expression in cultured rat aortic smooth muscle cells through transcriptional and post-transcriptional mechanisms. *J Biol Chem., 268*, 1987-1994.

[27] Noda,M., Katoh,T., Takuwa,N., Kumada,M., Kurokawa,K., and Takuwa,Y. (1994) Synergistic stimulation of parathyroid hormone-related peptide gene expression by mechanical stretch and angiotensin II in rat aortic smooth muscle cells. *J Biol Chem., 269*, 17911-17917.

[28] Welsch, S., Schordan, E., Coquard, C., Massfelder,T., Fiaschi-Taesch, N., Helwig, J.J., and Barthelmebs, M. (2006) Abnormal renovascular parathyroid hormone-1 receptor in hypertension: Primary defect or secondary to angiotensin II type 1 receptor activation? *Endocrinology, 147*, 4384-4391.

[29] Endlich, K., Massfelder, T., Helwig, J.J., and Steinhausen, M. (1995) Vascular effects of parathyroid hormone and parathyroid hormone-related protein in the split hydronephrotic rat kidney. *J Physiol, 483 (2)*, 481-490.

[30] Massfelder, T., Parekh, N., Endlich, K., Saussine, C., Steinhausen, M., and Helwig, J.J. (1996) Effect of intrarenally infused parathyroid hormone-related protein on renal blood flow and glomerular filtration rate in the anaesthetized rat. *Br J Pharmacol.,118*, 1995-2000.

[31] Maeda,S., Wu,S., Green,J., Kim,H., Bosch,R., Lee,I., Adams,J., Clemens,T.L., and Kurtz,I. (1998) The N-terminal portion of parathyroid hormone-related protein mediates the inhibition of apical Na+/H+ exchange in opossum kidney cells. *J Am Soc Nephrol., 9*, 175-181.

[32] Bringhurst, F.R., Juppner, H., Guo, J., Ureña, P., Potts, J.T., Jr., Kronenberg, H.M., Abou-Samra, A.B., and Segre, G.V. (1993) Cloned, stably expressed parathyroid hormone (PTH)/PTH-related peptide receptors activate multiple messenger signals and biological responses in LLC-PK1 kidney cells. *Endocrinology, 132*, 2090-2098.

[33] Guo,J., Iida-Klein, A., Huang, X., Abou-Samra, A.B., Segre, G.V., and Bringhurst, F.R. (1995) Parathyroid hormone (PTH)/PTH-related peptide receptor density modulates activation of phospholipase C and phosphate transport by PTH in LLC-PK1 cells. *Endocrinology, 136*, 3884-3891.

[34] Maeda,S., Wu,S., Juppner,H., Green,J., Aragay,A.M., Fagin,J.A., and Clemens,T.L. (1996) Cell-specific signal transduction of parathyroid hormone (PTH)-related protein through stably expressed recombinant PTH/PTHrP receptors in vascular smooth muscle cells. *Endocrinology, 137*, 3154-3162.

[35] Takasu, H., Guo,J., and Bringhurst,F.R. (1999) Dual signaling and ligand selectivity of the human PTH/PTHrP receptor. *J Bone Miner Res., 14*, 11-20.

[36] Friedman, P.A., Gesek, F.A., Morley, P., Whitfield, J.F., and Willick, G.E. (1999) Cell-specific signaling and structure-activity relations of parathyroid hormone analogs in mouse kidney cells. *Endocrinology, 140*, 301-309.

[37] Binswanger, U., Helmle-Kolb, C., Forgo, J., Mrkic,B., and Murer,H. (1993) Rapid stimulation of Na+/H+ exchange by 1,25-dihydroxyvitamin D3; interaction with parathyroid-hormone-dependent inhibition. *Pflugers Arch., 424*, 391-397.

[38] Burton, P.B., Moniz, C., and Knight,D.E. (1990) Parathyroid hormone related peptide can function as an autocrine growth factor in human renal cell carcinoma. *Biochem Biophys Res Commun 167*, 1134-1138.

[39] de Miguel,F., García-Cañero,R., and Esbrit,P. (1991) Co-purification of calcium transport-stimulating and DNA synthesis-stimulating agents with parathormone-like activity isolated from the hypercalcaemic strain of the Walker 256 tumour. *Eur J Cancer, 27*, 1022-1026.

[40] García-Ocaña, A., de Miguel, F., Peñaranda, C., Albar, J.P., Sarasa, J.L., and Esbrit, P. (1995) Parathyroid hormone-related protein is an autocrine modulator of rabbit proximal tubule cell growth. *J Bone Miner Res., 10*, 1875-1884.

[41] García-Ocaña, A., Gómez-Casero, E., Peñaranda, C., and Esbrit, P. (1998) Parathyroid hormone-related protein increases DNA synthesis in proximal tubule cells by cyclic AMP- and protein kinase C-dependent pathways. *Life Sci., 62*, 2267-2273.

[42] Ortega, A., Rámila, D., Ardura, J.A., Esteban, V., Ruiz-Ortega, M., Barat, A., Gazapo, R., Bosch, R.J., and Esbrit, P. (2006) Role of parathyroid hormone-related protein in tubulointerstitial apoptosis and fibrosis after folic acid-induced nephrotoxicity. *J Am Soc Nephrol., 17*, 1594-1603.

[43] Lieberthal, W. and Levine, J.S. (1996) Mechanisms of apoptosis and its potential role in renal tubular epithelial cell injury. *Am J Physiol, 271*, F477-F488.

[44] Humes,H.D., Lake,E.W., and Liu,S. (1995) Renal tubule cell repair following acute renal injury. *Miner Electrolyte Metab, 21*, 353-365.

[45] Vukicevic,S., Basic,V., Rogic,D., Basic,N., Shih,M.S., Shepard,A., Jin,D., Dattatreyamurty,B., Jones,W., Dorai,H., Ryan,S., Griffiths,D., Maliakal,J., Jelic,M., Pastorcic,M., Stavljenic,A., and Sampath,T.K. (1998) Osteogenic protein-1 (bone morphogenetic protein-7) reduces severity of injury after ischemic acute renal failure in rat. *J Clin Invest, 102*, 202-214.

[46] Matsumoto,K. and Nakamura,T. (2001) Hepatocyte growth factor: renotropic role and potential therapeutics for renal diseases. *Kidney Int., 59*, 2023-2038.

[47] Gobe,G., Zhang,X.J., Willgoss,D.A., Schoch,E., Hogg,N.A., and Endre,Z.H. (2000) Relationship between expression of Bcl-2 genes and growth factors in ischemic acute renal failure in the rat. *J Am Soc Nephrol., 11*, 454-467.

[48] Watson,P.H., Fraher,L.J., Hendy,G.N., Chung,U.I., Kisiel,M., Natale,B.V., and Hodsman,A.B. (2000) Nuclear localization of the type 1 PTH/PTHrP receptor in rat tissues. *J Bone Miner Res., 15*, 1033-1044.

[49] Ortega, A., Rámila, D., Izquierdo, A., González, L., Barat, A., Gazapo, R., Bosch, R.J., and Esbrit, P. (2005) Role of the renin-angiotensin system on the parathyroid hormone-related protein overexpression induced by nephrotoxic acute renal failure in the rat. *J Am Soc Nephrol., 16*, 939-949.

[50] García-Ocaña, A., Gómez-Casero, E., Peñaranda, C., Sarasa, J.L., and Esbrit, P. (1998) Cyclosporine increases renal parathyroid hormone-related protein expression in vivo in the rat. *Transplantation*, *65*, 860-863.

[51] Harris, R.C. and Martínez-Maldonado, M. (1995) Angiotensin II-mediated renal injury. *Miner Electrolyte Metab, 21*, 328-335.

[52] Egido, J. (1996) Vasoactive hormones and renal sclerosis. *Kidney Int., 49*, 578-597.

[53] Ruiz-Ortega, M. and Egido, J. (1997) Angiotensin II modulates cell growth-related events and synthesis of matrix proteins in renal interstitial fibroblasts. *Kidney Int., 52*, 1497-1510.

[54] Mezzano, S.A., Ruiz-Ortega, M., and Egido, J. (2001) Angiotensin II and renal fibrosis. *Hypertension, 38*, 635-638.

[55] Allred, A.J., Chappell, M.C., Ferrario, C.M., and Diz,D.I. (2000) Differential actions of renal ischemic injury on the intrarenal angiotensin system. *Am J Physiol Renal Physiol, 279*, F636-F645.

[56] Kontogiannis, J. and Burns,K.D. (1998) Role of AT1 angiotensin II receptors in renal ischemic injury. *Am J Physiol, 274*, F79-F90.

[57] Long, G.W., Misra, D.C., Juleff, R., Blossom, G., Czako, P.F., and Glover, J.L. (1993) Protective effects of enalaprilat against postischemic renal failure. *J Surg Res., 54*, 254-257.

[58] Abdulkader, R.C., Yuki, M.M., Paiva, A.C., and Marcondes, M. (1988) Prolonged inhibition of angiotensin II attenuates glycerol-induced acute renal failure. *Braz J Med. Biol Res., 21*, 233-239.

[59] Cook, J.L., Zhang, Z., and Re, R.N. (2001) In vitro evidence for an intracellular site of angiotensin action. *Circ Res, 89*, 1138-1146.

[60] Navar, L.G., Harrison-Bernard, L.M., Nishiyama, A., and Kobori, H. (2002) Regulation of intrarenal angiotensin II in hypertension. *Hypertension, 39*, 316-322.

[61] Frustaci, A., Kajstura, J., Chimenti, C., Jakoniuk, I., Leri, A., Maseri, A., Nadal-Ginard, B., and Anversa, P. (2000) Myocardial cell death in human diabetes. *Circ Res., 87*, 1123-1132.

[62] Remuzzi, G. and Bertani, T. (1998) Pathophysiology of progressive nephropathies. N. *Engl J Med., 339*, 1448-1456.

[63] Chevalier, R.L. (2006) Obstructive nephropathy: towards biomarker discovery and gene therapy. *Nat Clin Pract Nephrol., 2*, 157-168.

[64] Rees, A.J. (2006) The role of infiltrating leukocytes in progressive renal disease: implications for therapy. *Nat Clin Pract Nephrol., 2*, 348-349.

[65] Muller,G.A., Markovic-Lipkovski, J., Frank, J., and Rodemann, H.P. (1992) The role of interstitial cells in the progression of renal diseases. *J Am oc Nephrol., 2*, S198-S205.

[66] Strutz, F. and Neilson, E.G. (2003) New insights into mechanisms of fibrosis in immune renal injury. *Springer Semin Immunopathol., 24*, 459-476.

[67] Funk, J.L. (2001) A role for parathyroid hormone-related protein in the pathogenesis of inflammatory/autoimmune diseases. *Int Immunopharmacol., 1*, 1101-1121.

[68] Guillén, C., Martínez, P., de Gortázar, A.R., Martínez, M.E., and Esbrit, P. (2002) Both N- and C-terminal domains of parathyroid hormone-related protein increase

interleukin-6 by nuclear factor-kappa B activation in osteoblastic cells. *J Biol Chem., 277*, 28109-28117.

[69] Martín-Ventura, J.L., Ortego, M., Esbrit, P., Hernández-Presa, M.A., Ortega, L., and Egido, J. (2003) Possible role of parathyroid hormone-related protein as a proinflammatory cytokine in atherosclerosis. *Stroke, 34*, 1783-1789.

[70] Ishikawa, M., Akishita, M., Kozaki, K., Toba, K., Namiki, A., Yamaguchi, T., Orimo, H., and Ouchi, Y. (2000) Expression of parathyroid hormone-related protein in human and experimental atherosclerotic lesions: functional role in arterial intimal thickening. *Atherosclerosis, 152*, 97-105.

[71] Nakayama, T., Ohtsuru, A., Enomoto, H., Namba, H., Ozeki, S., Shibata,Y., Yokota, T., Nobuyoshi,M., Ito,M., Sekine,I. (1994) Coronary atherosclerotic smooth muscle cells overexpress human parathyroid hormone-related peptides. *Biochem Biophys Res Commun., 200*, 1028-1035.

[72] Rámila, D., Ardura, J.A., Esbrit, P. (2006) Parathyroid hormone-related protein (PTHrP): A new proinflammatory factor in renal disease. *Nephrol Dial Transplant 21* (Supl 4), 553 (Abstract).

[73] Kaushal, G.P., Basnakian, A.G., and Shah, S.V. (2004) Apoptotic pathways in ischemic acute renal failure. *Kidney Int., 66*, 500-506.

[74] Basnakian, A.G., Kaushal, G.P., and Shah, S.V. (2002) Apoptotic pathways of oxidative damage to renal tubular epithelial cells. *Antioxid Redox Signal., 4*, 915-924.

[75] Henderson, J.E., Amizuka, N., Warshawsky, H., Biasotto, D., Lanske, B.M., Goltzman, D., and Karaplis, A.C. (1995) Nucleolar localization of parathyroid hormone-related peptide enhances survival of chondrocytes under conditions that promote apoptotic cell death. *Mol Cell Biol., 15*, 4064-4075.

[76] Cebrián, A., García-Ocaña, A., Takane, K.K., Sipula, D., Stewart, A.F., and Vasavada, R.C. (2002) Overexpression of parathyroid hormone-related protein inhibits pancreatic beta-cell death in vivo and in vitro. *Diabetes, 51*, 3003-3013.

[77] Ortiz, A., Lorz, C., Catalán, M.P., Danoff, T.M., Yamasaki, Y., Egido, J., and Neilson, E.G. (2000) Expression of apoptosis regulatory proteins in tubular epithelium stressed in culture or following acute renal failure. *Kidney Int., 57*, 969-981.

[78] Fan, J.M., Ng, Y.Y., Hill, P.A., Nikolic-Paterson, D.J., Mu, W., Atkins, R.C., and Lan, H.Y. (1999) Transforming growth factor-beta regulates tubular epithelial-myofibroblast transdifferentiation in vitro. *Kidney Int., 56*, 1455-1467.

[79] Strutz, F., Zeisberg, M., Ziyadeh, F.N., Yang, C.Q., Kalluri, R., Muller, G.A., and Neilson, E.G. (2002) Role of basic fibroblast growth factor-2 in epithelial-mesenchymal transformation. *Kidney Int., 61*, 1714-1728.

[80] Ardura, J.A., Ortega, A., Rámila, D., Strutz, F., Esbrit, P. (2005). Parathyroid hormone-related protein (PTHrP): A new cytokine inducing epithelial-mesenchymal transition. *Nephrol Dial Transplant 20*(Supl 5), 206 (Abstract).

[81] Liu, Y. (2004) Epithelial to mesenchymal transition in renal fibrogenesis: pathologic significance, molecular mechanism, and therapeutic intervention. *J Am Soc Nephrol., 15*, 1-12.

[82] Li, Y., Yang, J., Dai, C., Wu, C., and Liu, Y. (2003) Role for integrin-linked kinase in mediating tubular epithelial to mesenchymal transition and renal interstitial fibrogenesis. *J Clin Invest, 112*, 503-516.

[83] Okada, H., Danoff, T.M., Kalluri, R., and Neilson, E.G. (1997) Early role of Fsp1 in epithelial-mesenchymal transformation. *Am J Physiol, 273*, F563-F574.

[84] Kalluri, R. and Neilson, E.G. (2003) Epithelial-mesenchymal transition and its implications for fibrosis. *J Clin. Invest, 112*, 1776-1784.

[85] Yang, J. and Liu, Y. (2001) Dissection of key events in tubular epithelial to myofibroblast transition and its implications in renal interstitial fibrosis. *Am J Pathol., 159*, 1465-1475.

[86] Ardura, J.A., Rámila, D., Berruguete, R., Alvarez-Arroyo, M.V., Esbrit, P. (2006) Parathyroid hormone-related protein interacts with transforming growth factor β, epidermal growth factor and vascular endothelial growth factor in epithelial-mesenchymal transition. *Nephrol Dial Transplant (Supl 4)*, 23 (Abstract).

[87] Cooper, M.E., Vranes, D., Youssef, S., Stacker, S.A., Cox, A.J., Rizkalla, B., Casley, D.J., Bach, L.A., Kelly, D.J., and Gilbert, R.E. (1999) Increased renal expression of vascular endothelial growth factor (VEGF) and its receptor VEGFR-2 in experimental diabetes. *Diabetes, 48*, 2229-2239.

[88] Katoh, M., Ohmachi, Y., Kurosawa, Y., Yoneda, H., Tanaka, N., and Narita, H. (2000) Effects of imidapril and captopril on streptozotocin-induced diabetic nephropathy in mice. *Eur J Pharmacol., 398*, 381-387.

[89] Yotsumoto,T., Naitoh,T., Shikada,K., and Tanaka,S. (1997) Effects of specific antagonists of angiotensin II receptors and captopril on diabetic nephropathy in mice. *Jpn J Pharmacol., 75*, 59-64.

[90] Izquierdo, A., López-Luna, P., Ortega, A., Romero, M., Guitiérrez-Tarres, M.A., Arribas, I., Alvarez, M.J., Esbrit, P., and Bosch, R.J. (2006) The parathyroid hormone-related protein system and diabetic nephropathy outcome in streptozotocin-induced diabetes. *Kidney Int., 69*, 2171-2177.

[91] Gross, M.L., Ritz, E., Schoof, A., Adamczak, M., Koch, A., Tulp, O., Parkman, A., El Shakmak, A., Szabo, A., and Amann, K. (2004) Comparison of renal morphology in the streptozotocin and the SHR/N-cp models of diabetes. *Lab Invest, 84*, 452-464.

[92] Wolf, G. and Ziyadeh, F.N. (1999) Molecular mechanisms of diabetic renal hypertrophy. *Kidney Int., 56*, 393-405.

[93] Burns, K.D. (2000) Angiotensin II and its receptors in the diabetic kidney. *Am J Kidney Dis., 36*, 449-467.

[94] Romero, M., Ortega, A., Izquierdo, A., Bover, J., Pemau, S., Rámila, D., Esbrit, P., and Bosch, R.J. (2006). Role of parathyroid hormone (PTH)-related protein in the mesangial hypertrophy associated to human diabetic nephropathy. *Nefrología 26* (Supl 6), 32 (Abstract).

[95] Benítez-Verguizas, J., Loarte, D., de Miguel, F., and Esbrit, P. (1999) Effects of transforming growth factor β1 on cell growth and parathyroid hormone-related protein in Walker 256 tumor cells. *Life Sci, 65*, 1807-1816.

[96] Alvarez, J., Sohn, P., Zeng, X., Doetschman, T., Robbins, D.J., and Serra, R. (2002) TGF β2 mediates the effects of hedgehog on hypertrophic differentiation and PTHrP expression. *Development, 129*, 1913-1924.

[97] Wolf, G., Sharma, K., Chen, Y., Ericksen, M., and Ziyadeh, F.N. (1992) High glucose-induced proliferation in mesangial cells is reversed by autocrine TGF-beta. *Kidney Int., 42*, 647-656.

[98] Fine, L.G., Holley, R.W., Nasri, H., and Badie-Dezfooly, B. (1985) BSC-1 growth inhibitor transforms a mitogenic stimulus into a hypertrophic stimulus for renal proximal tubular cells: relationship to Na+/H+ antiport activity. *Proc Natl Acad Sci U.S.A, 82*, 6163-6166.

[99] Hirschberg, R. (1996) Bioactivity of glomerular ultrafiltrate during heavy proteinuria may contribute to renal tubulo-interstitial lesions: evidence for a role for insulin-like growth factor I. *J Clin Invest, 98*, 116-124.

[100] D'Amico, G. and Bazzi, C. (2003) Pathophysiology of proteinuria. *Kidney Int., 63*, 809-825.

In: Novel Aspects of PTHrP Physiopathology
Editor: Claudio Luparello, pp. 115-141
ISBN: 978-1-60021-857-6

Chapter VI

EFFECTS OF TEMPORAL CHANGES IN PTHRP AND IHH EXPRESSIONS ON BONE GROWTH, STUDIED BY A THEORETICAL MODEL

C.C. van Donkelaar*

Department of Biomedical Engineering, Eindhoven University of Technology, 5600 MB Eindhoven, The Netherlands.

1. ABSTRACT

The rate of bone growth reduces in response to both short-term daily mechanical loading and irradiation therapy. The nature of these interventions and their distinct temporal effects suggest different mechanisms. Yet, both mechanical loading and irradiation therapy have been associated with changes in PTHrP. The question rises to what extent the observed effects can be assigned to the PTHrP-Ihh control system, which is probably the most important mechanism for regulating bone growth. This chapter addresses this question using a theoretical model in which bone growth is only controlled by the growth factors PTHrP, Ihh and VEGF.

To study the effects of mechanical loading on bone growth, first the expressions of PTHrP and Ihh by growth-plate chondrocytes in response to compressive loading are monitored. They decrease to 18% (PTHrP) and 44% (Ihh) of control levels. These values are used throughout the chapter to simulate both mechanical loading and irradiation therapy.

Simulations of daily loading periods reveal load-dependent variations in growth rate, without significant structural changes to the growth plate. Structural adaptation starts when multiple hours of loading are applied daily, therewith further reducing the growth rate. When twelve hours of activity are applied each day, a circadian growth-rhythm emerges. In simulations of irradiation therapy, it takes almost ten weeks to recover from

* Correspondence concerning this article should be addressed to: C.C. van Donkelaar, Department of Biomedical Engineering, Eindhoven University of Technology, WHoog 4.118, PO Box 513, 5600 MB Eindhoven, The Netherlands. c.c.v.donkelaar@tue.nl; http://www.mate.tue.nl/mate/showempcompl.php/65.

structural changes that are initiated during a one-week irradiation period. During this time the growth rate remains reduced and a bone-length difference develops which persists till adulthood.

These effects concur with experimental data. Therefore, it is concluded that a system with only PTHrP, Ihh and VEGF is sufficient to capture effects of temporal variations in growth factor expressions on bone growth. The most interesting insight from this study is that two effects with different time-constants determine the responses. The first one is the direct effect of these growth factors on the rates of proliferation and hypertrophy. The second one, acting on a longer time-scale, relates to the structural changes in the tissue, secondary to sustained changes in growth-factor expressions.

2. Introduction

Bone morphogenesis and longitudinal bone growth are importantly determined by the expansion of epiphyseal cartilage prior to mineralization. Cartilage expansion is the result of matrix synthesis, proliferation and chondrocyte hypertrophy. Matrix synthesis occurs throughout the cartilage, but proliferation and hypertrophy are concentrated in distinct regions in the developing fetal long bone. This gives rise to a zonal organization in which the zones are named according to the appearance of the chondrocytes as the reserve, proliferative, early hypertrophic, hypertrophic and mineralization zones. Processes in each of these zones need to be closely controlled, since inaccuracies in any of the zones may result in pathological longitudinal bone growth.

The best known feed-back mechanism for controlling bone growth over a larger working distance is without doubt the one involving PTHrP and Indian hedgehog (Ihh) [1-6]. Figure 1 contains a schematic representation of this control mechanism. Ihh, selectively expressed by early hypertrophic cells [2,7-10], has two important functions. First, it stimulates proliferation [1,2,11]. Thus, once a cell leaves the proliferative zone and becomes hypertrophic, it stimulates formation of a new cell in the proliferative zone by expressing Ihh. Second, Ihh stimulates dose-dependently the expression of PTHrP by periarticular perichondrium cells [10,12,13]. The pathway for the Ihh signal to travel the long way from the early hypertrophic zone to the periarticular region of the tissue is still unclear. It has been hypothesized that intermediate signaling by TGFβ or BMPs in the perichondrium is involved [5,7]. More recent evidence however, shows that Ihh itself may travel long distances through the cartilage matrix and accumulates rather close to the PTHrP expressing cells as a result of binding to heparin sulphate [8,14]. PTHrP transport is less disputed. It freely diffuses through the matrix towards the hypertrophic zone [15]. Its function is to keep cells in the proliferating pool [1,2]. A threshold PTHrP concentration has been identified above which proliferating cells cannot start hypertrophy. As soon as the PTHrP concentration drops below this threshold, cells may start to differentiate if they are triggered to do so [16,17]. A second effect of PTHrP is that it reduces the rate of hypertrophy dose-dependently [1,10,18,19].

Because the PTHrP-Ihh feedback loop spans the entire length of the epiphysis from the periarticular region to the hypertrophic zones, it is a very powerful control system. This is illustrated by pathologies caused by abnormal expressions of PTHrP or Ihh. Jansen's metaphyseal chondrodysplasia [20,21] and Blomstrand chondrodysplasia [22] are characterized by severe skeletal malformations. The same effects are seen in knock-out animal studies [11,19,20,23-26].

The control system is essentially dependent on a dynamic equilibrium in growth factor expressions. The concentration of PTHrP throughout the tissue varies with its expression by periarticular perichondrium cells, which depends on the local Ihh-concentration. The Ihh concentration in the periarticular region depends on the distance from the early hypertrophic zone, i.e. on the number of cells in the reserve and the proliferative zones, and on the expression of Ihh in the early hypertrophic region, which depends on the number of early hypertrophic cells and the expression per cell. These dynamic variations result in physiological variations in proliferation and hypertrophy during normal development.

The expressions of PTHrP and Ihh may also vary in time during normal development because their expressions depend on mechanical loading [27-29]. It can be argued that a mechano-sensing function of an important control system such as the PTHrP-Ihh feed-back loop may actually have an important regulating function in bone development. Such regulation may for instance be involved in the load-dependent decrease of longitudinal ulna growth in response to only a few minutes of axial compression per day [30-32]. Since the duration of loading in these experiments is very short, it is unlikely that the growth perturbation is a direct consequence of the applied strain. Changes in growth-factor expressions including PTHrP and/or Ihh may have caused these effects. Only VEGF expression was monitored. It was enhanced in the severest loading case, but this may be secondary to the tissue damage that was induced in this case [31].

Independent on these artificially applied diurnal loadings, growth is thought to follow a diurnal rhythm. Growth occurs during the night more than during the day and it can be speculated that the normal level of daily activity is partly responsible for this diurnal rhythm, acting in addition to systemic factors. This concurs with the finding that growth occurs predominantly during periods of relative unloading in goats [33]. A thorough explanation for this finding has however not yet been provided.

At the longer time-scale of weeks to months, an intriguing and clinically relevant growth reduction occurs as a severe side-effect of growth-plate irradiation during (bone)-tumor treatment. The growth rate of the irradiated bone lags behind on the contralateral bone for months and catch-up growth is generally insufficient [34-38]. Strongly reduced PTHrP expression is held responsible [36,39,40]. However, it is unexplained why the severest structural changes in growth plates occur a month after irradiation, while PTHrP expression has largely recovered within a week.

The decreased growth rate in rat ulnae which are loaded for only a few minutes daily, the physiological circadian growth rhythm and the response to irradiation therapy, occur at very different time-scales. Different time-scales suggest different mechanisms. However, appropriate mechanistic hypotheses for the transient effects in response to both diurnal loading and irradiation have not yet been provided, partly because of experimental limitations. Using a theoretical approach, this chapter will show that all aforementioned effects can in principle be explained by the PTHrP-Ihh control mechanism only.

The efficacy of the PTHrP-Ihh control loop has recently been evaluated with a simple analytical model, showing that Ihh primarily controls proliferation while a threshold level of PTHrP above which cells remain in the proliferative pool, is a key factor for controlling hypertrophy [41]. Another theoretical study shows that physiological fetal bone development can in principle be controlled by only three growth factors: PTHrP, Ihh and VEGF [42]. In the latter study, proliferation, hypertrophy and mineralization are dependent on local growth factor concentrations, which are functions of expression, degradation and transport through diffusion. PTHrP and Ihh are considered the only proteins responsible for controlling cartilage differentiation. VEGF was included to stimulate mineralization of the matrix around terminally differentiated chondrocytes (Figure 1). This simple three-growth-factor model [42] is able to simulate physiological bone development from the early embryonic cartilaginous anlage until birth [43-45]. In addition, predicted effects of pathological over- and under-expressions of PTHrP and Ihh agree very well with clinical data [20-22] and knock-out animal studies [11,19,23-26].

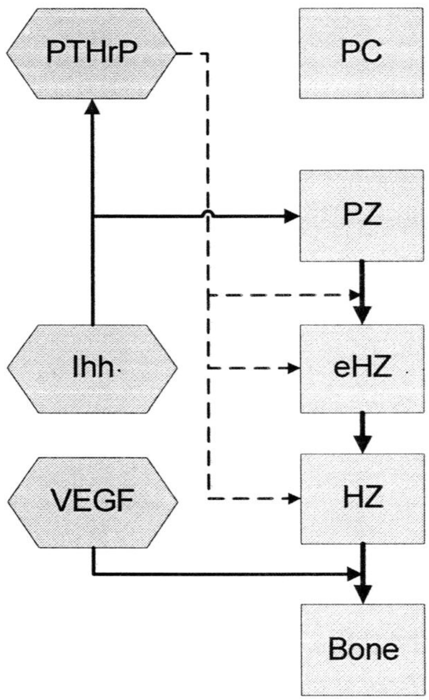

Figure 1. Schematic representation of the control mechanism that is considered in this chapter. The proteins PTHrP, Ihh and VEGF are expressed by the perichondrium (PC), early hypertrophic zone (eHZ) and hypertrophic zone (HZ), respectively. The proliferative zone and resting zone are together indicated as PZ. Solid lines represent stimulatory interactions, dotted lines represent inhibiting interactions.

The same three-growth-factor model is used in this chapter to evaluate the effects of diurnally applied loading and irradiation. The next paragraph provides an explanation of this model. For a more thorough description the reader is referred to the original publication [42]. Subsequently, an experiment is described that is performed to determine how PTHrP and Ihh expressions by fetal growth-cartilage cells change in response to compressive loading. These data are then used as input in simulations of diurnal loading with various durations and in simulations of one week of irradiation.

3. MODEL

3.1. Description

In the theoretical model used in this chapter, the three growth factors PTHrP, Ihh and VEGF interact by paracrine signaling to control bone growth in the longitudinal direction (Figure 1). PTHrP is expressed by cells in the periarticular region of the perichondrium, Ihh by early hypertrophic cells and VEGF by cells in the late hypertrophic zone. All effects of PTHrP, Ihh and VEGF depend on their local concentrations. To compute the growth factor concentration profiles, the location and phenotype of each individual cell are kept track of during the simulation. The concentrations are then defined by synthesis, transport and degradation, as

$$\frac{\delta c_{gf}}{\delta t} = S_{gf} + T_{gf} + D_{gf}, \text{ with } gf \in \{PTHrP, Ihh, VEGF\} \quad (1)$$

In this equation, c_{gf} represents the concentration of the corresponding growth factor, t represents time, and S_{gf}, T_{gf} and D_{gf} represent synthesis, transport and degradation rates, respectively.

3.1.1. Synthesis

Synthesis rates of Ihh and VEGF are assumed constant per cell. Hence, the total synthesis depends on the number of cells in these particular zones. Synthesis of PTHrP depends on the concentration of Ihh in the perichondrium, according to the Hill equation

$$S_{PTHrP} = a \frac{c_{Ihh}^4}{c_{Ihh}^4 + Km_{Ihh}^4}, \quad (2)$$

where a is the maximal synthesis rate and Km_{Ihh} the Ihh concentration at which half the maximal synthesis rate of PTHrP is reached. With this equation the PTHrP synthesis rate increases with the local Ihh concentration and levels off at higher Ihh concentrations. The number of PTHrP-expressing cells in the perichondrium is assumed constant.

3.1.2. Transport

Transport of all growth factors is assumed to occur through normal diffusion, as described by

$$T_{gf} = \nabla \cdot (d_{gf} \nabla c_{gf}) \quad (3)$$

The diffusion coefficient d_{gf} in the proliferative zone is assumed 63 $\mu m^2/s$ for both PTHrP and Ihh and 39 $\mu m^2/s$ for VEGF. These values scale with ECM/cell volumes in the other zones [42]. The approach to consider the proteins as freely diffusing molecules in the matrix is probably valid for VEGF and PTHrP [15]. Ihh transport is more complex as it binds to matrix components [8,14]. Accumulation of Ihh in the matrix may have an important beneficial consequence for the tissue. Yet, it will not qualitatively affect the control system, because regardless of accumulation the direction of signaling is always from the source, the early hypertrophic zone, toward the target area, the periarticular region of the perichondrium.

3.1.3. Degradation

Degradation of all growth factors is implemented as a constant half-life time τ_{gf} as

$$D_{gf} = \frac{-\ln(2)}{\tau_{gf}} c_{gf} \tag{4}$$

The half-life time is assumed 10 minutes for all growth factors, based on values previously used in another tissue differentiation model [46].

3.1.4. Differentiation

The rate of proliferation by cells in the proliferative zone increases with the actual concentration of Ihh in that zone. The minimum proliferation rate equals one cell per ten hours and this rate doubles in the presence of normal Ihh concentrations [11,16,47].

The rate of hypertrophy (H) is determined by the concentration of PTHrP as experienced by that cell, according to the Michaelis-Menten-like equation

$$H = f \frac{Km_{PTHrP}}{c_{PTHrP} + Km_{PTHrP}}, \tag{5}$$

where Km_{PTHrP} represents the concentration of PTHrP at which half the maximal hypertrophy rate is reached.

Differentiation of cells, i.e. the transition of cells between the proliferative, early hypertrophic and hypertrophic zones and ultimately the mineralization of the tissue, is defined as follows. Proliferative cells, 10.5 μm high, are kept in the proliferative pool as long as the concentration of PTHrP in the proliferative cell closest to the early hypertrophic zone remains above a threshold value [16]. Only when the concentration in this cell drops below the threshold, which is set at 0.1 nM based on an in vitro study [17], the cell starts to differentiate. It then becomes part of the early hypertrophic zone, i.e. it starts to increase size and expresses Ihh. Ihh expression stops when the cell leaves the early hypertrophic zone at a predefined cell height of 22.5 μm. It then turns into a late hypertrophic cell and expresses VEGF. The VEGF concentration is monitored in the mineralized zone. When the accumulated VEGF concentration reaches a threshold level, the matrix associated with the largest hypertrophic cell mineralizes and the cell becomes apoptotic. Note that VEGF is used as representative for many other factors expressed by hypertrophic cells, which stimulate in one way or the other the terminal differentiation of chondrocytes and matrix mineralization.

These factors include MMP's for matrix degradation and growth-factors that stimulate osteoclastic and osteoblastic activity and blood vessel invasion. For an excellent review on this topic see Ortega [48]).

3.2. Implementation

To solve this model it is implemented in Sepran finite-element software (Ingenieursbureau Sepra, Leidschendam, The Netherlands). For an accurate description of the implementation the reader is referred to the original publication [42]. A one-dimensional model is used as this suffices to model growth in the longitudinal direction, controlled by growth factors that diffuse in the same direction. The finite element model contains 1215 elements of fixed size. When cells proliferate, hypertrophy and differentiate, the cells change position relative to this fixed mesh. Each element is subsequently assigned properties as defined by the phenotype of the cell that is associated with the element. Simulations are performed with time-steps representing one hour of development. After time-step, the current growth factor distributions throughout the mesh are computed using a second-order Strang-operator splitting scheme [49]. Based on these concentration profiles it is then decided which structural changes occur in the tissue in this time-step, i.e. whether proliferation occurs, the magnitude of cell-growth in the hypertrophic zone, and which cells differentiate to another zone. These changes are applied in the next time-step when new concentration profiles are computed. This loop continues until the simulation is stopped (Figure 2).

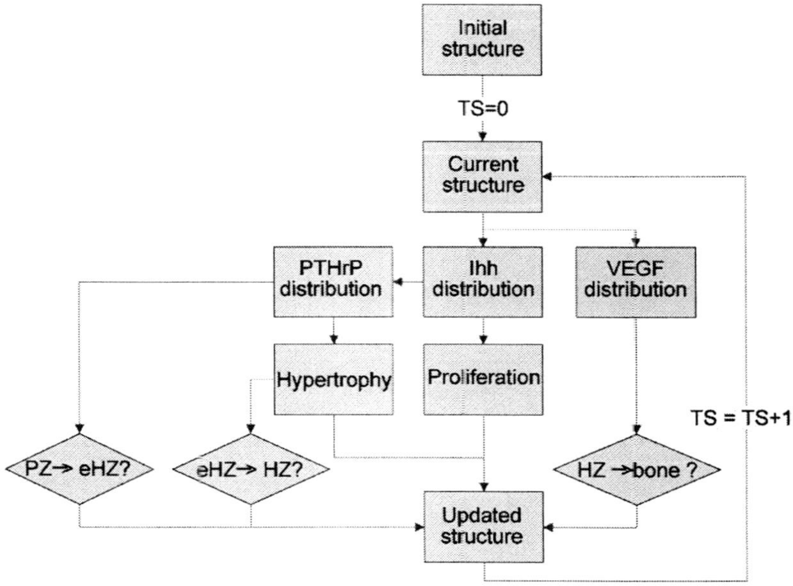

Figure 2. Flow chart of the model. Each time-step (TS) starts with computing the distributions of Ihh, PTHrP and VEGF throughout the tissue, based on the current structure, synthesis, degradation and transport. The local concentrations of these growth factors are then used to apply structural changes, i.e. to determine the rates of proliferation and hypertrophy and to decide upon differentiation of cells. The updated structure is then used in the next time-step.

3.3. Parameters

Many parameters can be derived from the literature. These are already mentioned in the above text. Unfortunately, several parameters remain unknown. These include for instance growth-factor synthesis rates. They are obtained from Brouwers et al [42], where they are inversely derived by assuring that, in a fully developed growth plate and given the aforementioned known parameters, concentration profiles, growth rates and zone widths are consistent with the literature. With these parameters, the model can explain normal and pathological bone growth from an early, unmineralized cartilaginous anlage to a mineralized bone at birth [42]. Total growth compares well to physiological bone growth [43-45]. Enhanced or reduced growth as a result of pathological growth-factor expressions concur with clinical data [20-22] and knock-out animal studies [11,19,23-26].

One set of parameters that has not yet been determined is how the expressions of PTHrP and Ihh change in response to mechanical compression. These parameters are determined in the next paragraph of this chapter.

3.4. Discussion

An obvious limitation of this model is that it only contains the three growth factors PTHrP, Ihh and VEGF, while many more regulating factors are involved in the control of bone development and cartilage differentiation. It is well possible to incorporate more growth factors in the model. However, quantitative parameters to describe the effect, synthesis, degradation and transport are required for each additional factor. Although these are all measurable quantities, such quantitative parameters are sparsely available and extremely difficult to obtain. Modern imaging techniques such as real-time multi-photon microscopy in combination with dedicated fluorescent probes may enable quantification of the distributions of PTHrP and Ihh concentrations throughout the growth plate in small animals and the variations thereof in time. Such data is ultimately necessary for model validation. At present however, the most suitable available data for validation are histological changes in response to interventions such as those described in this chapter.

An advantage of using a computational model is that it allows studying the control system by PTHrP, Ihh and VEGF in the exact way in which these three growth-factors are hypothesized to interact. If the model shows behavior that is in disagreement with experimental observations, either the hypothesis is false, or the model is incomplete and other aspects need to be added. This will lead to new insights in the behavior of the control mechanism under consideration. However, if predictions with the model concur with experimental data, the hypothesis is accurate enough to explain the observed phenomena. It can then be used for extrapolation of experimental observations, predicting outcomes of circumstances that are challenging to approach experimentally or ultimately for optimization of clinical treatment modalities within the boundaries of its applicability. To explore the boundaries of its use, the model should be corroborated to various experimental conditions.

One should always keep in mind, however, that even though experimental phenomena can be perfectly simulated with a model, this does not prove that the hypothesis behind the model is true. It is possible that a distinct hypothesis can explain the same phenomena as accurately. A model like the one used in this chapter therefore only shows that observed phenomena can (or cannot) be explained with the implemented hypothesis. Although this can provide very valuable insights, it does not by itself prove or disprove the hypothesis.

An interesting aspect of computational models such as this one is that it allows varying at any moment in time the expressions of any of the growth factors. This is a potentially valuable feature, for instance with regard to studying the effects of (temporal) clinical interventions. In this chapter, model predictions in which growth factor expressions are temporally and/or periodically changed are corroborated to experimental data. In this way the applicability of the three-growth-factor model to dynamic variations in growth-factor expressions is evaluated.

4. Effect of Mechanical Loading on PTHrP/IHH Expression

4.1. Introduction

PTHrP-mRNA expression in isolated rat growth-plate chondrocytes increases two- or four-fold in response to 7% or 12% cyclic 0.5 Hz stretching [27]. Similar effects are seen in bladder smooth muscle cells, which increase PTHrP-protein expression in response to mechanical stretching [28]. Ihh-mRNA expression in chick sternum growth-plate chondrocytes increases 18-fold in response to 1 Hz cyclic 5% stretching [29]. In vivo however, the cells which constitute growth plates are predominantly loaded in compression. Whether the expression decreases or increases in response to compressive loading has not yet been studied. However, given the Hueter-Volkmann principle that compression and tension have opposite effects on growth, it can be hypothesized that compression reduces the expressions of both PTHrP and Ihh. To confirm this hypothesis a short experiment is performed as explained below.

4.2. Method

Three approximately 80 days old porcine embryo's, weighing over 500 grams, are obtained from the local abattoir. All experiments are performed once per animal. The epiphyses of the femur, tibia, humerus and radius of one animal are dissected and growth plate cells are isolated by overnight incubation (37°C, 5%CO_2) in 50ml of DMEM (BioWhittaker BE12-707F), supplemented with 30 mg collagenase (Sigma, C0130)), 50 µg DNAse (Sigma, D4263) and antibiotics. Cell suspension is filtered (40 µm pores) to discard matrix remnants. This procedure results in a yield of approximately $20*10^6$ cells per animal.

Cells are separated by centrifuging for 5 minutes, 500G at room temperature through a percoll-gradient with densities varying from 1.07 to 1.01 g/ml in steps of 0.01 g/ml [50,51]. This separates growth plate cells from different zones, which vary in buoyant density from resting zone to hypertrophic cells as: 1.023, 1.032, 1.044 and 1.053 g/ml [6]. FACS analysis reveals differences in size and buoyancy between five groups of cells that are extracted from the percoll-gradient, with the least difference between the two groups with the smallest cells. These two groups also contain the lowest amounts of cells. Therefore, they are pooled in all experiments.

Each of the groups of cells is mixed in DMEM, supplemented with HEPES buffer. This solution is split into two stainless steel containers. One serves as the unloaded control. The other one is connected via a sterile air filter to an electronically controlled air pressure modulator. An air pressure varying between 0 and 0.1 MPa is applied at a frequency of 0.75 Hz (see Figure 3) to the cells for 90 minutes. Immediately thereafter the cells are frozen at -80°C and kept frozen until further processing.

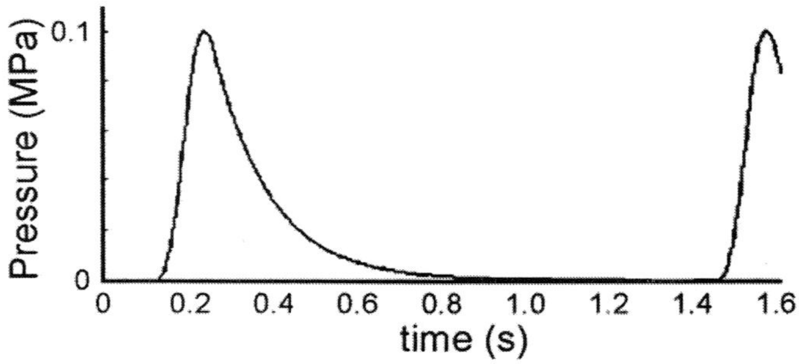

Figure 3. A pressure of 0.1 MPa is applied to the chondrocytes with a frequency of 0.7 Hz, for a total duration of 90 minutes. The pressure is applied by increasing the air pressure above the cell-suspension in a stainless-steel container.

4.2.1. Dot-Blotting

Thawed cells are washed and lysed using RIPA lysis buffer. Cell-remnants are paletted and 50µl of the supernatant is diluted 20x in PBS, 0.05% Tween 20 and kept on ice until further use.

Standard 2-fold dilution series are made with primary antibodies for PTHrP, Ihh and GAPDH (Santa Cruz 9680, 1190 and 20357), ranging from 2.0 to 0.0625 µg/ml PBS-Tween. Nitrocellulose dotblots are made using a Bio-Dot microfiltration apparatus (Bio-Rad). Each antibody dilution series is blotted in triplicate on a separate membrane. The diluted supernatant is blotted onto each membrane in triplicate.

The membranes are removed from the Bio-Dot apparatus and blocked for 60-90 min at room temperature in blocking buffer (5% blocking grade non-fat dry milk (Bio-Rad 960/607) in PBS-Tween). Subsequently the membranes are incubated with primary antibodies against GAPDH, Ihh, or PTHrP (1µg/ml antibody in blocking buffer) for 90 minutes at room temperature. The membranes are washed twice for 15 minutes in blocking buffer and subsequently incubated with HRP-coupled bovine-anti-goat (Santa Cruz 2350) secondary antibody (1µg/ml antibody in blocking buffer).

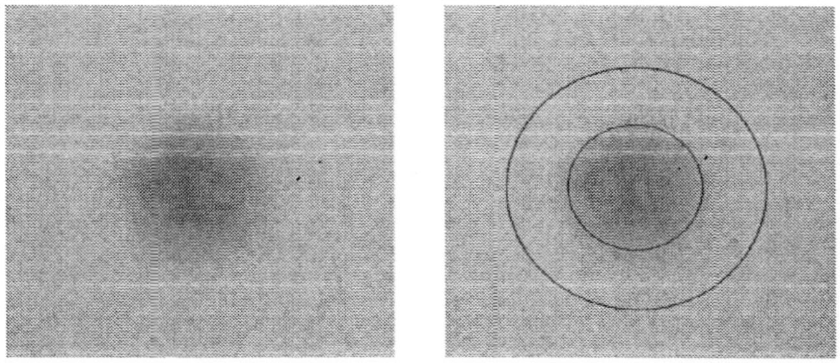

Figure 4. Example of a DOT-blot result. The signal equals the total intensity in the smallest circle, minus the intensity in the surrounding area as indicated by the larger circle, corrected for the areas under the circles.

After washing the membranes twice in blocking buffer, dots are visualized using enhanced chemiluminescence in a Versadoc system (Bio-Rad). The inner and outer contours of the wells of a 96-well frame are copied on the 10 minutes exposed images (circles in Figure 4). The signal equals the difference between the intensity (quantified with Quantity One software (Bio-Rad)) of the inner circle and the local background signal, as defined from the area between the circles, and corrected for the surface areas. Eventually, the PTHrP and Ihh signals are normalized against the GAPDH signal.

4.3. Results

PTHrP expression is most pronounced in the group containing the smallest cells, most likely representing the resting zone cells. The group with second-largest cells expresses most Ihh, confirming that these cells originate mainly from the early hypertrophic zone (Table 1).

PTHrP and Ihh expressions are reduced by hydrostatic loading in all groups. In the groups with the highest expressions of these proteins, dynamic hydrostatic loading reduces the expressions of PTHrP to 18% (±18%) and Ihh to 44% (±10%) of control levels (Table 1).

Table 1. Effects of hydrostatic compression on expressions of PTHrP and Ihh by cells originating from four different growth-plate zones. Values represent dot-blot intensities (standard deviations between brackets). As expected, the highest expressions for PTHrP and Ihh in the unloaded control situations are found in resting and early hypertrophic zones, respectively. In all zones, hydrostatic compression reduced the expressions of both PTHrP and Ihh, with the largest reductions in the aforementioned zones.

		RZ	PZ	eHZ	HZ
PTHrP	Control	3.865 (3.260)	1.102 (0.932)	1.971 (2.478)	0.575 (0.127)
	Loaded	0.706 (0.710)	0.334 (0.076)	0.630 (0.201)	0.325 (0.169)
	Ratio	0.18	0.30	0.32	0.56
Ihh	Control	0.683 (0.403)	0.696 (0.366)	1.067 (0.203)	0.889 (0.342)
	Loaded	0.619 (0.526)	0.442 (0.045)	0.473 (0.116)	0.511 (0.163)
	Ratio	0.91	0.63	0.44	0.58

4.4. Discussion

In agreement with the hypothesis, PTHrP and Ihh protein expressions decrease in response to dynamic hydrostatic compression. This fits well with the former finding that tensile loading enhances these expressions [27-29].

Caution is required when interpreting the data quantitatively. First, the standard deviations in the measurements are relatively large and the data result from only three animals. However, despite quantitative differences between animals, the tendencies are the same for each animal. Second, both PTHrP and Ihh are detected in all experimental groups, while they are supposed to be expressed selectively by the smallest and second-largest cell populations, respectively. Most likely, the cell-separation procedure with the percoll gradient did not completely separate cells per zone. Rather, Ihh-expressing cells from the early hypertrophic zone end up in the group containing the second largest cells, but also to a lesser extend in the adjacent groups. Third, the cells are frozen immediately after 90 minutes of 0.75Hz loading with 0.1MPa. Neither this time-point nor the loading protocol is optimized for maximum effects of hydrostatic compression on PTHrP or Ihh expressions. Fourth, total protein levels are measured rather than the level of active proteins.

To ultimately identify the exact responses of PTHrP and Ihh expressions to mechanical loading requires further study of the considerations above. Despite, the reduction of PTHrP to 18% and Ihh to 44% of control levels will be used throughout this chapter, as representative for the effect of mechanical loading on the expressions of these proteins.

5. Model Simulations

5.1. Introduction

Changes in growth rate and growth-plate structure are evaluated in response to temporal changes in growth factor expressions, which differ in duration and frequency.

All simulations in this chapter are performed with the same model parameters and start with the same initial situation to allow for maximum comparison between cases. Simulations start at an early developmental stage. Cells are present in the perichondrium, the resting zone and the proliferative zone, but early hypertrophic cells have not yet formed. The number of cells in this initial situation has been obtained from a longitudinal section of a 16-days old embryonic mouse metatarsal bone. In the reference conditions, all parameters are identical to those previously used [42]. These are assumed to represent the unloaded or control situation. With these conditions, a steady growth zone with an early and late hypertrophic zone and an appropriate number of cells per zone develops in approximately five days in the control situation [42]. To ensure a steady state situation has developed, experimental conditions are applied after 21 days of development.

The magnitude of the applied changes in growth factor expressions is the same for all simulations: PTHrP and Ihh expressions are decreased to 18% or 44% of the reference condition, respectively (see former paragraph in this chapter). To simulate decreased growth factor expressions as a result of daily mechanical loading in the next paragraph, these reduced expressions are applied each 24 hours for the duration of loading. To simulate the effects of irradiation therapy in the paragraph thereafter, PTHrP and Ihh expressions are reduced for 7 consecutive days. Thus, the frequency and duration of reduced growth factor expression are the only differences between simulations in this chapter.

5.2. Daily Loading

5.2.1. Introduction

Experimental data show a correlation between the magnitude of loading and growth retardation [30-32,52]. Only 10 minutes axial loading per day suffices to reduce the total longitudinal growth of rat ulnae at the compressed side by 8% [31]. Given this effect, it has been postulated that loading as a result of the normal activity during the day may give rise to the well-accepted diurnal growth rhythm in which growth at night exceeds growth during the day [53]. In support of this hypothesis it is known that approximately 90% of all bone elongation in lambs occurs during periods of recumbence [33]. Also, applying a compressive load to growing bones for 12 hours/day during the day induces the same growth retardation as when this loading is applied during the night [54]. These studies suggest that mechanical loading during the day and unloading during the night is stimulating a local mechanism that acts superimposed on the circadian systemic regulation. This systemic regulation is controlled by hormones such as PTH and GH, which are more expressed during the night than during the day [55-57].

This study evaluates whether decreased expressions of PTHrP and Ihh as a result of daily activity and elevated expressions of these proteins when the tissue is unloaded during the night, can explain the diurnal variations in bone lengthening. Also, growth-rate reduction in response to diurnal short term loading periods is studied.

5.2.2. Method

Load-dependent effects of diurnally applied short-term loading-periods on bone growth are evaluated by applying loading-induced decreased PTHrP and Ihh expressions for 10 and 20 minutes and two hours. To simulate the effects of daily activity and nightly rest, alternating periods of 12 hours of low (active) and high growth factor expression (rest) are applied. These perturbations are applied in the model when a steady growth has been reached after three weeks of growth. To further evaluate variations in growth rates over time, the accumulated bone growths per week, day and hour are monitored for a 20 weeks period, starting two weeks after the aforementioned perturbation started (i.e. between week 5 and 20 of simulation).

5.2.3. Results

Compression of only 10 or 20 minutes per day reduces average growth rate to 97% or 96% of control, respectively. When the daily loading period is extended to two or 12 hours, the average growth rate drops to 88% or 64% of control (Figure 5A). In the control situation and in the cases where 20 minutes and two hours of daily compression are applied, the proliferative zone is on the average 45, 44 and 41 cells wide. With 12 hours of activity the average number of cells in the proliferative zone decreases to only 24. The hypertrophic zones are less sensitive to daily loading; the total number of cells in the early and late hypertrophic zones equals 31 (control), 29 (20 minutes), 28 (two hours) and 28 (eight hours).

With 12 hours of loading a day-night growth rhythm prevails. Growth during the day is on the average 10-15% compared to nightly growth and growth rates vary per day (Figure 5B).

From the close-up in Figure 5B can be derived that predicted growth is not a smooth process. Rather, growth rate varies over and between days. This not only applies to diurnally loaded developing bones, but also to the development in the unloaded control. Periods of fast and slow grow alternate at the level of weeks, days and hours. This becomes apparent when the accumulated growth in such periods is monitored (Figure 6). The growth rates at all these time-scales vary, showing high and low rates, but the appearance is more or less the same.

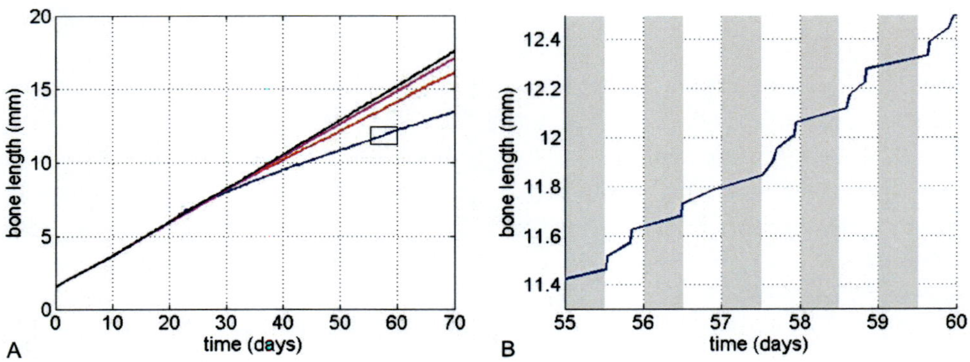

Figure 5. A) Bone growth decreases when diurnal loading is applied. Loading starts at day 21. (Black: no loading; Purple: 20 min/day; Red: 2 h/day; Blue: 12 h/day). The boxed area in the left figure is enlarged in the right figure. B) When 12 hours of loading are applied diurnally, most of the longitudinal bone growth occurs during the night (white lanes) when growth factor expressions are similar to control. During day-time (shaded lanes), when growth-factor expressions are reduced as a result of loading, growth decreases to 10-15% of the reference growth on the average.

5.2.4. Discussion

In agreement with experimental data, the bone growth rate decreases in response to mechanical compression. Even short durations of diurnal loading have an effect on the total bone length. Diurnal 12-hour loading seems to induce a synchronization of proliferation and tissue differentiation through the PTHrP-Ihh control system, resulting in a diurnal growth rhythm (Figure 5B). It should be kept in mind that effects of other factors such as PTH and GH, elevated during the night, are not included in the model and may overrule the PTHrP-Ihh system. Yet, the ten-fold difference in growth rates between loaded and unloaded periods concurs with the finding that 90% of growth occurs during periods of recumbence in lambs [33]. However, direct comparison with these data is to be done with care because the periods of rest and growth vary in the lamb-model, and because the growth monitored in the experiments results from the combination of growth and deformation due to compression.

With short-term daily loading regimes, growth is reduced during loading but recovers within one or two hours after the loading has stopped. However, when 12 hours of activity are applied daily, the growth rate during the unloaded periods is unable to recover to control levels. This is explained by adaptive reorganization of the growth plate. The widths of the various growth-plate zones vary around reference widths that are defined by the average concentrations of PTHrP and Ihh over a day. When the expression of PTHrP is low, the threshold level for cells to remain proliferating is reached relatively close to the site of PTHrP expression. Cells beyond this location will hypertrophy, which induces narrowing of the proliferative zone [41]. In the present simulations, proliferation during a 12-hour unloading period cannot restore the loss of proliferative cells that occurs during 12 hours of loading. Consequently, the width of the proliferative zone reduces from 45 to only 24 cells. These widths in the 20 minutes and two-hour loading cases are 44 and 41 cells, respectively. Quantitative data to compare simulations with is sparse. Proliferative zone width does not change in response to 10 minutes of daily loading [31] although less proliferative cells are reported when higher loading magnitudes are used [32]. In rats, a 12-hour loading period reduces the number of BrdU-labeled nuclei [54]. Both findings are in agreement with the simulations.

No significant changes to the hypertrophic zone are found experimentally when 12 hours of loading are applied daily, although a clear tendency towards decreased zonal height is observed [54]. This is in agreement with the modest decrease in the number of early and late hypertrophic cells predicted by the model. Interestingly, unlike model predictions, hypertrophic zone height increases in response to only 10 minutes of excessive diurnal loading [31,32]. This was accompanied by increased VEGF expression [32]. Increasing the VEGF-expression in the model will however induce to the opposite effect, suggesting a different mechanism. One explanation is that damage was induced in the experiments, as apparent from cracks in the tissue and compromised capillary invasion. As an alternative explanation, the threshold PTHrP-level for cells to remain proliferating may reduce in response to short-term mechanical loading or to biochemical stimuli. It is challenging to assess whether this threshold can adapt dynamically to changes in environmental conditions.

Proliferation, matrix synthesis and hypertrophy vary at the time-scales of hours, days and weeks due to varying numbers of cells per zone and fluctuations in local growth factor concentrations (Figure 6). The picture that emerges when accumulated growth is monitored per day or per hour is one of growth, varying slightly around distinct levels. These levels occur because in the model a proliferating cell instantly increases the total bone length by 12 μm. In vivo however, a proliferating cell splits horizontal to the longitudinal bone axis. Bone elongation subsequently occurs gradually when the two cells together rotate 90 degrees to end up on top of each other [58]. Thus, bone growth is less discontinuous than suggested in Figure 6C-F. Yet, the periodicity that seems to prevail in the order of 4 days is likely visible (Figure 6C). This is partly in agreement with a model that describes growth as a periodic phenomenon with uniform amplitudes and equal stasis increments [59-61]. However, the periodicity varies in amplitude and stasis increments. This agrees to some extent with the saltation model, although the simulated stasis times are not as long as those measured in humans [62-64]. Enhanced growth during the night as the result of normal daily activity, in combination with the saltation model, may explain the occurrence of incidental growing pains halfway during the night due to stretching of epiphyseal or periosteal pain receptors [64]. However, the etiology of growing pains is still unclear [33,65] and it is not sure that they are actually caused by growth.

In conclusion, despite differences in experimental conditions such as magnitudes and durations of loading, species and animal ages, model predictions concur largely with experimental observations in response to different durations of daily applied loading. In the model, the reduced expressions of PTHrP and Ihh are the only changes applied and the PTHrP-Ihh control system is the only mechanism involved in growth control. This indicates that the experimentally observed changes can theoretically be explained by changes to the PTHrP-Ihh system only. Obviously, PTHrP and Ihh act in synergy with many more factors that are involved in regulating bone development, some of which are known to respond to mechanical loading as well. It is well possible however, that the PTHrP-Ihh system plays a key-role in controlling load-dependent effects, because both PTHrP and Ihh respond load-dependently to mechanical perturbations, and because the control loop has the unique and powerful characteristic that it spans the entire length of the growing cartilage.

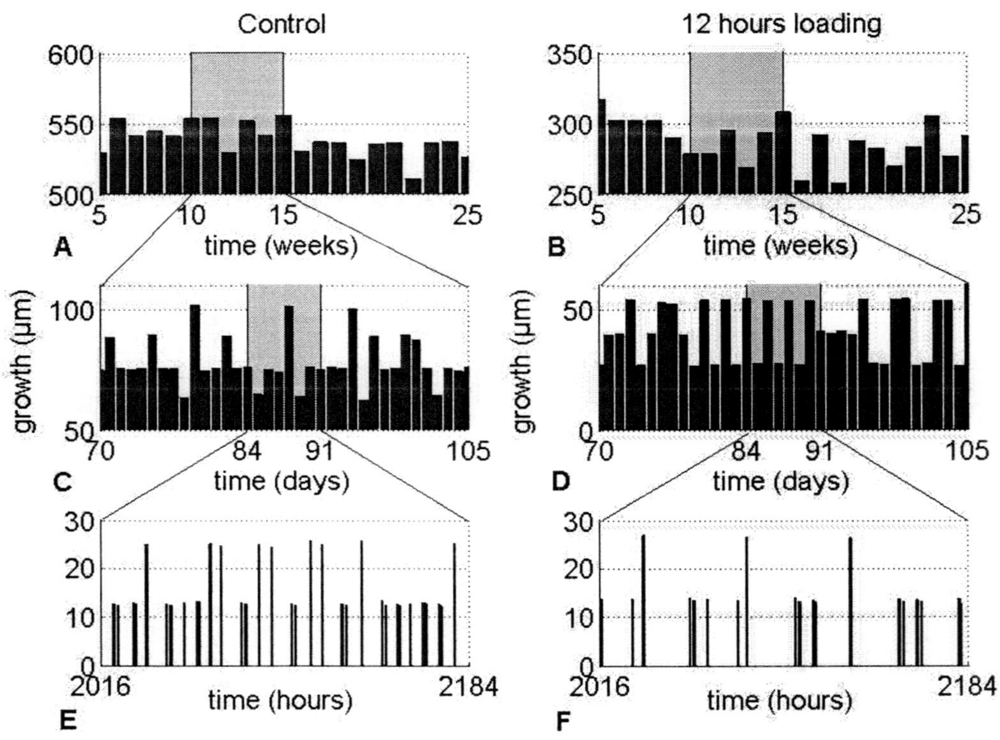

Figure 6. Bone growth per week (A,B), day (C,D) and hour (E,F) for the unloaded control (A,C,E) and the diurnal 12 hours loading case (B,D,F). The exact periods in the middle (C,D; total period five weeks) and bottom (E,F; total period seven days) graphs are shaded in the upper (A,B) and middle (C,D) graphs, respectively. Note that the axes of the right and left columns are different, representing the reduced growth rate when diurnal loading is applied (Figure 5A), but their scales are the same.

5.3. Irradiation Therapy

5.3.1. Introduction

Irradiation of an active growth plate in the leg as part of tumor treatment frequently results in severe limb length discrepancies and other bone deformities in patients [34,35] and this effect can be reproduced in rats [36-38]. Interestingly, most of the bone length difference develops in the few weeks after a one week irradiation period [66], with growth rates as low as 7% to 18% of control, one or two weeks post-irradiation [66,67]. To recover to 70% or 80% of the control growth rate takes at least four weeks [36,66]. Limb-length differences increase throughout the first 10 to 16 weeks after irradiation, after which bone-growth rates normalize but limb-length differences persist [36]. Consequently, several centimeters of limb length difference result are found in adult patients, causing a variety of secondary pathologies [35].

Most changes in growth plate development are pinpointed as being initiated in the proliferative activity of the growth-plate chondrocytes [39,40,66,67]. Proliferative activity decreases almost immediately after irradiation. The proliferative-zone height reduces by almost 50% within 48 hours after irradiation [39], and remains small for at least 12 days [67]. On the contrary, The width of the hypertrophic zone initially increases by 20% [39] before it decreases to 60% of control 7 days post irradiation [67].

It is hypothesized that strongly reduced PTHrP expression is the key factor in the response to irradiation [36,39,40]. There is no good consensus on the long-term transient changes in PTHrP expression, which are reported to recover within two weeks to values above normal [39,40], or to only partially recover after several weeks [36]. Similar changes were observed for Ihh [36], but unfortunately this quantitative analysis may be unreliable, according to the authors themselves. The best evidence for the importance of changes to PTHrP in this pathology is that selective inhibition of the decrease in PTHrP expression significantly reduces the pathological changes [68].

This pinpoints the initial cause of the pathology to changes in the expression of PTHrP. However, the question remains whether the long-term effects of irradiation can also be explained by the temporal changes in PTHrP expression.

5.3.2. Method

The effect of irradiation therapy is assessed using the theoretical model used throughout this chapter. The decreases in PTHrP [36,40] and Ihh expressions [36] are assumed to last for seven days post-irradiation. Therefore, decreased growth-factor expressions of the same magnitudes as used previously in this chapter (18% PTHrP and 44% Ihh) are applied between day 21 and 28 in the simulation. For easier interpretation of the response in time, however, the onset of irradiation is referred to as t=0 in this paragraph. Before and immediately after this seven-day period, the growth-factor expressions are assumed to equal control levels.

In addition to the simulation in which recovery after this seven-day period is evaluated, one simulation is performed in which the decreased growth-factor expression persists until the end of the simulation.

Growth rates as well as structural changes to the tissue, i.e. the sizes of the proliferative and hypertrophic zones, are monitored in time.

5.3.3. Results

Initially, the irradiated bone grows slightly faster than the control bone (Figure 7B). Within a few days the growth rate of the irradiated bone strongly reduces and a significant difference in bone length develops with the irradiated bone smaller than the control bone (Figure 7A,B). The initial increase in bone length is explained by a temporal increase in the number of hypertrophic zone cells (blue line in Figure 7C,D), which is the result of enhanced maturation of cells from the proliferative zone. Consequently, the number of cells in the proliferative zone rapidly drops to approximately half the normal number (red line in Figure 7C,D).

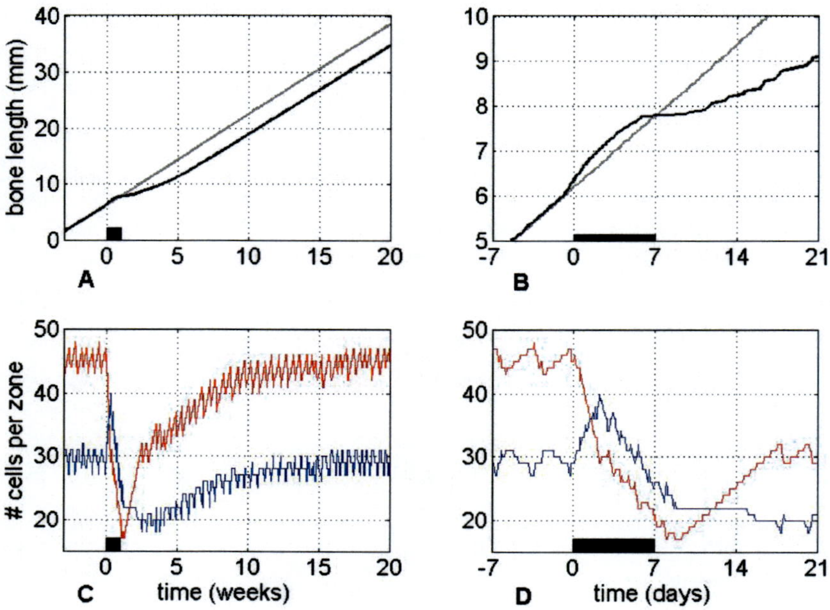

Figure 7. A,B: Bone length vs. time in weeks (A) and days (B). Grey: control bone growth; Black: bone growth when irradiation is applied, starting at t=0. After a short period of enhanced growth, the irradiated bone rapidly becomes smaller than the control bone. The bone length difference that develops in ten weeks persists until adulthood. C,D: The number of cells in the proliferative zone (red) rapidly decreases in time, resulting in a temporal increase in the number of hypertrophic cells (blue), which decreases after a few days. Recovery of the structure is slow and takes more than ten weeks. The thick black line near the bottom of each graph represents the duration of low growth factor expressions due to irradiation.

The initially enhanced bone growth is also seen in Figure 8, where the growth rate, normalized against the average growth in the control bone over ten weeks, is plotted against time. The minimal rate is reached after 12 days, i.e. five days after growth factor expressions are recovered. The growth rate remains below control for five weeks post-irradiation. Results of the simulations are compared with the literature in detail in Table 2.

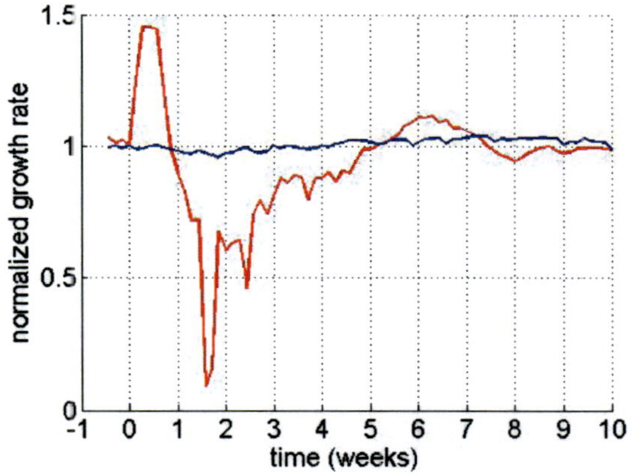

Figure 8. Growth rates in control (blue) and irradiated (red) growth plates, normalized against the average growth in the control limb over this period. Low growth factor expression was applied between weeks 0 and 1. Enhanced growth in the first few days is followed by a steep decline in growth rate which turns to less than 20% of control in between week 1 and 2 after irradiation. Then it slowly returns to normal at week 5 to eventually equilibrate after a short period of catch-up growth.

When the low growth factor expressions would persist after day seven, the numbers of cells in the proliferative and hypertrophic zones continue to reduce until almost none are left, and growth is fully arrested after 35 days (Figure 9). Interestingly, during the second week the bone growth rate in the low-expression group exceeds the growth rate in the irradiation group where growth factor expression is normalized after one week (Figure 9).

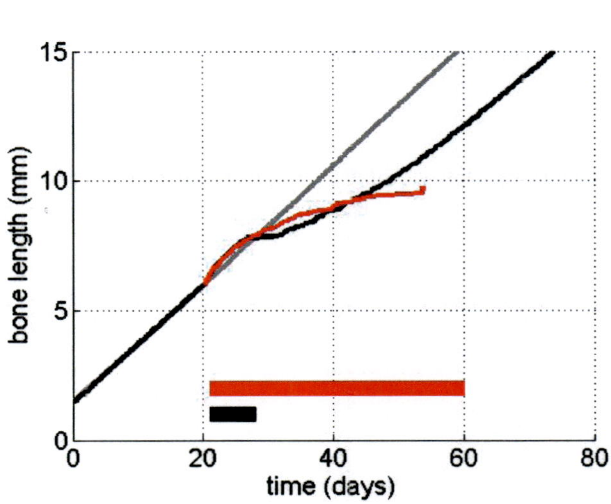

Figure 9. Total bone length vs. time during normal growth (grey), irradiation therapy between days 21 and 28 (black) and when reduced PTHrP and Ihh expressions persist, starting at day 21 (red), as indicated by the thick lines near the bottom of the graph. When low growth factor expressions persist, the growth rate reduces for approximately a month until growth is fully arrested.

Table 2. Comparison between experimental findings and computed predictions of growth, growth rates and histological changes in growing cartilage following irradiation

Experimental observations	Simulation
Bone length differences due to irradiation persist to adulthood in patients [34,35] and for more than 26 weeks post-irradiation in rats [36].	Bone length differences, which develop largely during the first five weeks post-irradiation, persist indefinitely (Figure 7A).
The difference in length between irradiated and control bones is only small after one week, but becomes obvious after two and four weeks when irradiated bones are 11 and 15% shorter than controls [66]. Length differences increase during the first 10 to 16 weeks, after which growth rate normalizes but length differences persist [36].	Bone length equals control after one week when it has recovered from a small initial elongation. After two weeks the irradiated bone is smaller than control and the difference increases for another few weeks (Figure 7A,B). At week five the growth rate has largely recovered (Figure), but only stabilizes when the proliferative and hypertrophic zones regain their original widths at weeks 10 and 15, respectively (Figure 7C,D).
Growth rates one or two weeks after irradiation vary between 7% and 18% of control [66,67]. The rate rebounds to 70% or 80% of control four weeks post-irradiation [36,66].	The normalized growth rate initially increases for four days and then decreased rapidly (Figure 8). The growth rate at day 7 is below normal and decreases to 10% of control in between one and two weeks post-irradiation. The rate rebounds to 70% of control after two weeks and slowly rises to normal at week five. It slowly oscillates around normal for ten more weeks (Figure 8) until the structure has fully recovered (Figure 7C,D).
Proliferation decreases immediately, resulting in almost 50% decrease of proliferative zone width in 48 hours [39]. The width remains below 60% for at least 12 days, with a minimum at day 7 of 45% [67].	Proliferation decreases immediately, resulting in 65% decrease of proliferative zone width in 48 hours. The width remains below 60% for 15 days, with a minimum at day 9 of 40% (Figure 8).
Hypertrophic zone width increases 20% within 12 hours and remains above control for at least 48 hours [39]. Then it drops to 60% of control in 7 days and remains low for the rest of the 12-day study [67]	Hypertrophic zone width increases 25% in 48 hours and remains above control for 5 days. Then it drops to 65% of control at day 7 and remains around 60% of control until week five, before it slowly increases. It does not reach control height until 16 weeks post-irradiation (Figure 7C,D).
The earliest signs that the growth rate catches up are visible after two weeks [36], when growth plate histology and width start to recover [40].	Growth rate starts to recover around day 10 (Figure 7B, Figure 8). Recovery of the proliferative zone height starts at day 9, but at this time the hypertrophic zone height still decreases and does not start to recover until 4 weeks post-irradiation (Figure 7D).

5.3.4. Discussion

In general, predicted responses to a seven-day period of reduced PTHrP and Ihh expressions agree remarkably well with experimental data both in magnitude and time. Examples include persisting bone length differences, growth retardation for several weeks, immediate decrease of proliferative zone height, and an initial increase in hypertrophic zone height followed by a rapid decrease. Since bone development in the model is only controlled by PTHrP and Ihh, this reinforces the original thought that irradiation induces severe effects on growth plate development through direct interaction with the PThrP-Ihh feedback system. Obviously, primary or secondary effects on expressions of other growth factors will also influence bone growth [39]. Yet, to understand many of the observed phenomena it is apparently sufficient to consider only the PTHrP-Ihh control system in combination with structural changes.

The long-term transient response in this study is largely caused by the difficulty to recover from the severe histological changes which occur during the first week. The recovery is particularly slow because resetting the growth factor expression per cell to normal expression levels does not automatically recover the growth factor concentrations throughout the tissue. To recover the normal tissue concentrations requires in addition that the same number of cells express the protein. Yet, because the number of cells per zone is decreased after one week of irradiation the total growth factor concentration throughout the tissue remains reduced. To recover the structure requires more cells and recovery is therefore dependent on proliferation. Proliferation in a column of cells depends on the number of cells available for proliferation and on Ihh concentration. Yet, the number of cells available for proliferation is low at day seven and only few early hypertrophic cells are available for Ihh synthesis. Taken together, an unfavorable situation has emerged in the growing tissue, which causes the slow recovery of its structure (Figure 7C).

When growth-factor expressions remain low, proliferating cells differentiate into hypertrophic cells until only very few are left. Hypertrophy continues until all cells are mineralized and the growth plate closes. An interesting effect in week two occurs (Figure 9). The growth rate when growth-factor expressions remain low exceeds the growth rate when expressions have recovered. The origin of this effect is the ongoing hypertrophy with persistent low expressions, compared to the temporal reduction in the number of cells entering the hypertrophic zone when growth factor expressions are recovered.

6. CONCLUSION

A one-dimensional theoretical model of bone development is used to explore the effects of transient changes in PTHrP and Ihh expressions on bone growth. In this model bone growth is determined by proliferation and differentiation (hypertrophy) of chondrocytes, and these processes are selectively controlled by PTHrP, Ihh and VEGF. It is known that this model can simulate steady state physiological and pathological bone growth [42]. The present chapter shows its applicability to dynamic responses in bone growth following transient changes in growth-factor expressions.

In response to hydrostatic compression, chondrocytes obtained from fetal epiphyseal cartilage decrease PTHrP and Ihh expressions by 18% and 44%, respectively (this chapter). More accurate data to describe the response to mechanical loading or irradiation therapy are not available in the literature. Therefore these values are used throughout this chapter. It should be kept in mind, however, that these magnitudes are probably not representative for all the different cases under examination. Hence, quantitative interpretation should be done with care, even though simulations may nicely fit experimental results.

Short-term and long-term applications of low growth-factor expressions show different responses in time. In agreement with the literature, the model predicts that short-term mechanical loading reduces bone growth rate in a dose-dependent way, but does not affect the structural organization of the tissue. When the period of daily loading is extended to twelve hours, a circadian growth rhythm develops in which growth occurs predominantly, but not selectively, during the night. Also, structural changes in the growth plate develop, leading to reduced bone growth even when the tissue is not loaded. When reduced growth factor expressions persist for seven days, which is the case when bones are subjected to irradiation, significant structural changes develop. Even though growth-factor expressions are restored to control after day seven, it takes multiple weeks to restore the structure of the growth plate, and hence to restore the rate of bone growth. The resulting difference in bone length persists until adulthood. These responses concur with the literature.

The insight obtained in this chapter is that a control system consisting of only PTHrP, Ihh and VEGF is very powerful. This system is sufficient to capture experimentally observed static and dynamic effects in the short-term (diurnal loading) as well as in the long-term (irradiation therapy). The short-term responses are directly due to dynamic changes in the concentrations of these three growth factors, while long-term dynamic responses are governed by structural changes in the growth plate, secondary to the changes in growth factor expressions.

It is extremely challenging to prove experimentally that a control mechanism by only three growth factors is in principal sufficient to capture these events. The theoretical evaluation in this chapter makes it possible to draw this conclusion.

7. Acknowledgements

I gratefully acknowledge M. Resink for performing the loading experiments and dr J. Brouwers and S. Witvoet-Braam for their contributions to the development of the theoretical model.

8. References

[1] Amizuka N, Davidson D, Liu H *et al.* Signalling by fibroblast growth factor receptor 3 and parathyroid hormone-related peptide coordinate cartilage and bone development. *Bone* 2004; 34(1):13-25.

[2] Kronenberg HM. Developmental regulation of the growth plate. *Nature* 2003; 423(6937):332-336.

[3] Minina E, Wenzel HM, Kreschel C *et al.* BMP and Ihh/PTHrP signaling interact to coordinate chondrocyte proliferation and differentiation. *Development* 2001; 128(22):4523-4534.

[4] Minina E, Kreschel C, Naski MC, Ornitz DM, Vortkamp A. Interaction of FGF, Ihh/Pthlh, and BMP signaling integrates chondrocyte proliferation and hypertrophic differentiation. *Developmental Cell* 2002; 3(3):439-449.

[5] Vortkamp A, Lee K, Lanske B *et al.* Regulation of rate of cartilage differentiation by Indian hedgehog and PTH-related protein. *Science* 1996; 273(5275):613-622.

[6] Weisser J, Riemer S, Schmidl M *et al.* Four distinct chondrocyte populations in the fetal bovine growth plate: highest expression levels of PTH/PTHrP receptor, Indian hedgehog, and MMP-13 in hypertrophic chondrocytes and their suppression by PTH (1-34) and PTHrP (1-40). *Experimental Cell Research* 2002; 279(1):1-13.

[7] Alvarez J, Sohn P, Zeng X *et al.* TGFbeta2 mediates the effects of hedgehog on hypertrophic differentiation and PTHrP expression. *Development* 2002; 129(8):1913-1924.

[8] Ehlen HWA, Buelens LA, Vortkamp A. Hedgehog signaling in skeletal develoment. *Birth Defects Research Part C - Embryo Today: Reviews* 2006; 78(3):267-279.

[9] Medill NJ, Praul CA, Ford BC, Leach RM. Parathyroid hormone-related peptide expression in the epiphyseal growth plate of the juvenile chicken: evidence for the origin of the parathyroid hormone-related peptide found in the epiphyseal growth plate. *Journal of Cellular Biochemistry* 2001; 80(4):504-511.

[10] Volk SW, Leboy PS. Regulating the regulators of chondrocyte hypertrophy. *Journal of Bone and Mineral Research* 1999; 14(4):483-486.

[11] Karp SJ, Schipani E, St Jacques B *et al.* Indian hedgehog coordinates endochondral bone growth and morphogenesis via parathyroid hormone related-protein-dependent and -independent pathways. *Development* 2000; 127(3):543-548.

[12] Lee K, Deeds JD, Segre GV. Expression of parathyroid hormone-related peptide and its receptor messenger ribonucleic acids during fetal development of rats. *Endocrinology* 1995; 136(2):453-463.

[13] Long F, Linsenmayer TF. Regulation of growth region cartilage proliferation and differentiation by perichondrium. *Development* 1998; 125(6):1067-1073.

[14] Hacker U, Nybakken K, Perrimon N. Heparan sulphate proteoglycans: The sweet side of development. *Nature Reviews Molecular Cell Biology* 2005; 6(7):530-541.

[15] Di Nino DL, Long F, Linsenmayer TF. Regulation of endochondral cartilage growth in the developing avian limb: cooperative involvement of perichondrium and periosteum. *Developmental Biology* 2001; 240(2):433-442.

[16] St Jacques B, Hammerschmidt M, McMahon AP. Indian hedgehog signaling regulates proliferation and differentiation of chondrocytes and is essential for bone formation. *Genes & Development* 1999; 13(16):2072-2086.

[17] Zhao Q, Brauer PR, Xiao L, McGuire MH, Yee JA. Expression of parathyroid hormone-related peptide (PthrP) and its receptor (PTH1R) during the histogenesis of cartilage and bone in the chicken mandibular process. *Journal of Anatomy* 2002; 201(2):137-151.

[18] Chung UI, Lanske B, Lee K, Li E, Kronenberg H. The parathyroid hormone/parathyroid hormone-related peptide receptor coordinates endochondral bone development by directly controlling chondrocyte differentiation. *Proceedings of the National Academy of Sciences of the United States of America* 1998; 95(22):13030-13035.

[19] Lee K, Lanske B, Karaplis AC *et al.* Parathyroid hormone-related peptide delays terminal differentiation of chondrocytes during endochondral bone development. *Endocrinology* 1996; 137(11):5109-5118.

[20] Ballock RT, O'Keefe RJ. The biology of the growth plate. *The Journal of Bone and Joint Surgery American Volume* 2003; 85-A(4):715-726.

[21] Schipani E, Langman C, Hunzelman J *et al.* A novel parathyroid hormone (PTH)/PTH-related peptide receptor mutation in Jansen's metaphyseal chondrodysplasia. *The Journal of Clinical Endocrinology and Metabolism* 1999; 84(9):3052-3057.

[22] Jobert AS, Zhang P, Couvineau A *et al.* Absence of functional receptors for parathyroid hormone and parathyroid hormone-related peptide in Blomstrand chondrodysplasia. *The Journal of Clinical Investigation* 1998; 102(1):34-40.

[23] Amizuka N, Warshawsky H, Henderson JE, Goltzman D, Karaplis AC. Parathyroid hormone-related peptide-depleted mice show abnormal epiphyseal cartilage development and altered endochondral bone formation. *The Journal of Cell Biology* 1994; 126(6):1611-1623.

[24] Karaplis AC, Luz A, Glowacki J *et al.* Lethal skeletal dysplasia from targeted disruption of the parathyroid hormone-related peptide gene. *Genes & Development* 1994; 8(3):277-289.

[25] Lanske B, Karaplis AC, Lee K *et al.* PTH/PTHrP receptor in early development and Indian hedgehog-regulated bone growth. *Science* 1996; 273(5275):663-666.

[26] Weir EC, Philbrick WM, Amling M *et al.* Targeted overexpression of parathyroid hormone-related peptide in chondrocytes causes chondrodysplasia and delayed endochondral bone formation. *Proceedings of the National Academy of Sciences of the United States of America* 1996; 93(19):10240-10245.

[27] Tanaka N, Ohno S, Honda K *et al.* Cyclic Mechanical Strain Regulates the PTHrP Expression in Cultured Chondrocytes via Activation of the Ca2+ Channel. *Journal of Dental Research* 2005; 84(1): 64-68.

[28] Steers WD, Broder SR, Persson K *et al.* Mechanical stretch increases secretion of parathyroind hormone-related protein by cultured bladder smooth muscle cells. *The Journal of Urology* 1998; 160(3, Part 1):908-912.

[29] Wu Q, Zhang Y, Chen Q. Indian hedgehog is an essential component of mechanotransduction complex to stimulate chondrocyte proliferation. *The Journal of Biological Chemistry* 2001; 276(38):35290-35296.

[30] Mosley JR, Lanyon LE. Growth rate rather than gender determines the size of the adaptive response of the growing skeleton to mechanical strain. *Bone* 2002; 30(1):314-319.

[31] Ohashi N, Robling AG, Burr DB, Turner CH. The effects of dynamic axial loading on the rat growth plate. *Journal of Bone and Mineral Research* 2002; 17(2):284-292.

[32] Robling AG, Duijvelaar KM, Geevers JV, Ohashi N, Turner CH. Modulation of appositional and longitudinal bone growth in the rat ulna by applied static and dynamic force. *Bone* 2001; 29(2):105-113.

[33] Noonan KJ, Farnum CE, Leiferman EM *et al.* Growing pains: are they due to increased growth during recumbency as documented in a lamb model? *Journal of Pediatric Orthopedics* 2004; 24(6):726-731.

[34] Goldwein JW. Effects of radiation therapy on skeletal growth in childhood. *Clinical Orthopaedics and Related Research* 1991; 262:101-107.

[35] Robertson WW, Butler MS, D'Angio GJ, Rate WR. Leg length discrepancy following irradiation for childhood tumors. *Journal of Pediatric Orthopedics* 1991; 11(3):284-287.

[36] Bakker B, van der Eerden BCJ, Koppenaal DW, Karperien M, Wit JM. Effect of x-irradiation on growth and the expression of parathyroid hormone-related peptide and Indian hedgehog in the tibial growth plate of the rat. *Hormone Research* 2003; 59(1):35-41.

[37] Spadaro JA, Baesl MT, Conta AC, Margulies BM, Damron TA. Effects of irradiation on the appositional and longitudinal growth of the tibia and fibula of the rat with and without radioprotectant. *Journal of Pediatric Orthopedics* 2003; 23(1):35-40.

[38] Damron TA, Spadaro JA, Tamurian RM, Damron LA. Sparing of radiation-induced damage to the physis: fractionation alone compared to amifostine pretreatment. *International Journal of Radiation Oncology, Biology, Physics* 2000; 47(4):1067-1071.

[39] Damron TA, Horton JA, Naqvi A *et al.* Decreased proliferation precedes growth factor changes after physeal irradiation. *Clinical Orthopaedics and Related Research* 2004;(422):233-242.

[40] Damron TA, Mathur S, Horton JA *et al.* Temporal Changes in PTHrP, Bcl-2, Bax, Caspase, TGF-[Beta], and FGF-2 Expression Following Growth Plate Irradiation with or Without Radioprotectant. *Journal of Histochemistry and Cytochemistry* 2004; 52(2):157-167.

[41] Van Donkelaar CC, Huiskes R. The PTHrP-Ihh feedback loop in the embryonic growth plate allows PTHrP to control hypertrophy and Ihh to regulate proliferation. *Biomechanics and Modeling in Mechanobiology* 2007; 6(1-2):55-62.

[42] Brouwers JEM, Van Donkelaar CC, Sengers BG, Huiskes R. Can the growth factors PTHrP, Ihh and VEGF, together regulate the development of a long bone? *Journal of Biomechanics* 2006; 39(15):2774-2782.

[43] Chitty LS, Altman DG. Charts of fetal size: limb bones. *BJOG: An International Journal of Obstetrics and Gynaecology* 2002; 109(8):919-929.

[44] Honarvar M, Allahyari M, Dehbashi S. Assessment of fetal weight based on ultrasonic femur length after the second trimester. *International Journal of Gynaecology and Obstetrics: The Official Organ of The International Federation of Gynaecology and Obstetrics* 2001; 73(1):15-20.

[45] Neufeld LM, Haas JD, Grajeda R, Martorell R. Ultrasound measurement of fetal size in rural Guatemala. *International Journal of Gynaecology and Obstetrics* 2004; 84(3):220-228.

[46] Bailon-Plaza A, van der Meulen MC. A mathematical framework to study the effects of growth factor influences on fracture healing. *Journal of Theoretical Biology* 2001; 212(2):191-209.

[47] Kember NF, Sissons HA. Quantitative histology of the human growth plate. *The Journal of Bone and Joint Surgery British Volume* 1976; 58-B(4):426-435.

[48] Ortega N, Behonick DJ, Werb Z. Matrix remodeling during endochondral ossification. *Trends in Cell Biology* 2004; 14(2):86-93.

[49] Sengers BG, Oomens CW, Baaijens FP. An integrated finite-element approach to mechanics, transport and biosynthesis in tissue engineering. *Journal of Biomechanical Engineering* 2004; 126(1):82-91.

[50] Alini M, Matsui Y, Dodge GR, Poole AR. The extracellular matrix of cartilage in the growth plate before and during calcification: changes in composition and degradation of type II collagen. *Calcified Tissue International* 1992; 50(4):327-335.

[51] Alini M, Carey D, Hirata S *et al.* Cellular and matrix changes before and at the time of calcification in the growth plate studied in vitro: arrest of type X collagen synthesis and net loss of collagen when calcification is initiated. *Journal of Bone and Mineral Research* 1994; 9(7):1077-1087.

[52] Stokes IAF. Mechanical effects on skeletal growth. *Journal of Musculoskeletal and Neuronal Interactions* 2002; 2(3):277-280.

[53] Russell JE, Grazman B, Simmons DJ. Mineralization in rat metaphyseal bone exhibits a circadian stage dependency. *Proceedings of the Society for Experimental Biology and Medicine* 1984; 176(4):342-345.

[54] Stokes IA, Gwadera J, Dimock A, Farnum CE, Aronsson DD. Modulation of vertebral and tibial growth by compression loading: diurnal versus full-time loading. *Journal of Orthopaedic Research* 2005; 23(1):188-195.

[55] Ahmad AM, Hopkins MT, Fraser WD *et al.* Parathyroid hormone secretory pattern, circulating activity, and effect on bone turnover in adult growth hormone deficiency. *Bone* 2003; 32(2):170-179.

[56] Fuleihan GE-H, Klerman EB, Brown EN *et al.* The Parathyroid Hormone Circadian Rhythm Is Truly Endogenous--A General Clinical Research Center Study. *Journal of Clinical Endocrinology & Metabolism* 1997; 82(1):281-286.

[57] Ahmad AM, Thomas J, Clewes A *et al.* Effects of Growth Hormone Replacement on Parathyroid Hormone Sensitivity and Bone Mineral Metabolism. *Journal of Clinical Endocrinology & Metabolism* 2003; 88(6):2860-2868.

[58] Aszodi A, Hunziker EB, Brakebusch C, Fassler R. {beta}1 integrins regulate chondrocyte rotation, G1 progression, and cytokinesis. *Genes and Development* 2003; 17(19):2465-2479.

[59] Heinrichs C, Munson PJ, Counts DR, Cutler GB, Jr., Baron J. Patterns of human growth. *Science* 1995; 268(5209):442-447.

[60] Hermanussen M, Geiger-Benoit K. No evidence for saltation in human growth. *Annals of Human Biology* 1995; 22(4):341-345.

[61] Klein KO, Munson PJ, Bacher JD, Cutler GB, Jr., Baron J. Linear growth in the rabbit is continuous, not saltatory. *Endocrinology* 1994; 134(3):1317-1320.

[62] Lampl M, Johnson ML, Frongillo EA, Jr. Mixed distribution analysis identifies saltation and stasis growth. *Annals of Human Biology* 2001; 28(4):403-411.

[63] Lampl M, Ashizawa K, Kawabata M, Johnson ML. An example of variation and pattern in saltation and stasis growth dynamics. *Annals of Human Biology* 1998; 25(3):203-219.

[64] Lampl M, Veldhuis JD, Johnson ML. Saltation and stasis: a model of human growth. *Science* 1992; 258(5083):801-803.

[65] Goodyear-Smith F, Arroll B. Growing pains. *British Medical Journal* 2006; 333(7566):456-457.

[66] Damron TA, Margulies BS, Strauss JA *et al.* Sequential histomorphometric analysis of the growth plate following irradiation with and without radioprotection. *The Journal of Bone and Joint Surgery American Volume* 2003; 85-A(7):1302-1313.

[67] Horton JA, Margulies BS, Strauss JA *et al.* Restoration of growth plate function following radiotherapy is driven by increase proliferative and synthetic activity of expansions of chondrocytic clones. *Journal of Orthopaedic Research* 2006; 24(10):1945-1956.

[68] Damron TA, Horton JA, Naqvi A *et al.* Combination radioprotectors maintain proliferation better than single agents by decreasing early parathyroid hormone-related protein changes after growth plate irradiation. *Radiation Research* 2006; 165(3):350-358.

In: Novel Aspects of PTHrP Physiopathology
Editor: Claudio Luparello, pp. 143-164
ISBN: 978-1-60021-857-6

Chapter VII

PTHrP/PTH1R: A Complex Crosstalk Among Different Signaling Pathways

Emanuela Maioli, Vittoria Fortino and Claudia Torricelli
Department of Physiology, University of Siena, Italy.

Abstract

Ligand-PTH/PTHrP type I receptor (PTH1R) interaction is followed by a number of signaling events which may work in isolation or, more often, may result in a complex integration among different signaling networks. Therefore, it is sometimes difficult to decipher the mechanism(s) mediating the several PTHrP biological effects.

In this chapter we will try to explain the versatility of N-terminal PTHrP, in terms of proliferative responses, through an updated overview of the signaling pathways triggered by the activated membrane receptor, mainly focused on 1) the several ways by which PTH1R signaling can modulate ERKs activity and cell cycle and 2) the cell type-specific outcomes of activated PKA and PKC.

Introduction

PTH and PTHrP share a common receptor, the PTH/PTHrP type I receptor (PTH1R), which is a class II G-protein coupled receptor (GPCR) [1]. The N-terminal 34 amino acids of both PTH and PTHrP are sufficient and necessary for PTH1R activation. Therefore, although the PTHrP family comprises at least three different secretory fragments [2], herein we will focus on the N-terminal PTHrP peptide, the only one able to transmit signals through the PTH1R.

Ligand-receptor interaction is followed by a number of signaling events which may work in isolation or, more often, may result in signal integration through crosstalk among complex signaling networks.

Our aim will be to try to clarify why and how PTHrP exhibits a great deal of variability in terms of biological responses, depending on the cell type and the biochemical context.

Classical PTH1R-Engaged Pathways

Tipically, PTHrP binding to GPCR stimulates the formation of cyclic 3', 5'-adenosine monophosphate (cAMP) by activating adenylate cyclase (AC) through the action of stimulatory G-alpha proteins (Gαs) coupled to the receptor. In turn, cAMP binds to the regulatory subunit of protein kinase A (PKA), which releases the active catalytic subunits of the enzyme. Vascular smooth muscle cells, enterocytes, kidney cells, chondrocytes and osteoblasts [3-7] represent well known examples of PTHrP-triggered cAMP pathway.

Conversely, in other target cells, such as squamous carcinoma cells, pancreatic islet cells, Walker 256 carcinoma cells and pancreatic insulinoma cells [8-11], PTHrP binding to GPCR mainly activates phospholipase C (PLC) β, by Gαq, leading to the formation of diacylglycerol (DAG), which activates protein kinase C (PKC) and 1,4,5 inositol triphosphate (IP3), which results in increased intracellular free Ca2+.

In certain cell types, both cAMP/AC/PKA and PLC/PKC routes are activated after PTHrP/PTH1R binding. Some examples are skin fibroblasts, MCF-7 breast cancer cells and Cos-7 cells [12-14,1].

As will be discussed below, the PTH1R classical transduction pathways can lead to very different biological outcomes, depending on the cell-specific biochemical background (Figure 1).

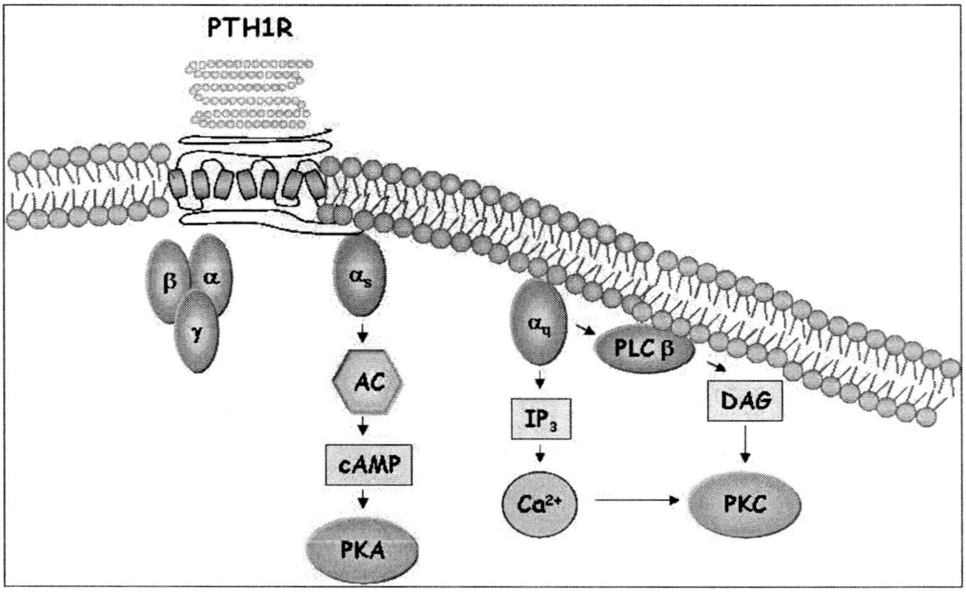

Figure 1. Classical PTHrP-engaged pathways.

NOVEL PTH1R-ENGAGED PATHWAYS

PTH1R stimulation, independently of PKA and PKC, can also result in a direct activation of Mitogen Activated Protein Kinases (MAPKs) by several alternative mechanisms.

The PTH1R Gβγ Dimer

The Ras/Raf/MAPK/ERK cascade, which usually links growth factor receptors (GFRs) at the plasma membrane to changes in gene expression in the nucleus, is a common pathway of both GFRs and GPCRs. There is significant heterogeneity in the ways in which GPCRs mediate activation of the MAPKs. Among the several mechanisms described, perhaps the most characterized is that involving the Gβγ dimer. Activation of the PTH1R releases Gβγ that, via Phosphatidyl Inositol 3-Kinase (PI3-kinase), regulates the phosphorylation of the adaptor molecule Shc, which then recruits a complex consisting of Grb2 and SOS, the Ras-specific guanine nucleotide exchange factor (GEF), to the membrane, resulting in Ras activation by exchanging GTP for GDP. GTP-bound Ras then binds directly to the serine-threonine kinase Raf, which in turn phosphorylates MEK, leading to the subsequent activation of extracellular signal-regulated kinase (ERK) 1/2; this pathway has been described in osteoblasts [15].

In rat enterocytes, an apparent variant has been reported, which also can interweave with the typical transduction pathway of GFRs and signal to ERK. This process is initiated by a direct association of the Gβγ dimer with the Src family of non-receptor tyrosine kinases [16].

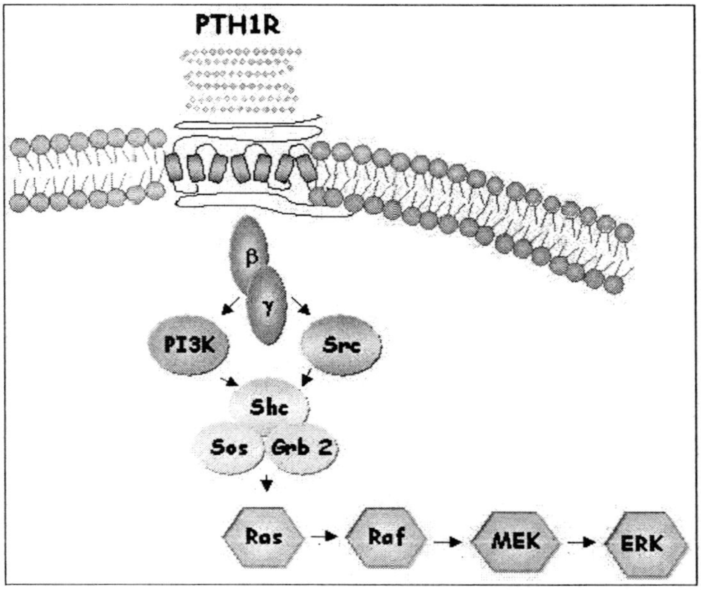

Figure 2. PTH1R Gβγ dimer signaling.

Because the Gβγ subunits of GPCRs can trigger tyrosine phosphorylation of the adapter protein Shc through Src kinases [17], signals arising from either Gβγ /IP3K or Gβγ /Src, both converging on Shc activation, likely belong to the same pathway (and lead to the same biological effects) (Figure 2).

PTHrP and Epidermal Growth Factor Receptor(EGFR) Transactivation

It has been shown that PTH1R can activate the ERK cascade in transgenic murine osteoblasts in an alternative manner, via the transactivation of the ubiquitously expressed EGF receptor through the metalloprotease-dependent shedding of endogenous EGF receptor ligands [18]. Also in human embryonic kidney HEK-293 cells, ERK activation can be achieved by PTH1R-mediated transactivation of EGF receptor, independently of second messenger pathways [19].

Although such data unequivocally demonstrate that PTH1R activation can lead to EGFR transactivation, the underlying molecular mechanisms are not well defined.

PTH1R and Arrestin

Recently, a new mechanism that directly links PTH1R to ERK has been described. After stimulation with agonist and phosphorylation by G protein-coupled receptor kinases (GRKs), PTH1R recruits cytosolic arrestin proteins to the cytoplasmic membrane. Binding of arrestin to the agonist-activated receptor causes uncoupling of receptor from G proteins, resulting in termination of agonist-mediated signaling and ligand-receptor-arrestin complex internalization [20]. The desensitization process, also called receptor downregulation, does not require the participation of second messengers [21], but it can be reinforced by the assembly of β arrestin and cAMP phosphodiesterase, which promotes cAMP degradation [22]. While this latter arrestin property has been documented thus far only after its recruitment by beta-2 adrenergic receptor, the general role of arrestin as agonist-regulated adaptor scaffold, able to trigger a second wave of signaling after internalization, has been expanded to several GPCRs. Among the known arrestin interacting proteins [23], ERK is the most documented [24-25].

By using elegant mutagenesis approaches, Ferrari and co-workers recently found that PTH1R, in its C-terminus, beares structural determinants able to reciprocally scaffold and anchor both Src and arrestin for ERK activation [26].

Thus, the PTH1R can activate Src in two independent ways: through the G βγ dimer (see above) and/or through arrestin acting as a scaffolding protein.

Regardless of the mechanism, Src activation is followed by Src-dependent tyrosine phosphorylation of Shc, Grb2-mediated recruitment of Sos, Ras activation and, ultimately, MEK/ERK phosphorylation (Figures 2-3).

An inevitable consequence of these different possibilities is that, following PTH1R activation, the time course of ERK phosphorylation often exhibits a characteristic biphasic pattern: an early transient peak, linked to the canonical Gs/q protein (and possibly to the Gβγ dimer) transduction, and a later prolonged peak, mediated by β arrestin [25].

Interestingly, although both pathways increase ERK phosphorylation, they inversely modulate cell proliferation. Indeed, the former leads to nuclear translocation of activated ERKs and possibly cell cycle progression; the latter results in the retention in the cytosol of activated ERK and hence in an attenuated proliferative response [27] (Figure 3).

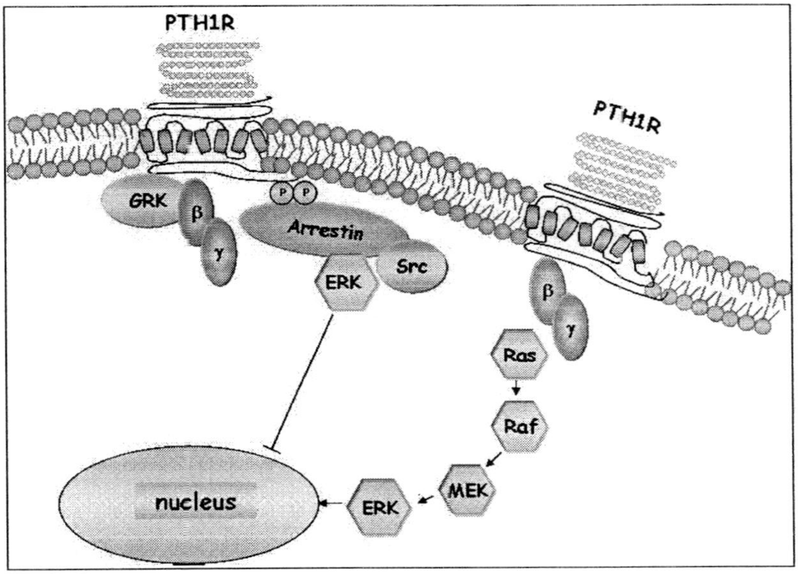

Figure 3. Opposite outcomes of ERK activation by βγ dimer and arrestin.

Therefore, although ERK phosphorylation can be achieved through multiple pathways, the ERK's mode of activation is likely the main determinant of its final biological effect [28].

Additional experimentation, however, will be required to determine whether the PTH1R/Arrestin-mediated ERK phosphorylation, as well as the several mentioned PTHrP interferences with growth factors, occurs broadly in PTHrP target cells.

Conversely, N-terminal PTHrP peptides always trigger a membrane signal through AC and/or PLC. These pathways, too, can produce very different biological outcomes, depending on the cell type and the biochemical context. In fact, because of the variable potentiality of the main second messengers, old and recent literature alike report conflict about the responsibility of PTHrP (then of PKA and PKC) in cell growth, with discordant results even in the same cell type, as in the case of MCF-7 breast cancer cells (discussed in ref 14).

Although the roles of the individual PKA and PKC signaling pathways, in mediating the downstream physiological effects of PTHrP are, in some respects, still obscure, the recently acquired knowledge explained below adds significant clarity.

Cell-Specific Responses to the PTH1R/AC Signal Transduction: ERK and the Isoform of Raf

The MAPK cascade usually transmits signals from GPCRs or GFRs to two members of the Ras family of small G proteins, Ras and Rap-1, which then stimulate the sequential activation of Raf, MEK and ERK 1/2. Ras works principally through Raf-1, whereas Rap-1 stimulates Raf-B isoform [29]. Downstream of the cAMP/PKA cascade, a dichotomy exists at the level of the different Raf-1 and Raf-B isoforms. The constitutively expressed Raf-1 isoform is phosphorylated in Ser 259 by PKA [30] and this site is one of the targets for 14.3.3 protein, which complexes to Raf-1 and prevents its recruitment to the plasma membrane (then its binding to Ras and signaling to ERK) [31].

Moreover, Rap-1 phosphorylated by PKA uncouples Raf-1 from Ras and sequestrates Raf-1 in a Rap-1/Raf-1 inactive complex. Both mechanisms, Raf-1 and Rap-1 phosphorylation, converge on blockage of ERK and lead to growth arrest in those cells where Raf-1 is the prevalent isoform [32] (Figure 4). Conversely, in Raf-B-expressing cells, the stimulation of ERK activity can be achieved through PKA-dependent Rap-1 phosphorylation, which allows the formation of an active Rap-1/Raf-B complex able to activate MEK [33].

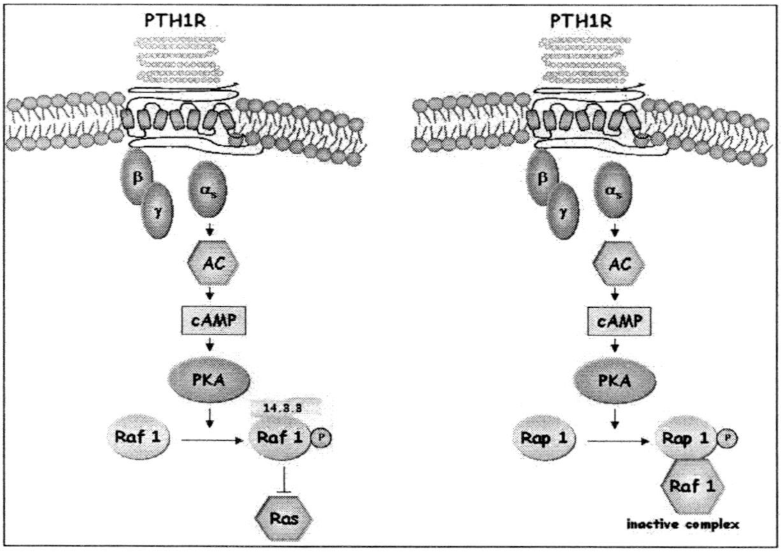

Figure 4. cAMP/PKA antiproliferative mechanism.

In addition to PKA, a second cAMP effector has been identified, the Rap-1-specific guanine nucleotide exchange factor cAMP-GEF (or Epac), the activation of which reinforces Rap-1/Raf-B signaling to ERK [34] (Figure 5).

Therefore, in Raf-B-expressing cells, cAMP has two potential mechanisms for activating ERKs, one via PKA-dependent phosphorylation of Rap-1 and another through direct activation of Rap-1-specific GEFs.

However, as already discussed, PKA-activated Rap-1 can be also an antagonist of Ras-dependent signaling, because of the competitive sequestration of Raf-1 that prevents its activation by Ras (Figure 4).

Hence, it is evident that the contingent Raf-1/Raf-B ratio plays a crucial role in determining the cAMP effects.

Consistently with the Raf isoform-based model, a PTHrP proliferative effect via the cAMP pathway has been described in rat enterocytes [35], which express Raf-B at high levels [36], whereas growth arrest is evoked in skin fibroblasts and in MCF-7 breast cancer cells [13-14], where the Raf-1 is the prevalent Raf isoform.

Nevertheless, it must be emphasized that, although this general scheme applies in several cellular models, additional cAMP effectors likely exist in the modulation of Rap-1 activity. For instance, in rat C 6 glioma cells, which express Raf isoform B, cAMP has been reported to inhibit Rap-1 in a PKA- and Epac- independent manner and to contribute to growth arrest through inhibition of ERK (and induction of p27) [37].

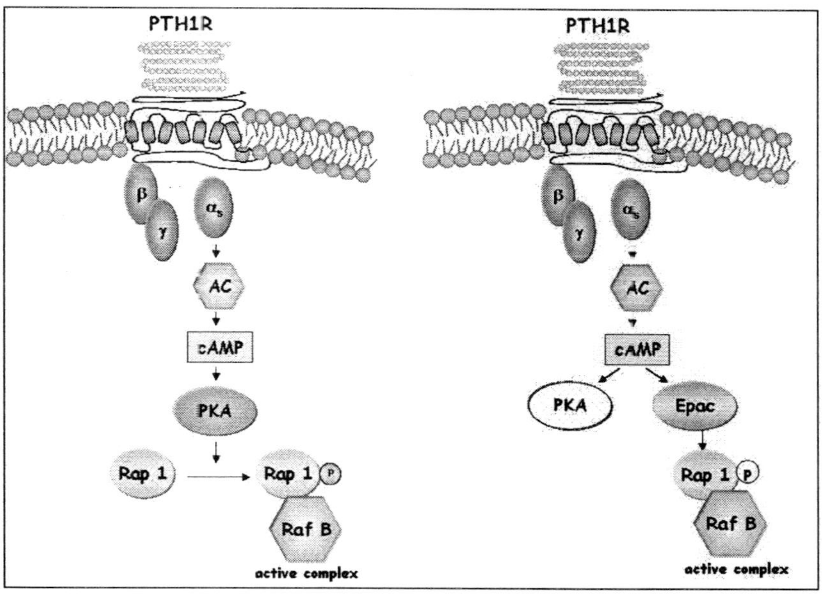

Figure 5. cAMP/PKA proliferative mechanism.

Cell-Specific Response to the PTH1R/PLC Signal Transduction: ERK and the Isoform of PKC

PKCs are a family of ubiquitous serine/threonine kinases, grouped according to their primary structure and activation requirements: the classical or conventional PKC isoforms (α, βI, βII, γ), the novel (δ, ε, η, θ) and the atypical (ζ, λ, ι). Only conventional and novel PKCs, bearing a DAG-binding site, can be pharmacologically activated by phorbol esters such as PMA. Both positive and negative roles have been ascribed to PKC in the control of cell life. The PKC transduction route can promote cell cycle progression [38-39], result in growth arrest [40] or even lead to apoptotic death [41]. Such contrasting effects are likely due to the cell-specific expression of different PKC isoforms that are thought to have non-redundant functions inside a cell.

It has long been accepted that the sequential activation of PKC/Raf-1/Ras/MEK/ERK leads to cell proliferation [42]. However, PKC stimulation can also result in the blockage of ERK phosphorylation and growth arrest [43].

The molecular switch, able to direct the PKC signal towards antiproliferative or mitogenic pathways, is the PKC isoform itself, combined with a discrete substrate specificity. Indeed, novel PKCs, similar to the action of PKA, directly phosphorylate (then inhibit) Raf-1 and prevent ERK activation.

Differently, classical and atypical PKCs phosphorylate a Raf kinase inhibitory protein (RKIP) on Ser-153, causing its dissociation from Raf-1 and thereby enhancing downstream signaling to ERK [44] (Figure 6).

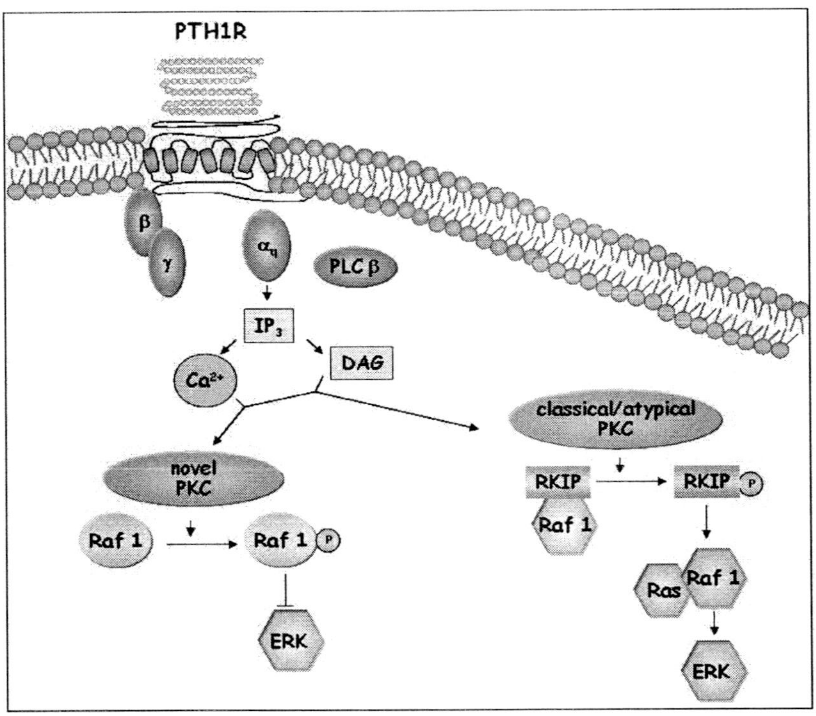

Figure 6. Isoform-based opposite PKC proliferative effects.

Evidence for these isoform-based different PKC outcomes can be found in the opposite proliferative effect of PMA in two widely used models of breast cancer cells (MCF-7 cells and MDA-MB-231 cells). In MCF-7 cells, where the novel PKCs are the prevalent isoforms, PMA evokes a growth arrest [45]; conversely, MDA-MB-231 cells that express mainly classical PKCs respond to PMA with an enhancement of their proliferation rate [46].

However, PKCs are pleiotropic kinase able to phosphorylate on Ser and Thr residues a number of different substrates. In particular, a new target of PKC has been recognized in a new class of serine/threonine protein kinases, the PKD family, originally described as a novel PKC and named PKCμ.

PTHrP and PKD (a Missing Link)

PKD is DAG/PMA sensitive, but it can be also activated by PKC-dependent phosphorylation. A recent study has demonstrated that PKCα is able to activate PKD in endothelial cells [47]. However, the bulk of research indicates that PKD activation is a prerogative of novel PKC isoforms. Several agents are known to activate PKD through PLC, leading to production of DAG and thereby activating PKC, which in turn phosphorylates (transphosphorylates) PKD. Therefore, although evidence for a direct association between PTH1R and PKD is still lacking, PKD regulation in response to other GPCRs has been demonstrated [48] and hence, there is no theoretical reason why PTH1R should not exhibit such a property.

The following sequential model of PKD activation has been proposed: GPCR activation leads to Gq-PLC-mediated production of DAG at the inner side of the plasma membrane. PKD interaction with this second messenger causes its translocation to the plasma membrane where the novel PKC, ε and/or η isoforms, are also translocated in response to DAG generation. PKC, allosterically activated by DAG, transphosphorylates PKD in Ser744 and Ser748 within the activation loop of the regulatory domain [49-50].

In turn, active PKD enhances Raf-1 kinase activity leading to MEK/ERK activation. In analogy with the classical PKCs (which act through RKIP), PKD does not directly phosphorylate Raf-1 [51] but it upregulates Ras activity by phosphorylating the Ras-binding protein RIN1. RIN1, phosphorylated at Ser 351, dissociates from Ras and is sequestered by 14.3.3 proteins. This event allows Ras to interact with Raf-1 and signal to the ERK cascade [52] (Figure 7). PKD can be the final mediator of PKC effects in many cases. The interplay between PKC and PKD is such that PKD is currently considered the crossing point between DAG and PKC [53].

These findings add a new twist to PKC signaling, as they suggest that novel PKC can have opposite effects on ERK, depending on the cell context; they can prevent ERK activation by directly phosphorylating Raf-1, but they can also activate ERK by transphosphorylating PKD This novel notion may help to reconcile the plethora of contradictory data about the effect of novel PKCs on ERK activity [54].

The phosphorylated and activated PKD moves from the plasma membrane to the cytosol and into the nucleus. Thus, PKD signals initiated at the cell surface, for example, in response to GPCR/PLC stimulation, might propagate into the interior of the cell where PKD functions as a communicator between different subcellular compartments. Indeed, PKD is implicated in a wide range of events in addition to cell proliferation, such as function and organization of the Golgi apparatus [55] and tumor cell metastatic invasion [56].

The pleiotropic effects of PKD probably depend also on its ability to control both ERK and the transcription factor nuclear factor kB (NFkB).

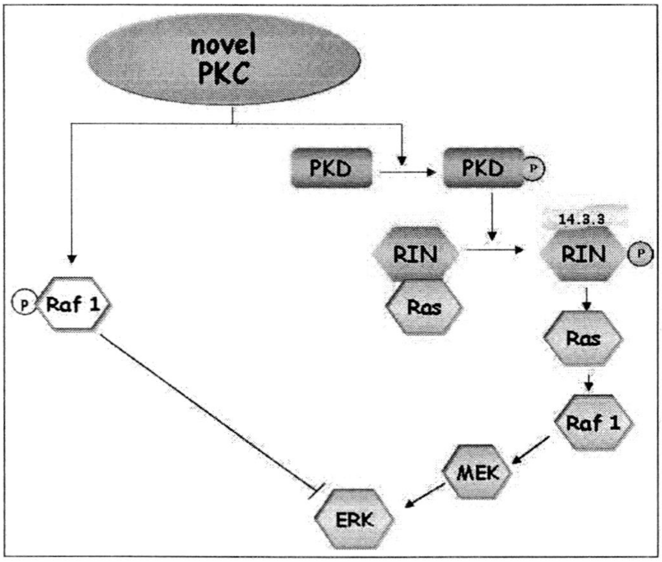

Figure 7. Novel PKC opposite effect on ERK.

PTHrP and NFkB

NFkB is an ubiquitous family of transcription factors that regulate the expression of various genes involved in inflammatory and immune responses, as well as in cell proliferation and/or apoptosis [57]. NFκB protein, mostly consisting of a heterodimer of one p50 subunit and one p65 subunit, resides in the cytoplasm, in complex with inhibitors belonging to the IκB family. Activation and nuclear migration of cytoplasmic NFκB complexes require ubiquitination and degradation of the associated IκB complex. Degradation of IκB is promoted by phosphorylation on Ser 32/36 by IkB kinase (IKK) α and β.

PKD induces NFkB translocation through activation of IKK β and subsequent degradation of IkB α [58].

Therefore, considering the determinant role in cell proliferation and survival of both ERK and NFkB, it is not surprising that, following PKC activation, conflicting results have been reported, because the different PKC isoforms can signal to ERK and NFkB through either independent or simultaneous ways (Figure 8).

It is worth mentioning here that, although the PTHrP signaling pathway to the NFkB cascade has not been clearly defined, both N- and C-terminal PTHrP domains promote NFkB activation in osteoblastic cells, as well as in vascular smooth muscle cells (VSMC) [59-60].

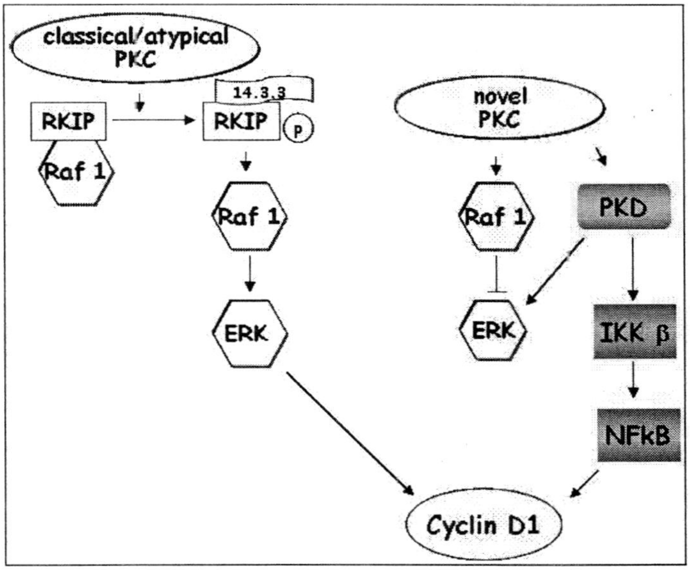

Figure 8. Double PKC signaling to ERK and NFkB.

Other PTHrP Molecular Targets in the Cell Cycle Control

PTHrP and Cyclin Dependent Kinase Inhibitors

As discussed before, activation of ERK1/2 has been described in various PTHrP target cells, and the molecular mechanisms used by PTH1R to control MAPK activity have demonstrated remarkable heterogeneity. A number of distinct mechanisms contribute to these responses, including signals mediated by second messenger-dependent protein kinases, signals mediated through cross-talk between PTH1R and receptor tyrosine kinases and signals mediated by the interaction of PTH1R-bound-arrestins with components of the MAPK cascade.

In general, activation of the ERK pathway is associated with increased proliferation. However, emerging evidence suggests that ERK activation beyond a proliferative threshold can also promote cell cycle arrest, especially in cancer cells.

Often, growth inhibition of tumor cells is dependent on expression of small inhibitory proteins, referred to as cyclin-dependent kinase inhibitors (CKIs). CKIs are grouped into two gene families, Ink4 and Cip/Kip, according to structural similarities [61]. INK4 proteins, such as p15 and p16, inhibit Cdk4 and Cdk6; Cip1/Kip1 proteins, such as $p21^{Cip1}$ and $p27^{Kip1}$, inhibit a broad range of Cdks, including Cdk2-cyclin E and Cdk2-cyclin A complexes.

In the human hepatoma HepG2 cells, enhanced ERK phosphorylation (by the classical isoform PKCα) has been shown to result in cell cycle arrest. This effect is dependent on the ERK transcriptional activity on p15 and p16 members of the INK4 family of CKIs [62].

In melanoma cells, activation of the ERK pathway leads to cell cycle arrest associated with dephosphorylation of the retinoblastoma protein (Rb) and transcriptional silencing of E2F-1. In this case, the antiproliferative effect is achieved through ERK-dependent induction of the p21 member of the Cip/Kip family of CKIs [63].

A few studies have reported the ability of PTHrP to modulate CKIs.

Datta *et al.* have shown that in differentiated osteoblastic cells, PTHrP 1-34 increases the levels of p16 protein. This effect, combined with inhibition of cyclin D1 protein expression, was responsible for cell cycle arrest [64].

In VSMC, PTHrP has been reported to inhibit cell proliferation through the cAMP pathway [65]. This effect has been ascribed to increased levels of p27.

Also in UMR-106 osteoblast-like cells, treatment with PTH (then activation of PTH1R) increases the levels of p27 and provokes growth arrest via the cAMP/PKA cascade [66].

Although in the latter two references, phospho-ERK levels were not detected, a cAMP/PKA/Raf-1-dependent inhibition of ERK phosphorylation is likely to occur both in VSMC and in UMR-106 osteoblast-like cells. Several other studies independently described an association between decreased ERK activity and enhanced p27 levels [67-68].

ERK indeed has a double effect on Cip/Kip family members, in that it induces p21 expression and promotes p27 protein degradation [63,69]. It follows that phosphorylated ERKs levels are directly proportional to p21 and inversely correlated to p27 protein (Figure 9).

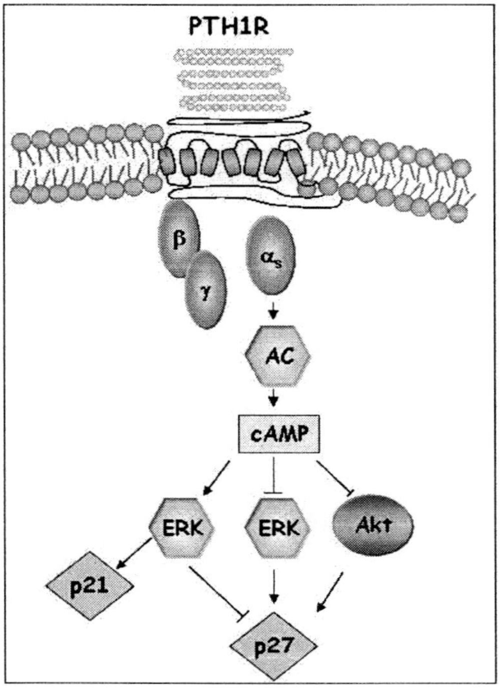

Figure 9. Triple cAMP effect on Cip/Kip CKIs.

Quite surprisingly, no study yet has demonstrated an association between PTHrP-evoked growth arrest and p21 induction.

An additional mechanism through which cAMP (and perhaps PTHrP) can control p27 levels has been described in mouse embryo fibroblasts. It is based on the ability of cAMP to inhibit Akt [70]. Akt is a serine/threonine kinase involved in cell survival, as well as in cell proliferation. One function of Akt is to negatively control the transcription factors FoxO. Because p27 is one of the FoxO targets, the cAMP pathway, via Akt inhibition, can result in p27 up-regulation [71].

Therefore, despite the fact that ERK inversely modulates p21 and p27 levels, both CKIs can be simultaneously upregulated in the same cell by cAMP: through enhanced ERK activity (p21) and through Akt inhibition (p27) (Figure 9).

PTHrP and Akt

As discussed before, the G βγ dimer of PTH1R can activate the Src/Shc/ERK pathway through PI3K. PI3K is a pleiotropic kinase, able to phosphorylate both proteins and lipids. The generation by PI3K of phosphatidylinositol 3,4,5-trisphosphate at the plasma membrane recruits Akt, the phosphorylation of which by phosphoinositide-dependent kinase (PDK), leads to its full activation.

PTH1R is known to activate the PI3K/Akt pathway in several osteoblastic cell lines and to promote cell survival [72]. In fact, among the many Akt targets, the pro-apoptotic protein Bad can be phosphorylated by this kinase and subsequently sequestrated in the cytoplasm by 14.3.3 protein [73].

The mechanism of PI3K activation in osteoblastic cells is based on a direct interaction of PTH1R with the p85 regulatory subunit of PI3K [72].

Other works described PTH1R-promoted Akt activation by different mechanisms.

In rat enterocytes, PTH1R mediates PI3K/Akt activation via Src kinase [74].

Also in breast cancer cell lines, PTHrP overexpression leads to increased levels of activated Akt. This event has been ascribed to enhanced integrin α6 β4 expression, which, in turn, triggers an integrin /PI3K/Akt pathway [75].

Further studies are required to determine whether these mechanisms linking PTHrP and Akt are actually distinct or in fact represent different starting points of a common pathway.

Additional evidence that further amplifies the number of possible combinations among different signaling pathways is the ability of Akt to phosphorylate IKK on Thr-23, thus allowing NFkB activation [76].

From this point of view, IKK/NFkB can be considered the crossroad of PKC/PKD (see above) and PI3K/Akt cascades, both of which can be (theoretically) under the control of PTH1R (Figure 10).

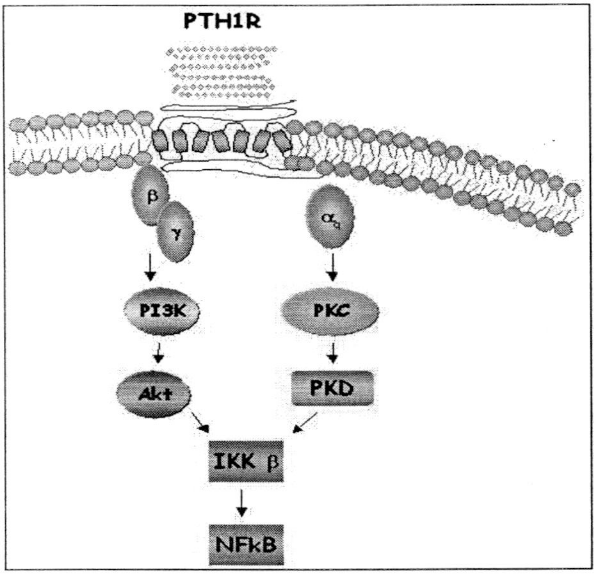

Figure 10. IKK/NFkB: the crossroad of PKC/PKD and PI3K/Akt pathways.

PTHrP and Cyclin D1

ERK, Akt and cyclin D1 are tightly connected in the control of the cell cycle [77-78].

Cyclin D1 is essential for G1/S progression. Cyclin D1 levels are the result of a balance between induction and degradation. The transcriptional induction of cyclin D1 is dependent on the Ras/Raf-1/MEK/ERK pathway [77]. Cyclin D1 turnover, i.e., its ubiquitination and proteasomal degradation, is regulated by cyclin phosphorylation on threonine 286 by glycogen sintase kinase (GSK)-3 β, which, in turn, is inactivated (by phosphorylation) via the Ras/PI3K/Akt axis [78].

PI3K indeed is also a downstream effector of Ras, by which it can be activated through a direct binding to its p110 catalytic subunit [79].

Growth Factors use this double mechanism to positively control the cyclin D1 levels and cell growth: they stimulate cyclin D1 transcription via Ras/ERK and inhibit its degradation via Ras/Akt/GSK. Therefore, in theory, PTHrP could behave as a conventional growth factor. Yet the final response to PTHrP appears to be much more complex and highly cell-specific. Indeed, PTHrP can also block cell cycle progression in a number of cell types.

Regarding the PTHrP modulation of cyclin D1, it has been recently reported that PTHrP signaling decreases cyclin D1 levels and induces growth arrest in osteoblasts [64]. On the other hand, PTHrP signaling through the PTH1R has also been reported to upregulate cyclin D1, in other cell types [80-81].

In an attempt to understand the origin of such heterogeneity, we should consider that cyclin D1 is under the transcriptional control of both ERK and NFkB [77,82-83]. Therefore, opposite PTHrP effects can be exerted on cyclin D1 levels, depending on which of the two pathways is the major target and how it is regulated by PTHrP in different cells (Figures 8, 11).

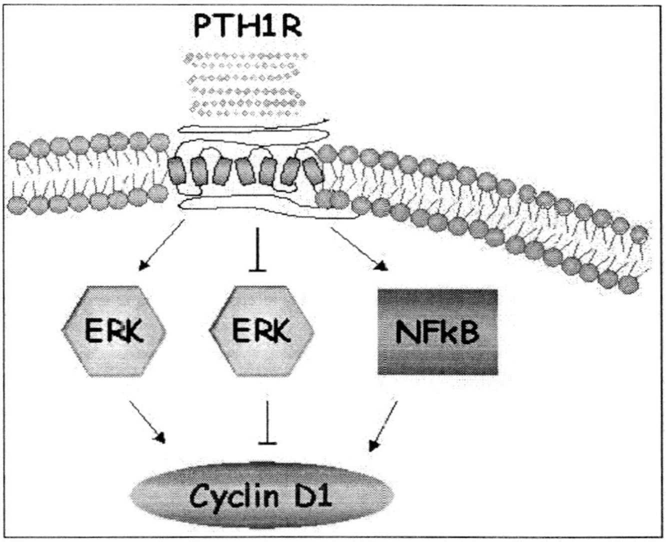

Figure 11. Antagonistic and/or synergistic PTH1R pathways on cyclin D1.

Conclusion

The number of molecular targets and biological events regulated by the activated membrane receptor has increased significantly in the past few years. The recently acquired notion that (overexpressed) PTHrP also acts as an intracrine with nuclear mitogenic and antiapoptotic effects [84], although profoundly expanding knowledge of the peptide's potentialities, somehow further confounded scientists. Indeed, mitogenic (through PKC/RKIP/ERK; PKA/Raf-B/ERK; Gβγ/Ras/ERK; Gβγ/Ras/PI3K/Akt; PKC/PKD/RIN/ERK) as well as survival effects (through p21, NFkB, Akt), similar to those ascribed to the intracrine PTHrP action in transfected cells, can also be obtained by the autocrine/paracrine PTHrP activity. With the current findings, it is very difficult to distinguish between the membrane and the nuclear PTHrP effects. In fact, although no study has ever demonstrated that the intracrine pathway is operative also in native cells, it has been shown that the exogenous peptide, even the N-terminal fragments [85], can reach the nucleus after internalization; thus it could have a "physiological" intracrine role. On this subject, Luparello and co-workers recently confirmed what was hypothesized before: exogenous PTHrP (the mid-region secretory form, so far) not only enters the nucleus of MDA-MB-231 cells but also has direct DNA-binding capability and likely transcriptional activity [86].

Moreover, the results from transfection studies do not unequivocally exclude the possibility that the overexpressed peptide, by entering into the secretory pathway, could signal through the membrane receptor, too. Therefore, infinite scenarios could be expected, depending on how the several signaling pathways interact with each other in different cell types and contexts.

To conclude, it is increasingly clear that the net functional consequences of the PTHrP activity are absolutely unpredictable and highly cell-specific.

For this reason, the scientific community should be very cautious about certain proposed strategies aimed at neutralizing autocrine/paracrine PTHrP activity in cancers, even if complicated by hypercalcemia and cachexia [87].

Indeed, no general conclusion can be drawn from any single study, and the whole chain of events has to be carefully reconstructed each time, step by step and cell by cell [88], before the real impact of PTHrP on the fate of cancer cells can be definitively established.

References

[1] Abou-Samra, A. B., Juppner, H., Force, T., Freeman, M. W., Kong, X. F., Schipani, E., Urena, P., Richards, J., Bonventre, J. V., Potts, J. T. Jr, Kronenberg, H. M. & Segre, G. V. (1992). Expression cloning of a common receptor for parathyroid hormone and parathyroid hormone-related peptide from rat osteoblast-like cells: a single receptor stimulates intracellular accumulation of both cAMP and inositol trisphosphates and increases intracellular free calcium. *Proc Natl Acad Sci USA, 89*, 2732-2736.

[2] Plawner, L. L., Philbrick, W. M., Burtis, W. J., Broadus, A. E. & Stewart, A. F. (1995). Cell type-specific secretion of parathyroid hormone-related protein via the regulated versus the constitutive secretion pathway. *J Biol Chem, 270*, 14078-14084.

[3] Maeda, S., Wu, S., Juppner, H., Green, J., Aragay, A. M., Fagin, J. A. & Clemens, T. L. (1996). Cell-specific signal transduction of parathyroid hormone (PTH)-related protein through stably expressed recombinant PTH/PTHrP receptors in vascular smooth muscle cells. *Endocrinology, 137*, 3154-3162.

[4] Gentili, C., Morelli, S. & de Boland A. R. (2003). Characterization of PTH/PTHrP receptor in rat duodenum: effects of ageing. *J Cell Biochem, 88*, 1157-1167.

[5] Yamamoto, Y., Fukase, M., Fujii, Y. & Fujita, T. (1989). The effects of human parathyroid hormone-related peptide on cytosolic free calcium and cAMP production in opossum kidney cell. *Bone Miner, 7*, 221-231.

[6] Loveys, L. S., Gelb, D., Hurwitz, S. R., Puzas, J. E. & Rosier R. N. (1993). Effects of parathyroid hormone-related peptide on chick growth plate chondrocytes. *J Orthop Res, 11*, 884-891.

[7] Rosol, T. J., Capen, C. C. & Horst, R. L. (1988). Effects of infusion of human parathyroid hormone-related protein-(1-40) in nude mice: histomorphometric and biochemical investigations. *J Bone Miner Res, 3*, 699-706.

[8] Orloff, J. J., Ganz, M. B., Ribaudo, A. E., Burtis, W. J., Reiss, M., Milstone, L. M. & Stewart, A. F. (1992). Analysis of PTHRP binding and signal transduction mechanisms in benign and malignant squamous cells. *Am J Physiol, 262*, E599-E607.

[9] Villanueva-Penacarrillo, M. L., Cancelas, J., de Miguel, F., Redondo, A., Valin, A., Valverde, I. & Esbrit, P. (1999). Parathyroid hormone-related peptide stimulates DNA synthesis and insulin secretion in pancreatic islets. *J Endocrinol, 163*, 403-408.

[10] Esbrit, P., Benìtez-Verguizas, J., de Miguel, F., Valin, A. & Garcia-Ocana, A. (2000). Characterization of parathyroid hormone/parathyroid hormone-related protein receptor and signaling in hypercalcemic Walker 256 tumor cells. *J Endocrinol, 166*, 11-20.

[11] Gaich, G., Orloff, J. J., Atillasoy, E. J., Burtis, W. J., Ganz, M. B. & Stewart, A. F. (1993). Amino-terminal parathyroid hormone-related protein: specific binding and cytosolic calcium responses in rat insulinoma cells. *Endocrinology, 132*, 1402-1409.

[12] Maioli, E., Fortino, V., Torricelli, C., Arezzini, B. & Gardi, C. (2002). Effect of parathyroid hormone-related protein on fibroblast proliferation and collagen metabolism in human skin. *Exp Dermatol, 11*, 302–310.

[13] Fortino, V., Torricelli, C., Gardi, C., Valacchi, G., Rossi Paccani, S. & Maioli, E. (2002). ERKs are the point of divergence of PKA and PKC activation by PTHrP in human skin fibroblasts. *Cell Mol Life Sci, 59*, 2165-2171.

[14] Maioli, E. & Fortino, V. (2004). PTHrP on MCF-7 breast cancer cells: a growth factor or an antimitogenic peptide? *Br J Cancer, 90*, 1293-1294.

[15] Carpio, L., Gladu, J., Goltzman, D. & Rabbani, S. A. (2001). Induction of osteoblast differentiation indexes by PTHrP in MG-63 cells involves multiple signaling pathways. Am J Physiol Endocrinol Metab, 281, E489-499.

[16] Gentili, C., Boland, R. & Russo de Boland, A. (2006). Implication of Gbetagamma proteins and c-SRC tyrosine kinase in parathyroid hormone-induced signal transduction in rat enterocytes. *J Endocrinol, 188*, 69-78.

[17] Luttrell, L. M., Hawes, B. E., van Biesen, T., Luttrell, D. K., Lansing, T. J., & Lefkowitz, R. J. (1996). Role of c-Src tyrosine kinase in G protein-coupled receptor- and Gbetagamma subunit-mediated activation of mitogen-activated protein kinases. *J Biol Chem, 271*, 19443-19450.

[18] Ahmed, I., Gesty-Palmer, D., Drezner, M. K. & Luttrell, L. M. (2003). Transactivation of the epidermal growth factor receptor mediates parathyroid hormone and prostaglandin F2 alpha-stimulated mitogen-activated protein kinase activation in cultured transgenic murine osteoblasts. *Mol Endocrinol, 17*, 1607-1621.

[19] Syme, C.A., Friedman, P. A. & Bisello, A. (2005). Parathyroid hormone receptor trafficking contributes to the activation of extracellular signal-regulated kinases but is not required for regulation of cAMP signaling. *J Biol Chem, 280*, 11281-11288.

[20] Vilardaga, J. P., Frank, M., Krasel, C., Dees, C., Nissenson, R. A. & Lohse M. J. (2001). Differential conformational requirements for activation of G proteins and the regulatory proteins arrestin and G protein-coupled receptor kinase in the G Protein-coupled receptor for parathyroid hormone (PTH)/PTH-related protein. *J Biol Chem, 276*, 33435-33443.

[21] Tawfeek, H. A., Che, J., Qian, F. & Abou-Samra, A. B. (2001). Parathyroid hormone receptor internalization is independent of protein kinase A and phospholipase C activation. *Am J Physiol Endocrinol Metab, 281*, E545-E557.

[22] Perry, S. J., Baillie, G. S., Kohout, T. A., McPhee, I., Magiera, M. M., Ang, K. L., Miller, W. E., McLean, A. J., Conti, M., Houslay, M. D. & Lefkowitz R. J. (2002). Targeting of cyclic AMP degradation to beta 2-adrenergic receptors by beta-arrestins. *Science, 298*, 834-836.

[23] Lefkowitz, R. J. & Shenoy, S. K. (2005). Transduction of receptor signals by beta-arrestins. *Science, 308*, 512-517.

[24] Gesty-Palmer, D., Chen, M., Reiter, E., Ahn, S., Nelson, C. D., Wang, S., Eckhardt, A. E., Cowan, C. L., Spurney, R. F., Luttrell, L. M. & Lefkowitz, R. J. (2006). Distinct beta-arrestin- and G protein-dependent pathways for parathyroid hormone receptor-stimulated ERK1/2 activation. *J Biol Chem, 281*, 10856-10864.

[25] Castro, M., Dicker, F., Vilardaga, J. P., Krasel, C., Bernhardt, M. & Lohse, M. J. (2002). Dual regulation of the parathyroid hormone (PTH)/PTH-related peptide receptor signaling by protein kinase C and beta-arrestins. *Endocrinology, 143*, 3854-3865.

[26] Rey, A., Manen, D., Rizzoli, R., Caverzasio, J. & Ferrari, S.L. (2006). Proline-rich Motifs in the Parathyroid Hormone (PTH)/PTH Related Protein-Receptor C-terminus Mediate Scaffolding of c-Src with beta-Arrestin2 for ERK1/2 activation. *J Biol Chem, 281*, 38181-38188.

[27] Tohgo A., Pierce K. L., Choy, E. W., Lefkowitz R. J. & Luttrell L. M. (2002). beta-Arrestin scaffolding of the ERK cascade enhances cytosolic ERK activity but inhibits ERK-mediated transcription following angiotensin AT1a receptor stimulation. *J Biol Chem, 277*, 9429-9436.

[28] Luttrell, D. K. & Luttrell, L. M. (2003). Signaling in time and space: G protein-coupled receptors and mitogen-activated protein kinases. *Assay Drug Dev Technol, 1*, 327-338.

[29] York, R. D., Yao, H., Dillon, T., Ellig, C. L., Eckert, S. P., McCleskey, E. W. & Stork, P. J. (1998). Rap1 mediates sustained MAP kinase activation induced by nerve growth factor. *Nature, 392*, 622-626.

[30] Kolch, W., Heidecker, G., Kochs, G., Hummel, R., Vahidi, H., Mischak, H., Finkenzeller, G., Marme, D. & Rapp, U. R. (1993). Protein kinase C alpha activates RAF-1 by direct phosphorylation. *Nature, 364*, 249-252.

[31] Dumaz, N. & Marais, R. (2003). Protein Kinase A blocks Raf-1 activity by stimulating 14-3-3 binding and blocking Raf-1 interaction with Ras. *J Biol Chem, 278*, 29819-29823.

[32] Fujita, T., Meguro, T., Fukuyama, R., Nakamuta, H. & Koida, M. (2002). New signaling pathway for parathyroid hormone and cyclic AMP action on extracellular-regulated kinase and cell proliferation in bone cells. Checkpoint of modulation by cyclic AMP. *J Biol Chem, 277*, 22191-22200.

[33] Erhardt, P., Troppmair, J., Rapp, U. R. & Cooper, G. M. (1995). Differential regulation of Raf-1 and B-Raf and Ras-dependent activation of mitogen-activated protein kinase by cyclic AMP in PC12 cells. *Mol Cell Biol, 15*, 5524-5530.

[34] Kawasaki, H., Springett, G. M., Mochizuki, N., Toki, S., Nakaya, M., Matsuda, M., Housman, D. E. & Graybiel, A. M. (1998). A family of cAMP-binding proteins that directly activate Rap1. *Science, 282*, 2275-2279.

[35] Gentili, C., Morelli, S., Boland, R. & de Boland, A. R. (2001). Parathyroid hormone activation of map kinase in rat duodenal cells is mediated by 3',5'-cyclic AMP and Ca(2+). *Biochim Biophys Acta, 1540*, 201-212.

[36] Alleaume, C., Eychene, A., Caigneaux, E., Muller, J. M. & Philippe, M. (2003). Vasoactive intestinal peptide stimulates proliferation in HT29 human colonic

adenocarcinoma cells: concomitant activation of Ras/Rap1-B-Raf-ERK signalling pathway. *Neuropeptides, 37*, 98-104.

[37] Wang, L., Liu, F. & Adamo, M. L. (2001). Cyclic AMP inhibits extracellular signal-regulated kinase and phosphatidylinositol 3-kinase/Akt pathways by inhibiting Rap1. *J Biol Chem, 276*, 37242-37249.

[38] Miao, D., Tong, X. K., Chan, G. K., Panda, D., McPherson, P. S. & Goltzman, D. (2001). Parathyroid hormone-related peptide stimulates osteogenic cell proliferation through protein kinase C activation of the Ras/mitogen-activated protein kinase signaling pathway. *J Biol Chem, 276*, 32204-32213.

[39] Huang, S., Maher, V. M. & McCormick, J. (1999). Involvement of intermediary metabolites in the pathway of extracellular Ca2+-induced mitogen-activated protein kinase activation in human fibroblasts. *Cell Signal, 11*, 263-274.

[40] Shanmugam, M., Krett, N. L., Maizels, E. T., Murad, F. M., Rosen, S. T. & Hunzicker-Dunn, M. (2001). A role for protein kinase C delta in the differential sensitivity of MCF-7 and MDA-MB 231 human breast cancer cells to phorbol ester-induced growth arrest and p21 (WAF1/CIP1) induction. *Cancer Lett, 172*, 43-53.

[41] Deng, Q., Liao, R., Wu, B. L. & Sun, P. (2004). High intensity ras signaling induces premature senescence by activating p38 pathway in primary human fibroblasts. *J Biol Chem, 279*, 1050-1059.

[42] Mackay, H. J. & Twelves, C. J. (2003). Protein kinase C: a target for anticancer drugs? *Endocr Relat Cancer, 10*, 389-396.

[43] Vucenik, I., Ramakrishna, G., Tantivejkul, K., Anderson, L. M. & Ramljak, D. (2005). Inositol hexaphosphate (IP6) blocks proliferation of human breast cancer cells through a PKCdelta-dependent increase in p27Kip1 and decrease in retinoblastoma protein (pRb) phosphorylation. *Breast Cancer Res Treat, 91*, 35-45.

[44] Corbit, K. C., Trakul, N., Eves, E. M., Diaz, B., Marshall, M. & Rosner, M. R. (2003). Activation of Raf-1 signaling by protein kinase C through a mechanism involving Raf kinase inhibitory protein. *J Biol Chem, 278*, 13061-13068.

[45] Falzon, M. & Du, P. (2000). Enhanced growth of MCF-7 breast cancer cells overexpressing parathyroid hormone-related peptide. *Endocrinology, 141*, 1882-1892.

[46] Jarzabek, K., Laudanski, P., Dzieciol, J., Dabrowska, M. & Wolczynski, S. (2002). Protein kinase C involvement in proliferation and survival of breast cancer cells. *Folia Histochem Cytobiol, 40*, 193-194.

[47] Wong, C. & Jin, Z. G. (2005). Protein kinase C-dependent protein kinase D activation modulates ERK signal pathway and endothelial cell proliferation by vascular endothelial growth factor. *J Biol Chem, 280*, 33262-33269.

[48] Romero, D. G., Welsh, B. L., Gomez-Sanchez, E. P., Yanes, L. L., Rilli, S. & Gomez-Sanchez, C. E. (2006). Angiotensin II-mediated protein kinase D activation stimulates aldosterone and cortisol secretion in H295R human adrenocortical cells. *Endocrinology, 147*, 6046-6055.

[49] Rykx, A., De Kimpe, L., Mikhalap, S., Vantus, T., Seufferlein, T., Vandenheede, J. R.,& Van Lint, J. (2003). Protein kinase D: a family affair. *FEBS Lett, 546*, 81-86.

[50] Rey, O., Reeve, J. R. Jr., Zhukova, E., Sinnett-Smith, J. & Rozengurt, E. (2004). G protein-coupled receptor-mediated phosphorylation of the activation loop of protein

kinase D: dependence on plasma membrane translocation and protein kinase Cepsilon. *J Biol Chem, 279*, 34361-34372.

[51] Hausser, A., Storz, P., Hubner, S., Braendlin, I., Martinez-Moya, M., Link, G. & Johannes F. J. (2001). Protein kinase C mu selectively activates the mitogen-activated protein kinase (MAPK) p42 pathway. *FEBS Lett, 492*, 39-44.

[52] Wang, Y., Waldron, R. T., Dhaka, A., Patel, A., Riley, M. M., Rozengurt, E. & Colicelli, J. (2002). The RAS effector RIN1 directly competes with RAF and is regulated by 14-3-3 proteins. *Mol Cell Biol. 22*, 916-926.

[53] Wang, Q. J. (2006). PKD at the crossroads of DAG and PKC signaling. *Trends Pharmacol Sci, 27*, 317-323.

[54] Maioli, E., Torricelli, C. & Fortino, V. (2006). Functional interactions of protein kinase A and C in signalling networks: a recapitulation. *Cell Mol Life Sci, 63*, 637-641.

[55] Liljedahl, M., Maeda, Y., Colanzi, A., Ayala, I., Van Lint, J. & Malhotra, V. (2001). Protein kinase D regulates the fission of cell surface destined transport carriers from the trans-Golgi network. *Cell, 104*, 409-420.

[56] Bowden, E. T., Barth, M., Thomas, D., Glazer, R. I., & Mueller, S. C. (1999). An invasion-related complex of cortactin, paxillin and PKCmu associates with invadopodia at sites of extracellular matrix degradation. *Oncogene, 18*, 4440-4449.

[57] Pahl, H. L. (1999). Activators and target genes of Rel/NF-kappaB transcription factors. *Oncogene, 18*, 6853-6866.

[58] Storz, P., Doppler, H. & Toker, A. (2004). Activation loop phosphorylation controls protein kinase D-dependent activation of nuclear factor kappaB. *Mol Pharmacol, 66*, 870-879.

[59] Guillén, C., Martínez, P., de Gortázar, A. R., Martínez, M. E. & Esbrit, P. (2002). Both N- and C-terminal domains of parathyroid hormone-related protein increase interleukin-6 by nuclear factor-kappaB activation in osteoblastic cells. *J Biol Chem, 277*, 28109-28117.

[60] Martin-Ventura, J. L., Ortego, M., Esbrit, P., Hernandez-Presa, M. A., Ortega, L. & Egido, J. (2003). Possible role of parathyroid hormone-related protein as a proinflammatory cytokine in atherosclerosis. *Stroke, 34*, 1783-1789.

[61] Vidal, A. & Koff, A. (2000). Cell-cycle inhibitors: three families united by a common cause. *Gene, 247*, 1-15.

[62] Wen-Sheng, W. (2006). Protein kinase C alpha trigger Ras and Raf-independent MEK/ERK activation for TPA-induced growth inhibition of human hepatoma cell HepG2. *Cancer Lett, 239*, 27-35.

[63] Cozzi, S. J., Parsons, P. G., Ogbourne, S. M., Pedley, J. & Boyle, G. M. (2006). Induction of senescence in diterpene ester-treated melanoma cells via protein kinase C-dependent hyperactivation of the mitogen-activated protein kinase pathway. *Cancer Res, 66*, 10083-10091.

[64] Datta, N. S., Chen, C., Berry, J. E. & McCauley, L. K. (2005). PTHrP signaling targets cyclin D1 and induces osteoblastic cell growth arrest. *J Bone Miner Res, 20*, 1051-1064.

[65] Stuart, W. D., Maeda, S., Khera, P., Fagin, J. A. & Clemens, T. L. (2000). Parathyroid hormone-related protein induces G1 phase growth arrest of vascular smooth muscle cells. *Am J Physiol Endocrinol Metab, 279*, E60-E67.

[66] Onishi, T. & Hruska, K. (1997). Expression of p27Kip1 in osteoblast-like cells during differentiation with parathyroid hormone. *Endocrinology, 138*,1995-2004.

[67] Betti, M. , Minelli, A., Canonico, B., Castaldo, P., Magi, S., Aisa, M. C., Piroddi, M., Di Tomaso, V. & Galli, F. (2006). Antiproliferative effects of tocopherols (vitamin E) on murine glioma C6 cells: homologue-specific control of PKC/ERK and cyclin signaling. *Free Radic Biol Med, 41*, 464-472.

[68] Hubina, E., Nanzer, A. M., Hanson, M. R., Ciccarelli, E., Losa, M., Gaia, D., Papotti, M., Terreni, M. R., Khalaf, S., Jordan, S., Czirjak, S., Hanzely, Z., Nagy, G. M., Goth, M. I., Grossman, A. B. & Korbonits. M. (2006). Somatostatin analogues stimulate p27 expression and inhibit the MAP kinase pathway in pituitary tumours. *Eur J Endocrinol, 155*, 371-379.

[69] Sakakibara, K., Kubota, K., Worku, B., Ryer, E. J., Miller, J. P., Koff, A., Kent, K. C. & Liu, B. (2005). PDGF-BB regulates p27 expression through ERK-dependent RNA turn-over in vascular smooth muscle cells. *J Biol Chem, 280*, 25470-25477.

[70] Kim, S., Jee, K., Kim, D., Koh, H. & Chung, J. (2001). Cyclic AMP inhibits Akt activity by blocking the membrane localization of PDK1. *J Biol Chem, 276*, 12864-12870.

[71] Kuiperij, H. B., van der Horst. A., Raaijmakers, J., Weijzen, S., Medema, R. H., Bos, J. L., Burgering, B. M. & Zwartkruis, F. J. (2005). Activation of FoxO transcription factors contributes to the antiproliferative effect of cAMP. *Oncogene, 24*, 2087-2095.

[72] Yamamoto, T., Kambe, F., Cao, X., Lu, X., Ishiguro, N. & Seo, H. (2006). Parathyroid hormone activates phosphoinositide 3-kinase-Akt-Bad cascade in osteoblast-like cells. *Bone, in press*.

[73] Datta, S. R, Brunet, A. & Greenberg, M. E. (1999). Cellular survival: a play in three Akts. *Genes Dev, 13*, 2905–2927.

[74] Gentili, C., Morelli, S & Russo De Boland, A. (2002). Involvement of PI3-kinase and its association with c-Src in PTH-stimulated rat enterocytes. *J Cell Biochem, 86*, 773–783.

[75] Shen, X. & Falzon, M. (2006). PTH-related protein upregulates integrin alpha6beta4 expression and activates Akt in breast cancer cells. *Exp Cell Res, 312*, 3822-3834.

[76] Ozes, O. N., Mayo, L.D., Gustin, J. A., Pfeffer, S. R., Pfeffer, L. M. & Donner, D. B. (1999). NF-kappaB activation by tumour necrosis factor requires the Akt serine-threonine kinase. *Nature, 401*, 82-85.

[77] Guillemot, L., Levy, A., Raymondjean, M. & Rothhut, B. (2001). Angiotensin II-induced transcriptional activation of the cyclin D1 gene is mediated by Egr-1 in CHO-AT(1A) cells. *J Biol Chem, 276*, 39394–39403.

[78] Shao, J., Sheng, H., DuBois, R. N. & Beauchamp, R. D. (2000). Oncogenic Ras-mediated cell growth arrest and apoptosis are associated with increased ubiquitin-dependent Cyclin D1 degradation. *J Biol Chem, 275*, 22916-22924.

[79] Rodriguez-Viciana, P., Warne, P. H., Dhand, R., Vanhaesebroeck, B., Gout, I., Fry, M. J., Waterfield, M. D. & Downward, J. (1994). Phosphatidylinositol-3-OH kinase as a direct target of Ras. *Nature, 370*, 527-532.

[80] Beier, F. & LuValle, P. (2002). The cyclin D1 and cyclin A genes are targets of activated PTH/PTHrP receptors in Jansen's metaphyseal chondrodysplasia. *Mol Endocrinol, 16,* 2163-2173.

[81] El-Hashash, A. H., Esbrit, P. & Kimber, S. J. (2005). PTHrP promotes murine secondary trophoblast giant cell differentiation through induction of endocycle, upregulation of giant-cell-promoting transcription factors and suppression of other trophoblast cell types. *Differentiation, 73,* 154-174.

[82] Guttridge, D. C., Albanese, C., Reuther, J. Y., Pestell, R. G. & Baldwin, A. S. Jr. (1999). NF-kappaB controls cell growth and differentiation through transcriptional regulation of cyclin D1. *Mol Cell Biol, 19,* 5785-5799.

[83] Wuerzberger-Davis, S. M., Chang, P. Y., Berchtold, C. & Miyamoto, S. (2005). Enhanced G2-M arrest by nuclear factor-{kappa}B-dependent p21waf1/cip1 induction. *Mol Cancer Res, 3,* 345-353.

[84] Tovar Sepulveda, V. A., Shen, X. & Falzon, M. (2002). Intracrine PTHrP protects against serum starvation-induced apoptosis and regulates the cell cycle in MCF-7 breast cancer cells. *Endocrinology, 143,* 596-606.

[85] Kumari, R., Robertson, J. F. & Watson, S. A. (2006). Nuclear targeting of a midregion PTHrP fragment is necessary for stimulating growth in breast cancer cells. *Int J Cancer, 119,* 49-59.

[86] Sirchia, R., Priulla, M., Sciandrello, G., Caradonna, F., Barbata, G. & Luparello, C. (2006). Mid-region parathyroid hormone-related protein (PTHrP) binds chromatin of MDA-MB231 breast cancer cells and isolated oligonucleotides "in vitro". *Breast Cancer Res Treat, in press.*

[87] Onuma, E., Sato, K., Saito, H., Tsunenari, T., Ishii, K., Esaki, K., Yabuta, N., Wakahara, Y., Yamada-Okabe, H. & Ogata, E. (2004). Generation of a humanized monoclonal antibody against human parathyroid hormone-related protein and its efficacy against humoral hypercalcemia of malignancy. *Anticancer Res, 24,* 2665-2673.

[88] Talon, I., Lindner, V., Sourbier, C., Schordan, E., Rothhut, S., Barthelmebs, M., Lang, H., Helwig, J. J. & Massfelder, T. (2006). Antitumor effect of parathyroid hormone-related protein neutralizing antibody in human renal cell carcinoma in vitro and in vivo. *Carcinogenesis, 27,* 73-83.

In: Novel Aspects of PTHrP Physiopathology
Editor: Claudio Luparello, pp. 165-190
ISBN: 978-1-60021-857-6

Chapter VIII

PTHrP and the Inflammatory Response

Janet L. Funk*
University of Arizona, Tucson, AZ, USA.

Abstract

The mystery of the identity of the PTH-like mediator of hypercalcemia of malignancy first proposed in 1941 was solved in the late 1980s with the isolation of parathyroid hormone-related protein (PTHrP) (Albright, 1941; Clements *et al.*, 2001; Philbrick *et al.*, 1996). Since that time, cloning of the classic PTH/PTHrP receptor (PTHR1) and the identification of other related receptors and ligands have revealed wider questions regarding the evolutionary and physiological significance of this family of proteins (Clements *et al.*, 2001; Phillbrick *et al.*, 1996). In working to unravel this complex area of study, multiple laboratories have identified key functions of PTHrP in different organs, such as bone, where PTHrP is now understood to have a significant developmental role (Kronenberg, 2006). My own research in this area, rather than focusing on the function of PTHrP in a particular organ, has sought instead to elucidate a potential role for PTHrP in the inflammatory response, a complex host defense that occurs at any site of tissue injury. A role for PTHrP in inflammation was in fact foreshadowed by the company that it keeps in the setting of malignancy; PTHrP production by malignant tumors derived from tissues where PTHrP normal acts in an autocrine fashion is frequently accompanied by the concomitant expression of multiple inflammatory cytokines, such as tumor necrosis factor (TNF), interleukin-1 (IL-1) and interleukin-6 (IL-6) (Esbrit, 2001; Nagai *et al.,* 1998; Sato *et al.,* 1989a; Mori *et al.,* 1996; Shobach & Funk, 2004). As will be discussed in this chapter, ongoing research in multiple laboratories has now revealed that PTHrP expression is indeed induced during the inflammatory response to tissue injury, and that this peptide plays a critical role in host defense and the pathophysiology of inflammatory disease.

* Correspondence concerning this article should be addressed to: Professor Janet L. Funk, University of Arizona, Tucson, AZ. e-mail: jfunk@u.arizona.edu.

INTRODUCTION

Inflammation is initiated locally in response to tissue injury. Certain early events in this process are fairly stereotypic, including the local production of cytokines and chemokines that facilitates the vascular adherence and subsequent extravasation of inflammatory cells at the site of injury (Taylor *et al.*, 2004). Other aspects of the local response are more specific to the nature of the injury (e.g. ischemia vs. bacteremia) and to the type of tissue injured (e.g. brain vs. joint) (Raz, 2007). In addition to these local responses, systemic events, such as the hepatic acute phase response, can also be triggered when locally produced inflammatory mediators spill out into the periphery (Magor & Magor, 2001). While the goal of these inflammatory processes is to limit further tissue damage, an excessive or inappropriate inflammatory response, as occurs with overwhelming sepsis or autoimmune disease, can instead be detrimental to the host.

Tumor necrosis factor-alpha (TNF-α) is recognized as an important inflammatory cytokine mediating key elements of the immune response (Dinarello, 2000; Ghezzi & Cerami, 2005). However, as its name implies, this protein and its first known biologic effect were actually identified in the setting of malignancy (Old, 1985). Parathyroid hormone-related protein (PTHrP) was similarly initially identified because of its systemic effects in malignancy (Philbrick *et al.,* 1996). However, a far more complex role for this protein in normal physiology has emerged from subsequent studies. In the absence of malignancy, PTHrP acts locally in various tissues at its site of production in a fashion more akin to a growth factor--or cytokine (Clemens *et al.*, 2004). Indeed, in the setting of inflammation, emerging evidence now supports a role for PTHrP as a local mediator of the inflammatory host response.

Many elements of the inflammatory response are due to activation of innate immunity, a macrophage and granulocyte-dependent arm of the immune system that is more developmentally primitive than the lymphocyte-dependent adaptive immune response (Delves & Roitt, 2000a; Medzhitov & Janeway, 2000). Known effects of PTHrP in both of these arms of the immune response will be reviewed here.

I. PTHRP AND INNATE IMMUNITY

Innate immunity is a rapid, immediate host reaction to pathogens that has been present throughout evolution in all plants and animals (Delves &Roitt, 2000a). In contrast, adaptive immunity rather abruptly appeared during evolution in cartilaginous fish (Janeway *et al.,* 2005). Interestingly, PTHrP, a highly conserved protein, is expressed in species more primitive than cartilaginous fish; using riboprobes and antisera against human PTHrP(1-14), constitutive expression of PTHrP has been identified in multiple tissues in lampreys (Danks *et al.*, 2001), primitive vertebrates whose only defense again injury is the innate immune response (Janeway *et al.,* 2005). While effects of PTHrP on immune function in lower vertebrates have not yet been studied in detail, it is interestingly to note that PTHrP does share with IL-1 the ability to stimulate cortisol production in these species (Holland *et al.,*

2002; Rotllant *et al.,* 2005; Guerreiro *et al.*, 2007). Specific roles of PTHrP in the innate immune response in higher vertebrates will be reviewed here (see Table 1 for summary).

Table 1. PTHrP and the Innate Immune Response

Category of Injury	Injury	Tissue	Cellular Source Inducible PTHrP	Function of Inducible PTHrP
Infection	endotoxin, low level	spleen	smooth muscle	Increase blood transit time through lymphoid organs (?)
	endotoxemia, lethal	vital organs (plus systemic)		Enhance lethality (hypotension?)
	endotoxemia or other systemic inflammation	liver	hepatocytes	Induce hepatic acute phase response
	granulomatous inflammation		epithelioid cells/vascular endothelium	Enhance granuloma formation/neutrophil influx
Nervous System Injury	kainic acid induced seizure	hippocampus	neuron (?)	Prevent excitotoxic neuronal death
	stab wound injury	brain	reactive astrocytes	Reactive gliosis (?)
	crush injury	peripheral nerve	Schwann cells	Axonal regeneration
Ischemia/ atheroma	ischemia	brain	vascular endothelium	Enhance blood flow/prevent infarction
	ischemia	heart	vascular endothelium	Vasodilate/preserve ventriciular function
	ischemia	kidney	proximal tubule/glomerular epithelium	?
	inflammation	vasculature	smooth muscle cells/macrophages	Enhance atheromatous lesion formation, destabilization, calcification
Autoimmune	RA	joint	synoviocytes/ vascular endothelium	Destroy periarticular bone and cartilage
Cancer	cachexia	systemic	tumor	Enhance catabolic state/suppress appetite (?)

I.A. PTHrP and Bacterial Sepsis

Defense against microbial pathogens is one of the most primitive functions of the immune response. One of the most ancient anti-bacterial defensive pathways, the Toll receptor system, remains the primary pathway in humans for activation of the immune response to endotoxin-bearing gram-negative bacteria (Medzhitov & Janeway, 2000; Magor & Magor, 2001). Interestingly, it was in investigating an animal model of endotoxemia that a possible role for PTHrP in the immune response was first discovered (Funk *et al.*, 1993). Very low levels of endotoxin were found to induce PTHrP mRNA expression and N-terminal PTHrP protein release from the spleen, an important site of inflammatory cytokine production during endotoxemia (Funk *et al.*, 1993). As these studies were performed soon after the initial isolation and identification of PTHrP from malignant tumors at a time when the role and regulation of PTHrP in normal physiology was not well understood, these findings led myself and my colleagues, Drs. Carl Grunfeld and Kenneth Feingold, to postulate that one possible physiologic function of this heretofore unknown protein would be to act as a member of the complex cascade of proteins induced locally in response to tissue injury. Additional studies confirmed this view. Induction of splenic PTHrP in response to endotoxin occurred subsequent to local increases in TNF and interleukin-1 (Funk *et al.*, 1993), pivotal cytokines that reside at the apex of the cascade of inflammatory mediators unleashed during the innate immune response (Dinarello, 2000; Ghezz & Cerami, 2005). Administration of either of these cytokines was also sufficient to induce splenic PTHrP expression (Funk *et al.*, 1993). As will be discussed throughout this review, this regulatory pathway for PTHrP expression in response to local injury (e.g. local injury stimulating induction of TNF and/or IL-1 which subsequently induce PTHrP) is recapitulated in numerous other tissues and in response to various types of injury (Figure 1).

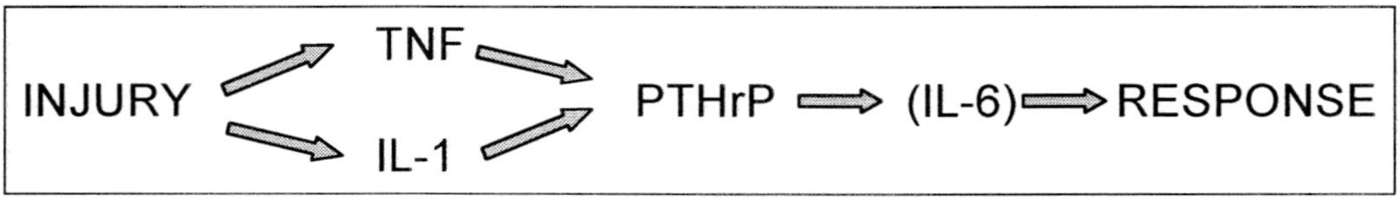

Figure 1. Common pathway of PTHrP induction during inflammation.

Based on earlier reports of lymphocyte PTHrP expression and binding, we initially postulated that PTHrP could function locally in the spleen during endotoxemia to modulate the adaptive immune response. However, this hypothesis was not supported by subsequent investigation. Endotoxin did not induce PTHrP in Toll-receptor deficient mice, nor in normal mice pretreated with a TNF inhibitor, thus demonstrating the central of role of inducible TNF in splenic PTHrP expression (Funk *et al.*, 1993). However, the ability of TNF to induce splenic PTHrP was unaltered in mice lacking T cells (nude), T and B cells (SCID), or depleted of NK cells, thus demonstrating that lymphocytes were not the source of inducible splenic PTHrP (Funk *et al.*, 1995). Moreover, PTHrP and PTHR1 were both detected only in the splenic stroma and not in splenic lymphocytes, thus making any direct effects of inducible PTHrP on lymphocyte function unlikely during endotoxemia (Funk *et al.*, 1995).

These initial studies, which were the first to identify a regulatory pathway for PTHrP expression during inflammation, were performed using very low levels of endotoxin that did not result in a detectable increase in circulating levels of PTHrP (Funk *et al.*, 1993). In contrast, in the face of a near lethal dose of endotoxin, a dose that models overwhelming sepsis, serum levels of PTHrP were induced, peaking at 2 hours and returning to baseline by 8 hours (Funk *et al.*, 1996), a pattern of secretion analogous to that of TNF in this model (Beutler *et al.*, 1985). PTHrP expression was induced in all vital organs examined (lung, heart, kidney, liver, and spleen) (Funk *et al.*, 1996). Peak induction of PTHrP mRNA expression in vital organs occurred just prior to the 2-hour time point, except in liver where expression peaked later (Funk *et al.*, 1996). These findings suggested that transient increases in systemic PTHrP levels during endotoxemia were the result of local changes in PTHrP protein production occurring in multiple tissues.

While the exact cause of death from gram-negative septic shock is not precisely known and is most likely multifactorial, profound hypotension due to extreme vasodilation is its hallmark (Parillo JE, 1993). Because PTHrP, a potent vasodilatory peptide (Clemens *et al.*, 2001), was induced in stroma cells, including smooth muscle cells, in the spleen in response to endotoxin (Funk *et al.*, 1995), we postulated that local and/or systemic effects of induced PTHrP on vascular resistance during sepsis could be contributing to organ failure, hypotension and, ultimately, lethality in this setting. Pretreatment of rodents with antisera directed against N-terminal PTHrP confirmed this; while almost half of mice receiving a control antibody were dead by 24 hours after lethal endotoxin administration and most did not survive beyond 36 hours, almost no animals treated with PTHrP neutralizing antisera had died at 24 hours, and lethality at 36 h was only 30% (Funk *et al.*, 1996). The precise cause or causes for this profound protective effect of PTHrP neutralization on survival during lethal endotoxemia, which is similar in magnitude to that reported for TNF blockade (Beutler *et al.*, 1985), is not known. However, the role of PTHrP in contributing to lethality in this model of septicemia is unequivocal.

I.B. PTHrP and the Hepatic Acute Phase Response

Early surveys documenting PTHrP expression in fetal but not adult livers had led to the general assumption that normal physiologic effects of hepatic PTHrP were primarily developmental (Philbrick *et al.*, 1996). However, this conclusion was hard to comprehend physiologically in an organ that was second only to the kidney in terms of the relative abundance of PTHR1 mRNA expression (Urena *et al.*, 1993). Therefore, in our endotoxemia studies, we found the gradual and prolonged induction of PTHrP in the liver in response to near lethal doses of endotoxin, which was quite distinct from the pattern of PTHrP induction in other vital organs, to be intriguing (Funk *et al.*, 1996). This finding takes on additional significance when one considers that that liver is the major site of production of the lipids and proteins that comprise the acute phase response (APR), which is a major arm of the innate immune response (Streetz *et al.*, 1999). Indeed, in response to endotoxin, hepatic PTHrP expression was primarily induced in the periportal hepatocytes that are a primary site of production of acute phase proteins (Funk *et al.*, 1997). The functional significance of inducible hepatic PTHrP during inflammation was proven *in vivo* in experiments in rodents demonstrating the dose-dependent ability of N-terminal PTHrP (but not a PTHR1 peptide antagonist) to (1) induce hepatic fatty acid synthesis and serum triglycerides (i.e. the release of hepatic VLDL) and to (2) stimulate hepatic expression and circulating serum levels of serum amyloid A (SAA), two important elements of the hepatic acute phase response (Funk *et al.*, 1997). Thus, rather than having no role in hepatic physiology, PTHrP may actually to be a critical regulator of the hepatic APR when its expression is induced locally during inflammation. This finding highlights the importance of regulated/inducible PTHrP expression when investigating its function during inflammation or other disease states, as will be seen again in this review when considering CNS injury; constitutive patterns of PTHrP expression are not a sufficient guide when postulating physiologic effects of PTHrP during the immune response.

The signaling pathways involved in PTHrP stimulation of the hepatic acute phase response (APR) have not yet been elucidated in the setting of inflammation. However, a large body of literature exists detailing the important role of IL-6 in induction of the APR (Gabay, 2006). Indeed, IL-6 is viewed as the primary regulator of the APR (Streetz *et al.*, 1999; Gabay, 2006). Interestingly, Mitnick *et al.* have demonstrated that perfusion of rat livers with N-terminal PTH rapidly stimulates hepatic production of IL-6 suggesting that a circulating level of PTHrP peptide similar to that achieved transiently during endotoxemia could generate 1 ng/min of IL-6 production by the liver (Mitnick *et al.*, 2001). While the focus of the Mitnick study was on possible systemic effects of these two proteins, these results are also most certainly consistent with the hypothesis that stimulatory effects of locally induced PTHrP on the APR could be mediated via local induction of IL-6 in the liver. IL-6 mediation of the effects of PTHrP during inflammation is a signaling pathway that occurs repeatedly in other sites and types of immune injury (Figure 1). Indeed, involvement of Il-6 in PTH/PTHrP signaling was first identified in the "classical", hormonal pathway of bone resorption mediated by PTH (Greenfield *et al.*, 1995).

I.C. PTHrP and Rheumatoid Arthritis

PTHrP has historically and physiologically been of great interest to bone researchers (Kronenberg, 2006). With its isolation and identification two decades ago, the mystery of the cause of the PTH-like syndrome of hypercalcemia of malignancy (HCM), a disease associated with profound bone resorption, was solved, and a new series of investigations began that have elegantly elucidated important functions of PTHrP in bone and cartilage development. However, not all aspects of HCM are yet understood, including the uncoupling of bone formation and resorption that is unique to this setting as compared to bone disease occurring with hyperparathyroidism (Stewart, 2002). One possible explanation that has been put forward to explain enhanced bone resorption in PTHrP-mediated HCM is the presence of "fellow travelers"; that is to say, tumors producing PTHrP also often produce prodigious amounts of other proteins, specifically TNF, IL-1 and IL-6, that also stimulate bone resorption (Esbrit, 2001; Mori *et al.,* 1996; Nagai *et al.,* 1998; Sato *et al.,* 1989a, b; de la Mata *et al.,* 1995; Uy *et al.,* 1997). Thus, even in the setting of malignancy, PTHrP retains its association with signaling pathways activated in innate immunity, a point that we will return to later in a discussion of PTHrP and cachexia.

Enhanced bone resorption contributes to morbidity in many chronic inflammatory diseases (Haynes, 2004; Bernstein, 2006). Therefore, to begin to examine possible bone effects of PTHrP in inflammation, my laboratory and others have focused on rheumatoid arthritis (RA). RA is notable among the arthritides for having as its basis an extreme activation of local inflammatory pathways that are also very destructive to bone (Choy & Panayi, 2001). The RA synovium grows to tumor-like proportions in the joint and acts as a local cytokine-producing "factory" that not only fuels the traditional *dolor, rumor color* and *tumor* associated with inflammation, but also facilitates the local invasion and extreme erosion of periarticular cartilage and bone (Choy & Panayi, 2001). In examining N-terminal PTHrP release from fresh explants of synovial tissue obtained from RA patients undergoing joint replacement surgery vs. patients diagnosed with the less inflammatory but more common osteoarthritis (OA), PTHrP production was detected in fewer than half of the OA specimens, while being produced by all but one RA sample (Funk *et al.*, 1998). Moreover, we identified a 10-fold increase in PTHrP production per weight of tissue from RA vs. OA synovial tissue, a finding is even more dramatic when one considers that the mass of synovial tissue in RA joints far exceeds that in present in OA (Funk *et al.*, 1998). Other laboratories have similarly measured increased levels of PTHrP peptides in rheumatoid synovial fluid (Okano *et al.*, 1996; Kohno *et al.*, 1997; Horiuchi *et al.*, 1999), levels that correlate locally with increased IL-6 levels (Horiuchi *et al.*, 1999) and systemically with increased circulating levels of C-reactive protein (Okano *et al.*, 1996), an acute phase protein.

Synoviocytes, the cytokine-producing cells within in the human rheumatoid synovium (Choy & Panayi, 2001), are immunoreactive for PTHrP (Okano *et al.*, 1996; Kohno *et al.*, 1997; Funk *et al.*, 1998; Horiuchi *et al.*, 1999), a finding confirmed by *in vitro* studies evaluating PTHrP expression in primary cultures of rheumatoid synoviocytes (Funk *et al.*, 1998). TNF and IL-1, but not IL-6, stimulate PTHrP gene expression and protein release from rheumatoid synoviocytes (Funk *et al.*, 1998). PTHrP in turn, stimulates production of IL-6 from the PTHR1-expressing synoviocytes (Funk *et al.*, 1998), thus replicating signaling pathways previously identified during endotoxemia (Funk *et al.*, 1993) (Figure 1). Moreover, because IL-6 mediates bone resorption induced by PTH/PTHrP (Greenfield *et al.*, 1995), this finding suggested that locally produced PTHrP could also be contributing to local bone destruction in RA. Consistent with this postulate, Yoshida *et al.* have also demonstrated that PGE_2, yet another mediator of inflammatory bone resorption, also induces PTHrP production in rheumatoid synoviocytes (Yoshida *et al.*, 2001).

Endothelial cells in the human rheumatoid synovial microvasculature, which supports the tumor-like growth of synovium (Firestein, 1999), are also immunoreactive for PTHrP (Funk *et al.*, 1998). This finding was also confirmed *in vitro* by documentation of N-terminal PTHrP secretion from cultured rheumatoid microvascular endothelial cells (Funk *et al.*, 2002). Contrasting with the endothelial location of PTHrP in the vasculature, its cognate receptor was expressed on adjacent smooth muscle cells and pericytes (Funk *et al.*, 2002). Given the known vasodilatory effects of N-terminal PTHrP (Clemens *et al.*, 2001), this suggested that PTHrP may regulate blood flow in the chronically hypoxic synovium. In addition, identification of PTHrP in the high endothelial venules that are that are a primary site of entry of inflammatory cells also suggested a possible luminal role for PTHrP in the vasculature (Funk *et al.*, 2002). In light of results from our laboratory and others demonstrating chemotaxic properties of PTH/PTHrP peptides (Ritchie *et al.*, 1997; Halstead *et al.*, 2001; Funk *et al.*, 2003c), this finding suggested that PTHrP could also enhance the local recruitment of inflammatory cells into the rheumatoid joint.

To address these postulates regarding the functional significance of PTHrP production in the rheumatoid synovium, an animal model of RA was employed (Funk *et al.*, 2003c). Interestingly, and contrary to our initial postulate that PTHrP may enhance inflammation in RA by stimulating inflammatory cell influx and supporting the growth of the cytokine-producing synovium, treatment of animals with the same PTHrP neutralizing antisera employed in our endotoxemia studies had no effect on joint inflammation (Funk *et al.*, 2003c). In contrast, however, PTHrP blockade had a major inhibitory impact on periarticular bone destruction. Treatment with N-terminal PTHrP neutralizing antisera preventing 30-50% of periarticular bone destruction as measured by bone mineral density (which decreases a remarkable 50% in arthritic animals), biomarkers of bone resorption and periarticular osteoclast formation (Funk *et al.*, 2003c). Thus, it would appear that PTHrP could be a major mediator of the periarticular bone destruction that complicates rheumatoid arthritis. Indeed, the pathophysiologic parallel between the local bone resorptive effects of PTHrP--and other cytokines—produced locally by bone metastases vs. the tumor-like rheumatoid synovium is striking.

I.D. PTHrP and Granulomatous Inflammation and Neutrophil Function

The lack of anti-inflammatory effect of PTHrP blockade on joint inflammation in our pre-clinical rheumatoid arthritis studies can be contrasted to its profound, and completely unanticipated, inhibitory effect on granulomatous inflammation in the same model (Funk *et al.*, 2003c). In the animal model that we employed, streptococcal cell wall (SCW)-induced arthritis, the inflammatory but non-vital SCW product stimulates a RA-like inflammatory response at its site of deposition in the joint, while a classic granulomatous response is mounted at sites of SCW deposition in liver and spleen (Geratz *et al.*, 1990). In this model, the majority of untreated animals administered SCW form hepatic and splenic granulomas. In contrast, treatment with N-terminal PTHrP neutralizing antisera reduced the incidence of granuloma formation by 40-60% in these organs and also reduced the size of lesions that did occur (Funk *et al.*, 2003c). In addition, in parallel with its suppressive effects on granuloma formation, PTHrP blockade suppressed the neutrophil influx into these tissues that is thought to be a critical early event in granuloma formation (Funk *et al.*, 2003c).

Immunohistochemical assessment of PTHrP and PTHR1 expression in the granulomatous organs revealed a remarkable finding; neutrophils within the granulomas, parenchyma and vasculature of untreated animals were strongly immunoreactive for PTHR1, while PTHrP was identified in the macrophage-derived epithelioid cells of the granulomas and in the associated vasculature (Funk *et al.*, 2003c). Macrophages and neutrophils are the two key immune cells in the innate immune response (Delves & Roitt, 2000a). This striking juxtaposition of PTHrP and its cognate receptor in these two cell types in a classic granulomatous lesion suggests that PTHrP produced by epithelioid cells (whose periarticular accumulation precedes neutrophil influx in this model) and/or the vasculature may recruit PTHR1-expressing neutrophils into the affected organs (Funk *et al.*, 2003c). Consistent with this postulate, we demonstrated through the use of a classic Boyden chamber technique that picomolar amounts of N-terminal PTHrP peptides are as effective as the classic neutrophil activator, fMLP, in stimulating neutrophil chemotaxis (Funk *et al.*, 2003c).

In human granulomatous diseases, much less is known about PTHrP function. For example, in the case of sarcoidosis, one retrospective series evaluating PTHrP expression in lymph node biopsies taken from patients with sarcoidosis, including 2 cases with PTHrP-mediated hypercalcemia, reported 85% positivity for immunoreactive PTHrP, while PTHrP mRNA was detected in 58% of specimens (Zeimer *et al.*, 1998). No increase in circulating levels of PTHrP in sarcoidosis was detected in two other series examining PTHrP production in patients with various disorders of calcium metabolism that included sarcoid patients with or without hypercalcemia, (Bucht *et al.*, 1992; Pandian *et al.*, 1992). However, the existence of additional case reports documenting PTHrP-mediated hypercalcemia in patients with sarcoidosis (Morii *et al.*, 1998) suggests that PTHrP and 1,25-dihydroxyvitamin D should both be considered as possible culprits mediating hypercalcemia in this disease. Moreover, the expression of PTHrP in sarcoid lesions even in the absence of hypercalcemia (Zeimer *et al.*, 1998) suggests the possibility, given our demonstration of the remarkable suppressive effect of PTHrP neutralizing antisera on granuloma formation, that PTHrP blockade could also prove effective in the treatment of sarcoidosis even in the absence of PTHrP-mediated hypercalcemia.

As compared to sarcoidosis, granuloma formation in response to infectious agents is physiologically advantageous. Therefore, inhibition of granulomatous inflammation in this setting, as has been reported with TNF blockade in patients with quiescent tuberculosis (Keane *et al.*, 2001), would be detrimental. While PTHrP expression in infectious granulomatous disease in humans has not been well documented, there are case reports in other vertebrates, such as dogs infected with schistosomiasis (Fradkin *et al.*, 2001). The functional significance of PTHrP expression in this setting is not known. However, one could postulate, for example, that PTH/PTHrP peptide treatment of osteoporotic patients with co-existing infectious granulomatous disease may, at least in theory, have protective effects in addition to those established for bone.

I.E. PTHrP and Nervous System Injury

Upon its discovery as the tumor product responsible for the clinical syndrome of hypercalcemia of malignancy, surveys were undertaken to identify organs and cell types expressing PTHrP under normal physiologic conditions. In the case of the central nervous system (CNS), neurons were identified as a primary site of PTHrP expression within the brain (Weir *et al.*, 1990; Weaver *et al.*, 1995). A series of elegant *in vitro* and *in vivo* studies by Dr. Arthur Broadus and colleagues provided the first insight into PTHrP function in the CNS, suggesting that neuronal PTHrP produced as a result of depolarization-driven L-channel calcium influx can feed back to dampen this influx, thus protecting against resultant neurotoxicity and neuronal death, such as that which occurs in response to kainic acid-induced seizures (Holtz *et al.*, 1996; Brines *et al.*, 1999; Chatterjee *et al.*, 2002). In contrast, there was no evidence for PTHrP expression in normal glial cells in brain (Weir *et al.*, 1990; Weaver *et al.*, 1995), the cellular "glue" that maintains neuronal health and is the primary site of the CNS immune response (Hauwel *et al.*, 2005). However, following a report by Esbrit and colleagues of immunoreactive PTHrP in human astrocytomas, but not normal astrocytes (de Miguel *et al.*, 1998), my laboratory examined PTHrP and PTHR1 expression in malignant and fetal human astrocytes *in vitro*, verifying their co-expression and an inducible effect of TNF on PTHrP expression (Shankar *et al.*, 2000). Because so-called "reactive" astrocytes, cytokine-producing cells that are activated within the brain during CNS inflammation, often express markers consistent with dedifferentiation (Lin *et al.*, 1995), we postulated that the TNF-mediated expression of PTHrP that we documented *in vitro* in immature and transformed human astrocytes could also be an important element of the repertoire of inflammatory mediators produced by normal astrocytes in response to CNS injury. To address this question, we collaborated with Dr. Seymour Reichlin to investigate PTHrP expression in rodents in response to brain stab wound injury, a classic model of reactive gliosis (Funk *et al.*, 2001). Indeed, while neurons were the primary site of PTHrP expression in normal brain and in brain tissue immediately following brain stab wound injury, as reactive gliosis developed over several days at the site of the wound, PTHrP expression was induced in these reactive astrocytes and in the neighboring vasculature (Funk *et al.*, 2001). Primary cultures of rat astrocytes verified the ability of TNF, an important product of reactive astrocytes, to induce PTHrP expression in these normal cells (Funk *et al.*, 2001). Moreover, recapitulating pathways described earlier for rheumatoid synoviocytes, N-terminal PTHrP synergized with TNF to induce interleukin-6 expression in these PTHR1-positive cells and in normal mixed glial cell cultures, while a PTHR1 peptide antagonist was without effect (Funk *et al.*, 2001) (Figure 1). Interestingly and in keeping with the site-specific effects of immune mediators during inflammation, while IL-6 plays a destructive role in bone, this PTHrP-inducible CNS cytokine has neuroprotective effects in the brain (Loddick *et al.*, 1996).

In human disease, ischemia is a prevalent cause of CNS injury that is also a major source of mortality and morbidity (Thom *et al.*, 2006). Moreover, IL-6 has been shown to be neuroprotective in animal models of focal stroke, an injury characterized by tissue infarction in a focal area surrounded by a penumbra of at-risk, inflamed tissue (Loddick *et al.*, 1996). In work performed in collaboration with Dr. Leslie Ritter (Funk *et al.*, 2003a), we therefore turned to an animal model of this clinically relevant disease to determine whether PTHrP could similarly be induced—and play a protective role—in focal stroke induced by occlusion of the middle cerebral artery. Consistent with our hypothesis and with our previous findings in other models of inflammation, PTHrP was indeed produced in response to focal ischemic injury, being induced in damaged brain tissue subsequent to local inductions in TNF and IL-1, while achieving peak levels of expression prior to peak induction of IL-6 (Funk *et al.*, 2003a) (Figure 1). Ischemia increased PTHrP expression primarily in the endothelium of the microvessels in the area of injury (Funk *et al.*, 2003a), suggesting that vasodilatory effects of this peptide could help to limit further penumbral damage by enhancing blood flow to the at-risk area. *In vitro* evidence reported by other laboratories already supported this hypothesis as TNF and IL-1 had been demonstrated to induce PTHrP expression in vascular endothelial cells (Fergusen *et al.*, 1995; Eto *et al.*, 1998), and PTHrP synergizes with IL-1 in the vascular endothelium to induce nitric oxide synthase (Jiang *et al.*, 1997). Vasodilatory effects of PTHrP in the CNS vasculature were verified *in vivo* by demonstrating a 30% increase in vessel diameter when the pial microcirculation, a surrogate for the CNS microvasculature, was superfused with N-terminal PTHrP, an effect that could increase blood flow 3-fold according to the Poiseuille equation (Funk *et al.*, 2003a). Thus, locally produced PTHrP should be able to protect brain during focal ischemia by enhancing blood flow.

To test whether the identification of this endogenous protective pathway could be translated into a potential clinical treatment, the effect of N-terminal PTHrP peptide treatment on infarction size was assessed in the same animal model (Funk *et al.*, 2003a). PTHrP reduced infarct size by almost 50% in the cortex, an area that is amenable to rescue by increased blood flow, while having no effect on infarction volume in the less easily reperfused striatum (Funk *et al.*, 2003a). These findings are consistent with the theory that ischemia-induced endothelial PTHrP is neuroprotective due to effects on blood flow, while not ruling out the possibility that it may also stimulate other neuroprotective pathways, such as those mediated by IL-6. Consistent with the theory that induction of PTHrP in the brain in response to ischemia serves a protective vascular function, inducible endothelial PTHrP was also identified in the vasculature of the hippocampus in response to transient global ischemia in rats (Funk *et al.*, 2003b), a second model of cerebral ischemia analogous to near drowning or near fatal MI where focal ischemic damage to the hippocampus can result in defects of memory (Smith *et al.*, 1984). Thus, induction of PTHrP in the cerebral microcirculation may be a universal response to different types of localized ischemic injury that helps to limit brain damage by enhancing blood flow (Macica & Broadus, 2003).

Moving away from the CNS to the peripheral nervous system (PNS), recent studies by Macica *et al.* have also documented a protective role for inducible PTHrP expression in PNS glial cells (Schwann cells) in response to nerve crush injury (Macica *et al.*, 2006). Thus, just as PTHrP is induced in reactive, "dedifferentiated" astrocytes at the site of CNS stab wound injury (Funk *et al.*, 2001), PTHrP expression is induced in Schwann cells in response to sciatic nerve crush injury (Macica *et al.*, 2006). PTHrP expression in Schwann cells, which are also postulated to dedifferentiate in response to injury, appears critical for axonal regeneration (Macica *et al.*, 2006). More specifically, blockade of endogenous N-terminal PTHrP production in an *ex vivo* model of nerve regeneration prevented the migration of Schwann cells along regenerating axons as well as the normal rebundling of axons that occurs during repair (Macica *et al.*, 2006).

Common to all of these models of nervous system injury is the inducible expression of PTHrP. Beyond this, these studies also nicely demonstrate the importance of the type and site of injury in determining the cellular source of PTHrP and its related local function. Thus, even within a single tissue type, one can see that the functional significance and site of inducible PTHrP expression varies with injury, including vasodilation when induced in the vascular endothelium in response to CNS ischemia or axonal regeneration following PNS crush injury when induced in Schwann cells.

1.F. PTHrP and Non-CNS Ischemic Injury

Our finding of ischemia-induced PTHrP in the brain recapitulates earlier findings from other laboratories that identified PTHrP induction in response to ischemic injury in the kidney and heart. Soifer *et al.* were the first to demonstrate effects of ischemia on PTHrP expression, documenting induced expression of PTHrP following ischemia-reperfusion injury in the rat kidney (Soifer *et al.*, 1993). Immunohistochemical staining localized increased PTHrP expression in proximal tubulular cells and glomerular epithelial cells (Soifer *et al.*, 1993). The biological significance of this increase remains unknown. One additional report examining the effects of transgenic over-expression of PTHrP in the proximal tubules found no effect of a focal increase in constitutive PTHrP expression on recovery from acute ischemic injury (Fiaschi-Taesch *et al.*, 2004). A discussion of additional effects of PTHrP in other types of renal injury can be found in the chapter by Dr. Pedro Esprit and colleagues.

In isolated perfused rat hearts, Schluter and colleagues have demonstrated that ischemia induces an increase in the release of PTHrP in the absence of cardiac damage as measured by CPK (Schluter *et al.*, 2000). It is postulated that coronary endothelial cells are the source of this increased PTHrP (Schluter *et al.*, 2000). A protective role for this increase in PTHrP expression in myocardial ischemia has been demonstrated. Following myocardial ischemia-reperfusion injury in pigs, infusion of N-terminal PTHrP reduces coronary resistance and improves ventricular function (Jansen *et al.*, 2003), an effect postulated to be due to direct effects on PTHR1-positive ventricular cardiomyocytes (Lutteke *et al.*, 2005). Moreover, a similar vasodilatory, protective role for endogenous PTHrP was also demonstrated in isolated rat hearts subjected to ischemia-reperfusion where treatment with a PTHR1 peptide antagonist attenuated recovery of left ventricular function (Jansen *et al.*, 2003). Interestingly, experiments in rats also suggest that the myocardial effects of PTHrP may be sex-specific, having more of a vasodilatory effect in normal hearts and a more dramatic effect on improving post-ischemic cardiac function in females than in males (Grohe *et al.*, 2004).

I.G. PTHrP and Atherosclerosis

Clinically, myocardial ischemia most commonly occurs in the setting of coronary atherosclerosis. Here, too, there is evidence of a pathogenic role for PTHrP. Inflammation is increasingly understood to play a significant role in vascular injury and the development of vascular lesions in atherosclerotic disease (Hansson, 2005). Indeed, extravasation of macrophages, one of the key cells of the innate immune response, is one of the first steps leading to the development of mature atheroma (Hansson, 2005). In one of the first reports examining PTHrP in atherosclerosis, Nakayama and colleagues reported over-expression of PTHrP in atherosclerotic, but not normal, smooth muscle cells at sites of atheroma formation in humans (Nakayama *et al.*, 1994). They further demonstrated that denudation of rat carotid arteries led to a similar marked increase in PTHrP expression at these sites of increased smooth muscle cell proliferation (Ozeki *et al.*, 1996). A functional role for PTHrP in atherosclerotic lesion formation was described in a later study by Ishikawa *et al.* who also reported increased PTHrP expression in both smooth muscles and macrophages within the thicken intima of lesions in human coronary artery lesions or lesions induced in rats by cuff placement on the femoral artery (Ishikawa *et al.*, 2000). Furthermore, in the rat cuff injury model, local application of an N-terminal PTHrP-containing gel inhibited intimal thickening and stenosis, while a PTHR1 peptide antagonist enhanced this process (Ishikawa *et al.*, 2000). In contrast, other investigators have suggested a pro-inflammatory effect of PTHrP in atherosclerotic lesions, reporting a co-localization of PTHrP and monocyte chemoattractant protein-1 (MCP-1) in human carotid atherosclerotic plaques and demonstrating *in vitro* N-terminal PTHrP peptide stimulation of MCP-1 expression in vascular smooth muscle cells via activation of NF-κB (Martin-Ventura *et al.*, 2003). Clearly, while the detailed functional role of PTHrP in atherosclerosis remains to be clarified, the enhanced expression of PTHrP in inflammatory atherosclerotic lesions is not in doubt. Also intriguing is the report by Shao and colleagues suggesting that N-terminal PTH/PTHrP peptides may also prevent the vascular calcification that enhances plaque instability and/or limits vascular compliance (Shao *et al.*, 2003). Thus, *in toto*, existing evidence primarily suggests a protective function for PTHrP when induced locally in the vasculature at sties of atheroma formation.

I.H. PTHrP and Cachexia

To end this discussion of possible effects of PTHrP during inflammation and the innate immune response, we return again to the setting in which PTHrP was discovered, cancer, and to analogies that can be drawn between TNF and PTHrP. However, in this case, the focus will be on the severe weight loss (cachexia) associated with cancer or with overwhelming inflammation. In these settings, profound metabolic changes, exacerbated by decreased appetite, lead to muscle wasting. The role of TNF, also known as cachexin when first discovered, as a key mediator of cachexia as been the focus of intense study since its cloning several years prior to PTHrP (Old, 1985). While effects of TNF on both muscle wasting and appetite have been demonstrated, it is thought that the metabolic syndrome of cachexia may only be explained by the combine effects of TNF and other cytokines (Spiegelman & Hotamisligli, 1993). Interestingly, initial reports documenting the ability of PTHrP blockade to prevent hypercalcemia of malignancy in PTHrP-producing tumor models also documented a prevention of weight loss (Sato *et al.*, 1993). However, a direct causal cachexia-inducing effect of PTHrP, rather than hypercalcemia itself, could not be deduced from these studies. This point has now been clarified by two more recent studies: (1) a report by Capparelli *et al.* (2000) documenting normalization of serum calcium levels but no prevention of cachexia in animals with PTHrP-producing neoplasms treated with OPG; and (2) a second report by Iguchi *et al.* (2006) evaluating effects of PTHrP neutralizing antibody and OPG as single or combined treatments suggesting that PTHrP blockade may ameliorate cachexia independent of its effects on calcium metabolism and in the absence of any effects on tumor size. Possible mechanisms of PTHrP-induced cachexia have yet to be reported (i.e. catabolic effects and/or appetite suppression). It should be noted, however, that hypertriglyceridemia induced by both TNF and PTHrP appears to be mediated by increased hepatic lipogenesis (Spiegelman & Hotamisligli, 1993; Funk *et al.*, 1997). Thus, as with TNF, hypertriglyceridemia is not likely to be a marker of PTHrP-induced catabolic activity.

II. PTHrP and the Acquired Immune Response

The innate immune response is an immediate response mediated by germ line-encoded receptors that recognize invariant structures common to entire classes of pathogens, such as endotoxin (Medzhitov & Janeway, 2000). In contrast, the T and B cell receptors that are central to the delayed, adaptive immune response are somatically generated and therefore have the potential to recognize "other" and well as "self" (Medzhitov & Janeway, 2000). However, certain proteins, such as cytokines and chemokines whose existence as part of the innate response can be traced back even to protozoa, still have a role in adaptive immunity. There is also considerable cross talk between the two systems (Kabelitz & Madzhitov. 2007). A classic example of this is IL-6, a macrophage product that stimulates the clonal expansion of B cells (Gabay, 2006). Moreover, inducible proteins produced by macrophages that are central to the innate immune response, such as TNF, can also be produced by lymphocytes (Weitzmann & Pacifici, 2006). Evidence to date suggests that PTHrP, analogous to the effects of other cytokines, may contribute in a similar way to the adaptive immune response.

Thus, PTHrP is more likely to be involved in the propagation rather than initiation of autoimmune disease, a postulate supported by our findings in RA (Funk *et al.*, 2003c). A brief summary of the body of knowledge regarding PTHrP in lymphocyte biology is presented here.

II.A. PTHrP and Lymphocytes

Over 100 case reports and series in the literature have documented PTHrP expression by various types of leukemias and lymphomas. Transactivation of PTHrP expression by Tax in human T cell leukemia virus (HTLV-1)-induced adult T cell leukemia or lymphoma, and the resultant hypercalcemia that occurs in the majority of these patients, is well documented (Ejima *et al.*, 1995). In addition, there are also reports of PTHrP-mediated hypercalcemia occurring in association with non-Hodgkin's lymphomas, particularly B cell lymphomas, and acute lymphoblastic leukemia (Shoback & Funk, 2004). What, then, is the evidence for PTHrP expression by normal, non-transformed lymphocytes? Soon after the isolation of PTHrP and identification of PTHrP expression in HTLV-1 infected T cells (Motokura *et al.*, 1988), Adachi *et al.* examined PTHrP expression in normal human lymphocytes. In this report, using human mononuclear cell preparations depleted of macrophages which, in some cases, were also enriched for T cells, PTHrP(1-34) release was detected in PHA- or ConA-stimulated, but not in unstimulated, cells (Adachi *et al.*, 1990). However, we are not aware of any subsequent *in vitro* evidence of PTHrP production by non-transformed lymphocytes, including unpublished studies by our own laboratory examining PTHrP expression in resting or ConA-stimulated rat thymocytes or T cell-enriched rat splenocytes (Funk *et al.*, unpublished). Interestingly, in a recent report by Godler *et al.* investigating PTHrP expression in murine collagen-induced arthritis, an arthritis model where B cell-produced immunoglobulins play an important pathogenic role (van den Berg, 2001), immunohistochemical PTHrP expression was reported at early time points in small numbers of scattered lymphocytes in draining lymph nodes (Godler *et al.*, 2005). Given this level of evidence, however, the physiological significance of PTHrP expression by lymphocytes remains uncertain.

While questions thus remain about lymphocyte PTHrP expression, effects of PTH and PTHrP peptides on lymphocyte function have been repeatedly documented. A body of literature predating the discovery of PTHrP has documented effects of PTH on various lymphocyte preparations, beginning in 1969 with a report by Whitfield *et al.* of PTH stimulation of rat thymocyte proliferation (Whitfield *et al.*, 1969). While PTH peptides can stimulate cAMP in rat thymocytes (Whitfield *et al.*, 1970; Atkinson *et al.*, 1987), PTH-induced thymocyte proliferation appears to occur independent of this and require extracellular calcium (Atkinson *et al.*, 1987). In contrast, in circulating human lymphocytes, cAMP-stimulating N-terminal PTH peptides have the opposite effect on cell growth, inhibiting proliferation (Adachi *et al.*, 1990; Elias *et al.*, 1988; Hoette *et al.*, 1977; Klinger *et al.,* 1990; Perry *et al.*, 1984; Shasha *et al.*, 1988; Yamamoto *et al.*, 1983). In B cells, binding of PTH peptides is also reported to inhibit immunoglobulin production (Bialasiewicz *et al.*, 1979; Gaciong *et al.*, 1991, Jiang Y *et al.*, 1992). We are only aware of 3 studies reporting effects of PTHrP (vs. PTH) peptides on lymphocytes. These studies suggest that N-terminal PTHrP peptides stimulate protein kinase C (PKC) (McCauley *et al.*, 1992; Whitfield *et al.*, 1994) and not cAMP (McCauley *et al.*, 1992) in lymphocytes and inhibit their proliferation (Adachi *et al.*, 1990; McCauley *et al.*, 1992).

While the exact reason for discrepancies in effects of N-terminal PTH vs. PTHrP peptides in lymphocyte preparations or of PTH in rat thymocytes vs. circulating human lymphocytes is not known, these differences may be explained by the presence of both PTHR1 and PTHR2 receptors in these cells (McCauley *et al.*, 1992; Funk *et al.*, 2000; Seelinger *et al.*, 2003) and the increased selectivity of PTHR2 for PTH effects in humans vs. rats (Hoare *et al.*, 1999). In addition, evidence of PTHrP stimulation of PKC but not cAMP in HTLV-1 infected lymphocytes (McCauley *et al.*, 1992) has led to speculation that the PTHR1 receptor in lymphocytes is atypical, analogous to similar receptors on keratinocytes and squamous cell carcinoma cells (Orloff *et al.*, 1995; Clemens *et al.*, 2001). In these later cells, the existence of a different gene or differential splice variants of the PTHR1 have been postulated based on the identification of RNA transcripts that are smaller (1-1.5 kB) or larger (3.5-5 kB) than the 2.3 kB transcript of the classic PTHR1 (Orloff *et al.*, 1995). Interestingly, in our own fractionation experiments examining PTHR1 mRNA expression the stromal vs. lymphocyte fractions of rat thymus, while the 2.3 kB PTHR1 mRNA is only present in thymic stromal cells, a faint band consistent with a 5kB mRNA species is detected in the thymocyte fraction by Northern analysis when probed with PTHR1 cDNA (Funk *et al.*, 2000).

II.B. PTHrP and the Spleen

As previously discussed, during endotoxemia, splenic PTHrP expression is induced in the stromal elements of this lymphoid organ, an effect that is mediated by TNF (Funk *et al.*, 1993; Funk *et al.*, 1995). Constitutively, PTHrP and 2.3 kB PTHR1 mRNA are both only detected in the stromal elements of the spleen, and not in the splenic lymphocytes (Funk *et al.*, 1995). Interestingly, in T and B cell deficient SCID mice, constitutive levels of PTHrP and TNF are both 10-fold lower than in wild-type spleens, suggesting the possibility that TNF may also regulate constitutive PTHrP expression in this organ (Funk *et al.*, 1995). Both constitutive and inducible PTHrP were expressed in smooth muscle cells located within the splenic capsule as well as in an unidentified subpopulation of rounded, non-lymphoid stromal cells located immediately below the capsule (Funk *et al.*, 1995). Given the ability of capsular contraction or relaxation to alter splanchnic blood flow, the colocalization of a smooth muscle relaxing peptide and its cognate receptor at this site suggests that local splenic effects of induced PTHrP during inflammation may, analogous to its effects during CNS ischemia, primarily relate to local blood flow regulation (Hartwig & Hartwig, 1985; Withrington *et al.*, 1969). By this means, it is possible that PTHrP may indirectly alter elements of the innate and/or adaptive immune response by prolonging the transit time of blood through this lymphoid organ during invasion by pathogenic microorganisms (Delves & Roitt, 2000b).

II.C. PTHrP and the Thymus

Intrigued by our finding that PTHrP and its cognate receptor were primarily expressed in the splenic stroma, and not in the splenic lymphocytes, we worked in collaboration with Dr. Marian Kendall to determine whether—and where—PTHrP might be expressed in the thymus, an organ that plays a critical role in T cell development and therefore, adaptive immunity (Funk *et al.*, 1999). Earlier surveys of PTHrP expression in human organs had identified immunoreactive PTHrP in thymic epithelial cells (TECs) in the medulla of human fetal thymus (Kramer *et al.*, 1991). In rodents, immunoreactive N-terminal PTHrP in adult rat thymus was similarly only located in TECs, primarily those in the medullary and subcapsular areas (Funk *et al.*, 1999). In contrast, rat thymocytes did not express PTHrP (Funk *et al.*, 1999). Immunoreactive PTHR1 was also only found in TEC, again primarily in medullary TEC, and not in thymocytes (Funk *et al.*, 1999). Consistent with these findings, mRNA for PTHrP and the 2.3 kB PTHR1 were also primarily expressed in the stromal fraction, and not the thymocyte fraction, of rat thymus (Funk *et al.*, 2000). Immunohistochemical staining of primary cultures of rat TEC confirmed TEC expression of PTHrP and the PTHR1 (Funk *et al.* 1999). Moreover, IL-1, but not TNF, induced TEC PTHrP expression *in vitro* (Funk *et al.*, 2000) (Figure 1). A subsequent examination of adult human thymus by Gessi *et al* also documented the co-expression of PTHrP and PTHR1 in TEC (primarily medullary) and not in thymocytes (Gessi *et al.*, 2005). Interestingly, PTHrP also stimulated IL-6 production from human TEC *in vitro* (Gessi *et al.*, 2005) (Figure 1). IL-6, a cytokine that also colocalized with PTHrP in the thymic stroma in rats (Funk *et al.*, 2000), may influence thymocyte differentiation (Ritter & Boyd, 1993). Indeed, the medullary TECs that are a primary site of expression of PTHrP and its cognate receptor are known to play an important role in negative selection (i.e. deletion of self reactive T cells) (Naquet *et al.*, 1999). The importance of TECs in T cell development is also underscored in the SCID mouse model where a primary defect in TECs leads to severe T cell deficiency (Naquet *et al.*, 1999). Therefore, research to date suggests that PTHrP could influence T cell development indirectly via induction of IL-6 or directly via binding to putative atypical PTHR1 receptors that may be present in thymocytes (Funk *et al.,* 2000). However, the functional significance of PTHrP in T cell development is not known. Case reports of naturally-occurring over-expression of PTHrP by TEC in the setting of thymoma are primarily notable for systemic effects of PTHrP (hypercalcemia) (Suzuki *et al.*, 1998; Yoshiike *et al.*, 2004; Yoshikawa *et al.*, 1994). Moreover, in transgenic mice with over-expression of PTHrP driven by CK-14 (Wysolmerski *et al.*, 1994, 1995), a promoter that is active in medullary TEC (Klug *et al.*, 1998), the general microarchitecture of the thymus is no different from that of wild-type animals (Wysolmerski JJ and Funk J, unpublished observation).

CONCLUSION

Investigation of the effects of PTHrP in inflammation is not an organ-specific endeavor, nor will it likely yield a unified hypothesis on the global effect of PTHrP in this disease setting (i.e. protective vs. harmful). For, as with the immune response itself, local effects of induced PTHrP in inflammation are both organ and injury specific. Thus, for example, inducible expression of PTHrP in the vascular endothelium may be protective in the setting of stroke, yet contribute to lethality during overwhelming sepsis. Clearly, though, the physiologic effects of PTHrP, once induced in a particular tissue or cell type, are dictated by the PTH/PTHrP receptor-mediated pathways present at that site. Thus, research aimed at discovering the effects of these signaling pathways in the absence of inflammation will continue to inform and guide the discovery of as yet unidentified roles for PTHrP during the inflammatory response. Moreover, while current inflammation research has focused on identifying the function of N-terminal PTHrP peptides, it is possible, and indeed, likely, that other translational products of PTHrP may also subserve other important functions when produced locally at sites of inflammation. Indeed, consistent with this postulate, other laboratories have also reported evidence of increased levels of C-terminal PTHrP peptides in rheumatoid synovial fluid (Okano *et al.*, 1996; Kohno *et al.*, 1997).

Our view and understanding of the role of inflammation itself in disease processes continues to evolve. For example, it has only been in the last two decades that certain common chronic diseases not previously thought of as inflammatory have been demonstrated to have a strong pathophysiologic basis in the activation of the immune response (e.g. peptic ulcer disease (Crowe, 2005), atherosclerosis (Hansson, 2005) and osteoporosis (Weitzmann *et al.*, 2006)). Therefore, it should be anticipated that our understanding of the function of PTHrP in the pathophysiology of inflammatory diseases will also similarly continue to evolve. Lastly, evolution itself and analysis of PTH/PTHrP peptide expression and function in phylogenetically distinct species may hold additional keys that will enhance our understanding of the complex biology of this family of proteins. For example, research suggests that the structure and function of PTH/PTHrP peptides continued to evolve in fish after their evolutionary divergence from mammals such that these peptides have a complex role in calcium homeostasis distinct from that in mammals (Gensure *et al.*, 2004). Given the ancient evolutionary origin and fundamental biological importance of the innate immune response, perhaps future research evaluating the evolutionary development of non-calcitrophic aspects of PTH/PTHrP peptide biology will uncover additional information relevant to immune function that will not only enhance our understanding of human disease, but also potentially identify new uses for the PTH/PTHrP signaling pathway as a target for treatment of these diseases.

References

Adachi N. Yamaguchi K. Miyake Y. Honda S. Nagasak K. Akiyama Y. Adachi I. Abe K. Parathyroid hormone-related protein is a possible autocrine growth inhibitor for lymphocytes. *Biochem. Biophys. Res. Commun. 166*:1088-1094, 1990.

Albright F. Case records of the Massachusetts General Hospital (Case 27461). *New Eng J Med 225*:789-91, 1941.

Atkinson MJ. Hesch HD. Cade C. Wadwah M. Perris AD. Parathyroid hormone stimulation of mitosis in rat thymic lymphocytes is independent of cyclic AMP *J. Bone Min. Res. 2*:303-309, 1987.

Bernstein CN. Inflammatory bowel diseases as secondary causes of osteoporosis. *Curr Osteoporos Rep. 4(3)*:116-23, 2006.

Beutler B. Milsark IW. Cerami AC. Passive immunization against cachectin/tumor necrosis factor protects mice from lethal effect of endotoxin. *Science. 229*:869-71, 1985.

Bialasiewicz AA. Jüppner H. Diehl V. Hesch RD. Binding of bovine parathyroid hormone to surface receptors of cultured B-lymphocytes. *Biochim. Biophys. Acta 584*:467-478, 1979.

Brines ML. Ling Z. Broadus AE. Parathyroid hormone-related protein protects against kainic acid excitotoxicity in rat cerebellar granule cells by regulating L-type channel calcium flux. *Neurosc Letters. 274*:13-6, 1999.

Bucht E. Eklund A. Toss G. Lewensohn R. Granberg B. Sjostedt U. Eddeland R. Torring O. Parathyroid hormone-related peptide, measured by a midmolecule radioimmunoassay, in various hypercalcaemic and normocalcaemic conditions. *Acta Endocrinologica. 127*:294-300, 1992.

Capparelli C. Kostenuik PJ. Morony S. Starnes C. Weimann B. Van G. Scully S. Qi M. Lacey DL. Dunstan CR. Osteoprotegerin prevents and reverses hypercalcemia in a murine model of humoral hypercalcemia of malignancy. Canc Res. 60:783-7, 2000.

Chatterjee O. Nakchbandi IA. Philbrick WM. Dreyer BE. Zhang JP. Kaczmarek LK. Brines ML. Broadus AE. Endogenous parathyroid hormone-related protein functions as a neuroprotective agent. *Brain Res. 930*:58-66, 2002.

Choy EH. Panayi GS. Cytokine pathways and joint inflammation in rheumatoid arthritis. *New Eng J Med. 344*:907-16, 2001.

Clemens TL. Cormier S. Eichinger A. Endlich K. Fiaschi-Taesch N. Fischer E. Friedman PA. Karaplis AC. Massfelder T. Rossert J. Schluter KD. Silve C. Stewart AF. Takane K. Helwig JJ. Parathyroid hormone-related protein and its receptors: nuclear functions and roles in the renal and cardiovascular systems, the placental trophoblasts and the pancreatic islets. *Brit J Pharmacol. 134*:1113-36, 2001.

Crowe SE. Helicobacter infection, chronic inflammation, and the development of malignancy. *Curr Opin Gastroenterol. 21*:32-8, 2005.

Danks JA. Trivett MK. Power DM. Canario AV. Martin TJ. Ingleton PM. Parathyroid hormone-related protein in lower vertebrates. *Clin Exp Pharmacol Physiol. 25*:750-2, 1998.

de la Mata J. Uy HL. Guise TA. Story B. Boyce BF. Mundy GR. Roodman GD. IL-6 enhances hypercalcemia and bone resorption mediated by PTHrP *in vivo*. *J. Clin. Invest. 95*:2846-2852, 1995.

de Miguel F. Sarasa JL. Lopez-Ferro O. Esbrit P. Immunohistochemical detection of PTHrP in human astrocytomas, *J. Histochem. Cytochem., 46*:277-279, 1998.

Delves PJ. Roitt IM. The immune system; Part I. 343:37-49. 2000.

Delves PJ. Roitt IM. The immune system; Part II. 343:108-117, 2000.

Dinarello CA. Proinflammatory cytokines. *Chest. 118*:503-8, 2000.

Dinarello CA. The paradox of pro-inflammatory cytokines in cancer. *Canc Metas Rev. 25*:307-13, 2006.

Ejima E. Rosenblatt JD. Ou J. Prager D. Parathyroid hormone-related protein gene expression and human T cell leukemia virus-1 infection. *Min Electrolyte Metabol. 21*:143-7, 1995.

Elias AN. Sharma BS. Valenta LJ. Kyaw T. Immunomodulatory effect of bovine PTH extract on lymphocyte response to plant mitogens. *J Med 19*, 109-17, 1988.

Esbrit P. Hypercalcemia of malignancy--new insights into an old syndrome. *Clin Laboratory. 47(1-2)*:67-71, 2001.

Eto M. Akishita M. Ishikawa M. Kozaki K. Yoshizumi M. Hashimoto M. Ako J. Sugimoto N. Nagano K. Sudoh N. Toba K. Ouchi Y. Cytokine-induced expression of parathyroid hormone-related peptide in cultured human vascular endothelial cells. *Biochem Biophys Res Commun. 249*:339-43, 1998.

Ferguson JE. Seaner RM. Bruns DE. Bruns ME. Interleukin-1 beta and interleukin-4 increase parathyroid hormone-related protein secretion by human umbilical vein endothelial cells in culture. *Amer J Obstet Gynecol. 173*:448-55, 1995.

Fiaschi-Taesch NM. Santos S. Reddy V. Van Why SK. Philbrick WF. Ortega A. Esbrit P. Orloff JJ. Garcia-Ocana A. Prevention of acute ischemic renal failure by targeted delivery of growth factors to the proximal tubule in transgenic mice: the efficacy of parathyroid hormone-related protein and hepatocyte growth factor. *J Amer Soc Nephrol. 15*:112-25, 2004.

Firestein G. Starving the synovium: angiogenesis and inflammation in RA, *J. Clin. Invest. 103*:3-4, 1999.

Fradkin JM. Braniecki AM. Craig TM. Ramiro-Ibanez F. Rogers KS. Zoran DL. Elevated parathyroid hormone-related protein and hypercalcemia in two dogs with schistosomiasis. *J Amer Animal Hosp Assoc. 37*:349-55, 2001.

Funk JL. KruL EJT. Moser AH. Shigenaga JK. Strewler GJ. Grunfeld C. Feingold KR. Endotoxin increases parathyroid hormone-related protein mRNA levels in mouse spleen: mediation by tumor necrosis factor. *J. Clin. Invest. 92*:2546-2552, 1993.

Funk JL. Lausier J. Moser AH. Shigenaga JK. Huling S. Nissenson RA. Strewler GJ. Grunfeld C. Feingold KR. Endotoxin induces parathyroid hormone-related protein gene expression in splenic stromal cells--not in splenic lymphocytes. *Endocrinol 136*:3412-21, 1995.

Funk JL. Moser AH. Strewler GJ. Feingold KR. Grunfeld C. Parathyroid hormone-related protein is induced during lethal endotoxemia and contributes to endotoxin-induced mortality in rodents. *Molec Med 2*:204-210, 1996.

Funk JL. Moser AH. Grunfeld C. Feingold KR. Parathyroid hormone related protein is induced in the adult liver during endotoxemia and stimulates hepatic acute phase response. *Endocrinol, 138*:2665-2673, 1997.

Funk JL. Cordaro LA. We H. Benjamin JB. Yocum DE. Synovium as a source of increased amino terminal parathyroid hormone-related protein expression in rheumatoid arthritis: a possible role for PTHrP in the pathogenesis of rheumatoid arthritis. *J. Clin. Invest. 101*:1362-1371,1998.

Funk JL. Jones GV. Botham CA. Morgan G. Wooding P. Kendal MD. Expression of PTHrP and the PTH/PTHrP receptor in rat thymic epithelial cells. *J. Anat. 194*:255-264, 1999.

Funk JL. Davee SM. Stafford G. PTHrP Expression in Rat Thymus. *J. Bone Min. Res., 15(S1)*: S569, 2000.

Funk JL. Trout CR. Wei H. Stafford G. Reichlin S. PTHrP induction in reactive astrocytes following brain injury: a possible mediator of CNS inflammation. *Brain Res. 915*:195-209, 2001.

Funk JL. Wei H. Downey KJ. Yocum D. Benjamin J. Carley W. Expression of PTHrP and its cognate receptor in the rheumatoid synovial microcirculation. *Biochem. Biophys. Res. Comm. 297*:890-897, 2002.

Funk JL. Migliat Ei. Chen G. Wei H. Wilson J. Downey KJ. Mallarky P. Coull BM. McDonagh PF. Ritter L. PTHrP induction in focal stroke: a neuroprotective vascular peptide. *Amer. J. Physiol. Regul. Integr. Comp. Physiol. 284*:R1-21-R1030, 2003.

Funk JL. Downey KJ. Migliati E. Wilson J. Ritter L. Increase in PTHrP Immunoreactivity in Rat Brain at Site of Neuronal Death Following Transient Global Ischemia. *Endocrine Soc. Annual Meeting*, 2003.

Funk JL. Chen J. Downey KJ. Davee S. Stafford G. Blockade of PTHrP prevents joint destruction and granuloma formation in streptococcal cell wall-induced arthritis. *Arthritis Rheum. 48*:1721-1731, 2003.

Gabay C. Interleukin-6 and chronic inflammation. *Arth Res Ther. 8 Suppl 2*:S3, 2006.

Gaciong Z. Alexiewicz JM. Linker-Israeli M. Shulman IA. Pitts TO. Massry SG. Inhibition of immunoglobulin production by parathyroid hormone. Implications in chronic renal failure. *Kidney Internat. 40*:96-106, 1991.

Gensure RC. Ponugoti B. Gunes Y. Papasani MR. Lanske B. Bastepe M. Rubin DA. Jüppner H. Identification and characterization of two parathyroid hormone-like molecules in zebrafish. *Endocrinol. 145*:1634-9, 2004.

Geratz JD. Tidwell RR. Schwab JH. Anderl SK. Pryzwansky KB. Sequential events in the pathogenesis of SCW-induced arthritis and their modulation by bis(5-amidino-2-benzimidazolyl)methane. *Amer. J. Pathol. 136*:909-21, 1990.

Gessi M. Monego G. Lauriola L. Maggiano N. Ranelletti FO. Parathyroid hormone-related peptide (hPTHrP) and parathyroid hormone-related peptide receptor type 1 (PTHR1) expression in human thymus. *J Histochem Cytochem. 53*:955-62, 2005.

Ghezzi P. Cerami A. Tumor necrosis factor as a pharmacological target. *Mol Biotechnol. 31*:239-44, 2005.

Godler DE. Stein AN. Bakharevski O. Lindsay MM. Ryan PF. Parathyroid hormone-related peptide expression in rat collagen-induced arthritis. *Rheumatol. 44*:1122-31, 2005.

Greenfield EM. Shaw SM. Gornik SA. Banks MA. Adenyl cyclase and IL-6 are downstream effectors of PTH resulting in stimulation of bone resportion. *J. Clin. Invest. 96*:1238-1244, 1995.

Grohe C. van Eickels M. Wenzel S. Meyer R. Degenhardt H. Doevendans PA. Heinemann MP. Ross G. Schluter KD. Sex-specific differences in ventricular expression and function of parathyroid hormone-related peptide. *Cardiovas Res. 61*:307-16, 2004.

Guerreiro PM. Renfro JL. Power DM. Canario AVM. The parathyroid hormone family of peptides: structure, tissue distribution, regulation, and potential functional roles in calcium and phosphate balance in fish. *Am J Physiol Integ Comp Physiol 292*:679-696, 2007.

Halstead LR. Lai CF. Cheng SL. PTH stimulates chemotaxis of human osteoblasts via protein kinase C pathway. *J. Bone Min. Res. 16(S1)*:S498, 2001.

Hansson GK. Inflammation, atherosclerosis, and coronary artery disease. *New Eng J. Med 352*:1685-95, 2005.

Hartwig H. Hartwig HG. Structural characteristics of the mammalian spleen indicating storage and release of red blood cells. Aspects of evolutionary and environmental demands. *Experientia 41*:159-163, 1985.

Hauwel M. Furon E. Canova C. Griffiths M. Neal J. Gasque P. Innate (inherent) control of brain infection, brain inflammation and brain repair: the role of microglia, astrocytes, "protective" glial stem cells and stromal ependymal cells. *Brain Res - Brain Res Rev. 48*:220-33, 2005.

Haynes DR. Bone lysis and inflammation. *Inflamm Res. 53*:596-600, 2004.

Hoare SR. Bonner TI. Usdin TB. Comparison of rat and human parathyroid hormone 2 (PTH2) receptor activation: PTH is a low potency partial agonist at the rat PTH2 receptor. *Endocrinology. 140*:4419-25, 1999.

Hoette M. Kalany A. Lundin AP. Gottlieb MN. Suthanthiran M. Carpenter CB. Strom TB. *In vitro* modulation of phytohemagglutinin-P induced blastogenesis by parathyroid hormone. In: *Regulatory Mechanisms in Lymphocyte Activation*, DO Lucas (ed.), 1977, Academic Press, New York, pp 453-555.

Holland JW. Pottinger TG. Secombes CJ. Recombinant interleukin-1 beta activates the hypothalamic-pituitary-interrenal axis in rainbow trout, Oncorhynchus mykiss. *J Endocrinol. 175*:261-7, 2002.

Holt EH. Broadus AE. Brines ML. Parathyroid hormone-related peptide is produced by cultured cerebellar granule cells in response to L-type voltage-sensitive Ca2+ channel flux via a Ca2+/calmodulin-dependent kinase pathway. *J Biol Chem. 271*:28105-11, 1996.

Horiuchi T. Yoshida T. Koshihara Y. Sakamoto H. Kanai H. Yamamoto S. Ito H. The increase of parathyroid hormone-related peptide and cytokine levels in synovial fluid of elderly rheumatoid arthritis and osteoarthritis. *Endo J. 46(5)*:643-9, 1999.

Iguchi H. Aramaki Y. Maruta S. Takiguchi S. Effects of anti-parathyroid hormone-related protein monoclonal antibody and osteoprotegerin on PTHrP-producing tumor-induced cachexia in nude mice. *J Bone Min Metabol. 24*:16-9, 2006.

Ishikawa M. Akishita M. Kozaki K. Toba K. Namiki A. Yamaguchi T. Orimo H. Ouchi Y. Expression of parathyroid hormone-related protein in human and experimental atherosclerotic lesions: functional role in arterial intimal thickening. *Atherosclerosis. 152*:97-105, 2000.

Janeway CA. Travers P. Walport M. Shlomchik M. Evolution of the Innate Immune System. In: *Immunobiology: the immune system in health and disease.* Garland Science Publishing, New York, NY, 2005.

Jansen J. Gres P. Umschlag C. Heinzel FR. Degenhardt H. Schluter KD. Heusch G. Schulz R. Parathyroid hormone-related peptide improves contractile function of stunned myocardium in rats and pigs. *Amer J Physiol - Heart Circu Physiol. 284*:H49-55, 2003.

Jiang B. Morimoto S. Yang J. Fukuo K. Hirotani A. Kitano S. Ogihara T. Parathyroid hormone-related protein upregulates interleukin-1beta-induced nitric oxide synthesis. *Hypertension. 30*:922-7, 1997.

Jiang Y. Yoshida A. Ishioka C. Imata H. Mikawa H. PTH inhibits immunoglobulin production without affecting cell growth in human B cells. *Clin Immunol Immunopath 65*:286-93, 1992.

Kabelitz D. Medzhitov R. Innate immunity--cross-talk with adaptive immunity through pattern recognition receptors and cytokines. *Curr Opin Immunol. 19*:1-3, 2007.

Keane J. Gershon S. Wise RP. Mirabile-Levens E. Kasznica J. Schwieterman WD. Siegel JN. Braun MM. Tuberculosis associated with Infliximab, a TNF-α neutralizing agent. *New Eng. J. Med. 15*:1098-1104, 2001.

Klinger M. Alexiewicz JM. Linker-Israeli M. Pitts TO. Gaciong Z. Fadda GZ. Massry SG. Effect of parathyroid hormone on human T cell activation. *Kidney International 37*:1543-1551, 1990.

Klug DB. Carter C. Crouch E. Roop D. Conti CJ. Richie ER. Interdependence of cortical thymic epithelial cell differentiation and T-lineage commitment. *Proc Nat Acad Sci USA. 95(20)*:11822-7, 1998.

Kohno H. Shigeno C. Kasai R. Akiyama H. Iida H. Tsuboyama T. Sato K. Konishi J. Nakamura T. Synovial fluids from patients with osteoarthritis and rheumatoid arthritis contain high levels of parathyroid hormone-related peptide. *J. Bone Min. Res. 12*:847-854, 1997.

Kramer S, FH Reynolds, Jr., M Castillo, DM Valenzuela, M Thorikay and JM Sorvillo. Immunological identification and distribution of parathyroid hormone-like protein polypeptides in normal and malignant tissues. *Endocrinol 128*:1927-1937, 1991.

Kronenberg HM. PTHrP and skeletal development. *Annals New York Acad Sci. 1068*:1-13, 2006.

Lin RCS, Matesic DF, Marvin M, McKay RD, Brustle O. Re-expression of the intermediate filament nestin in reactive astrocytes. *Neurobiol. Dis. 2*:79-85, 1995.

Loddick SA. Turnbull AV. Rothwell NJ. Cerebral IL-6 is neuroprotective during permanent focal cerebral ischemia in the rat. *J. Cerebral Bld. Flow Met. 18*:176-179, 1998.

Lutteke D. Ross G. Abdallah Y. Schafer C. Piper HM. Schluter KD. Parathyroid hormone-related peptide improves contractile responsiveness of adult rat cardiomyocytes with depressed cell function irrespectively of oxidative inhibition. *Basic Res Cardiol. 100*:320-7, 2005.

Macica CM. Broadus AE. PTHrP regulates cerebral blood flow and is neuroprotective. *Amer J Physiol - Regulatory Integ Comp Physiol. 284*:R1019-20, 2003.

Macica CM. Liang G. Lankford KL. Broadus AE. Induction of parathyroid hormone-related peptide following peripheral nerve injury: role as a modulator of Schwann cell phenotype. *GLIA. 53*:637-48, 2006.

Martin-Ventura JL. Ortego M. Esbrit P. Hernandez-Presa MA. Ortega L. Egido J. Possible role of parathyroid hormone-related protein as a proinflammatory cytokine in atherosclerosis. *Stroke. 34*:1783-9, 2003.

McCauley LK. Rosol TJ. Merryman JI. Capen CC. PTHrP binding to human T-cell lymphotropic virus type I-infected lymphocytes. *Endocrinol 130*:300-306, 1992.

Magor BG. Magor KE. Evolution of effectors and receptors of innate immunity. *Dev Comp Immunol. 25*:651-82, 2001.

Medzhitov R. Janeway C. Innate Immunity. *New Eng J Med 343*:338-344, 2000.

Mitnick MA. Grey A. Masiukiewicz U. Bartkiewicz M. Rios-Velez L. Friedman S. Xu L. Horowitz MC. Insogna K. Parathyroid hormone induces hepatic production of bioactive interleukin-6 and its soluble receptor. *Amer J Physiol – Endocrinol Metabol. 280*:E405-12, 2001.

Mori H. Aoki K. Katayama I. Nishioka K. Umeda T. Humoral hypercalcemia of malignancy with elevated plasma PTHrP, TNF alpha, and IL-6 in cutaneous squamous cell carcinoma. *J. Dermatol. 136*:3412-21. 1996.

Morii S. Oka K. Naoi Y. Kotsuji T. Nihei T. Nagayama R. Kashimura K. Kameta S. Yatabe Y. Mori N. Coexisting primary early gastric plasmacytoma and sarcoidosis with hypercalcaemia. *Virchows Archiv. 432(5)*:473-6, 1998.

Motokura T, Fukumoto S, Takahashi S, Watanabe T, Matsumoto T, Igarashi T, Ogata E. Expression of parathyroid hormone-related protein in a human T cell lymphotrophic virus type 1-infected T cell line. *Biochem. Biophys. Res. Comm. 154*:1182-1188, 1988.

Nagai Y. Yamato H. Akaogi K. Hirose K. Ueyama Y. Ikeda K. Matsumoto T, Fujita T. Ogata E. Role of IL-6 in uncoupling of bone *in vivo* in a human squamous carcinoma coproducing PTHrP and IL-6. *J Bone Min. Res. 13*:664-72, 1998.

Naquet P, Maspetti M, Boyd R Development, organization and function of the thymic medulla in normal , immunodeficient or autoimmune mice. *Seminars Immunol. 11*:47-55, 1999.

Nakayama T. Ohtsuru A. Enomoto H. Namba H. Ozeki S. Shibata Y. Yokota T. Nobuyoshi M. Ito M. Sekine I. *et al.* Coronary atherosclerotic smooth muscle cells overexpress human parathyroid hormone-related peptides. *Biochem Biophys Res Comm. 200*:1028-35, 1994.

Okano K. Tsukazaki T. Ohtsuru A. Namba H. Osak Mi. Iwasaki K. Yamashita S. Parathyroid hormone-related peptide in synovial fluid and disease activity of rheumatoid arthritis. *British J. Rheumatol. 35*:1056-1062, 1996.

Old LJ. Tumor necrosis factor (TNF). *Science 230*:630-2, 1985.

Orloff JJ. Kats Y. Urena P. Schipani E. Vasavada RC. Philbrick WM. Behal A. Abou-Samra AB. Segre GV. Jüppner H. Further evidence for a novel receptor for amino-terminal parathyroid hormone-related protein on keratinocytes and squamous carcinoma cell lines. *Endocrinol. 136*:3016-23, 1995.

Ozeki S. Ohtsuru A. Seto S. Takeshita S. Yano H. Nakayama T. Ito M. Yokota T. Nobuyoshi M. Segre GV. Yamashita S. Yano K. Evidence that implicates the parathyroid hormone-related peptide in vascular stenosis. Increased gene expression in the intima of injured carotid arteries and human restenotic coronary lesions. *Arterio, Thromb Vasc Biol. 16*:565-75, 1996.

Pandian MR. Morgan CH. Carlton E. Segre GV. Modified immunoradiometric assay of parathyroid hormone-related protein: clinical application in the differential diagnosis of hypercalcemia. *Clin Chem. 38*:282-8, 1992.

Parrillo JE. Pathogenetic mechanisms of septic shock. N. Engl. J. Med. 328:1471-1477, 1993.

Perry HM. Chappel JC. Bellorin-Font E. Tamao J. Martin KJ. Teitelbaum SL. Parathyroid hormone receptors in circulating human mononuclear leukocytes. *J. Biol. Chem. 259*:5531-5535, 1984.

Philbrick WM. Wysolmerski JJ. Galbraith S. Holt E. Orloff JJ. Yang KH. Vasavada RC. Weir EC. Broadus AE. Stewart AF. Defining the roles of parathyroid hormone-related protein in normal physiology. *Physiol Rev 76*:127-173, 1996.

Raz E. Organ-specific regulation of innate immunity. *Nat Immunol. 8*:3-4, 2007.

Ritchie CK. Thomas KG. Andrews LR. Tindall DJ. Fitzpatrick LA. Effects of calciotropic peptides calcitonin and PTH on prostate cancer growth and chemotaxis. *Prostate 30*:183-187, 1997.

Ritter MA. Boyd RL. Development in the thymus: it takes two to tango. *Immunol Today 14*:462-469, 1993.

Rotllant J. Guerreiro PM. Anjos L. Redruello B. Canario AV. Power DM. Stimulation of cortisol release by the N terminus of teleost parathyroid hormone-related protein in interrenal cells *in vitro*. *Endocrinol 146*:71–76, 2005.

Sato K. Fujii Y. Kakiuchi T. Kasono K. Imamura H. Kondo Y. Mono H. Okabe T. Asano S. Takaku F. *et al.* Paraneoplastic syndrome of hypercalcemia and leukocytosis caused by squamous carcinoma cells (T3M-1) producing PTHrP, IL-1alpha, and G-CSF. *Cancer Res. 49*:4740-6, 1989.

Sato K. Fujii Y. Kasono K. Ozawa M. PTHrP and IL-1 synergistically stimulate bone resorption *in vitro* and increase the serum calcium concentration in mice *in vivo*. *Endocrinol. 124*:2172-2176, 1989.

Sato K. Yamakawa Y. Shizume K. Satoh T. Nohtomi K. Demura H. Akatsu T. Nagata N. Kasahara T. Ohkawa H. *et al.*. Passive immunization with anti-parathyroid hormone-related protein monoclonal antibody markedly prolongs survival time of hypercalcemic nude mice bearing transplanted human PTHrP-producing tumors. *J Bone Min Res. 8*:849-60, 1993.

Schluter K. Katzer C. Frischkopf K. Wenzel S. Taimor G. Piper HM. Expression, release, and biological activity of parathyroid hormone-related peptide from coronary endothelial cells. *Circulation Res. 86*:946-51, 2000.

Seeliger S. Hausberg M. Eue I. Usdin T. Rahn KH. Kosch M. The parathyroid hormone-2 receptor is expressed on human leukocytes and down-regulated in hyperparathyroidism. *Clin Nephrol. 59*:429-35, 2003.

Shankar PP. Wei H. Davee SM. Funk JL. PTHrP is expressed by transformed and fetal human astrocytes and inhibits cell proliferation. *Brain Res. 868*:230-240, 2000.

Shao JS. Cheng SL. Charlton-Kachigian N. Loewy AP. Towler DA. Teriparatide (human parathyroid hormone (1-34) inhibits osteogenic vascular calcification in diabetic low density lipoprotein receptor-deficient mice. *J Biol Chem. 278(50)*:50195-202, 2003.

Shasha SM. Kristal B. Barzilai M. Makov UE. Shkolnik T. *In vitro* effect of PTH on normal T cell functions. *Nephron 50*:212-216, 1988.

Shoback D. Funk J. 2004. Humoral Manifestions of Malignancy. In: Greenspan FS, Gardner DG, editors. *Basic and Clinical Endocrinology*. New York , NY: Lange; 2004; 814-829.

Smith ML. Bendek G. Dahlgren N. Rosen I. Wieloch T. Siesjo BK. Models for studying long-term recovery following forebrain ischemia in the rat. 2. A 2-vessel occlusion model. *Acta Neurolog Scand 69*:385-401, 1984.

Soifer NE. Van Why SK. Ganz MB. Kashgarian M. Siegel NJ. Stewart AF. Expression of parathyroid hormone-related protein in the rat glomerulus and tubule during recovery from renal ischemia. *J Clin Invest. 92*:2850-7, 1993.

Spiegelman BM. Hotamisligli GS. Through thick and Thin: wasting, obesity and TNFalpha. *Cell 73*, 625-627, 1993.

Stewart AF. Hyperparathyroidism, humoral hypercalcemia of malignancy, and the anabolic actions of parathyroid hormone and parathyroid hormone-related protein on the skeleton. *J Bone Miner Res. 17*:758-62, 2002.

Streetz KL. Wustefeld T. Klein C. Manns MP. Trautwein C. Mediators of inflammation and acute phase response in the liver. *Cellular Molec Biol. 47*:661-73, 2001.

Ramadori G. Christ B. Cytokines and the hepatic acute-phase response. *Sem Liver Dis. 19*:141-55, 1999.

Suzuki K. Tanaka H. Shibusa T. Shibuya Y. Inuzuka M. Fujishima T. Abe S. Parathyroid-hormone-related-protein-producing thymic carcinoma presenting as a giant extrathoracic mass. *Respiration. 65*:83-5, 1998.

Taylor PC. Williams RO. Feldmann M. Tumour necrosis factor alpha as a therapeutic target for immune-mediated inflammatory diseases. *Curr Opin Biotechnology. 15*:557-63, 2004.

Thom T. Haase N. Rosamond W. Howard V. *et al.* Heart disease and stroke statistics--2006 update. A report from the American Heart Association statistics committee and stroke statistics subcommittee. *Circulation 113*:1-67. 2006.

Urena P. Kong XF. Abou-Samra A-B. Jüppner H. Kronenberg HM. Potts Jr JT. Segre GV. Parathyroid hormone/parathyroid hormone-related peptide receptor mRNAs are widely distributed in rat tissues. *Endocrinol 133*:617-623, 1993.

Uy H. Mundy GR. Boyce BF. Story BM. Dunstan CR. *et al.* Tumor necrosis factor enhances parathyroid hormone-related protein-induced hypercalcemia and bone resorption without inhibiting bone formation *in vivo*. *Cancer Res. 57*:3194-9, 1997.

van den Berg WB. Anti-cytokine therapy in chronic destructive arthritis. *Arthritis Res. 3*:18-26, 2001.

Wada S. Kitamura H. Matsuura Y. Katayama Y. Ohkawa H. Kugai N. Motoyoshi K. Fuse Y. Nagata N. Parathyroid hormone-related protein as a cause of hypercalcemia in a B-Cell type malignant lymphoma. *Int. Med. 31*:968-972, 1992.

Weaver DR. Deeds JD. Lee K. Segre GV. Localization of parathyroid hormone-related peptide (PTHrP) and PTH/PTHrP receptor mRNAs in rat brain. Brain Research. *Molecular Brain Res. 28*:296-310, 1995.

Weir EC. Brines ML. Ikeda K. Burtis WJ. Broadus AE. Robbins RJ. Parathyroid hormone-related peptide gene is expressed in the mammalian central nervous system. *Proc Nat Acad Sci USA. 87*:108-12, 1990.

Weitzmann MN. Pacifici R. Estrogen deficiency and bone loss: an inflammatory tale. *J Clin Invest. 116*:1186-94, 2006.

Whitfield JF. Perris AD. Youdale T. The calcium-mediated promotion of mitotic activity in rat thymocyte populations by growth hormone, neurohormones, parathyroid hormone and prolactin. *J Cellular Physiol. 73*:203-11, 1969.

Whitfield JF. MacManus JP. Rixon RH. The possible mediation by cyclic AMP of parathyroid hormone-induced stimulation of mitotic activity and DNA synthesis in rat thymic lymphocytes. *J. Cell. Physiol. 75*:213-224, 1970.

Whitfield JF. Isaacs RJ. Chakravarthy BR. Durkin JP. Morley P. Neugebauer W. Williams RE. Willick G. Rixon RH. C-terminal fragments of parathyroid hormone-related protein, PTHrP-(107-111) and (107-139), and the N-terminal PTHrP-(1-40) fragment stimulate membrane-associated protein kinase C activity in rat spleen lymphocytes. *J. Cell. Physiol. 158*:518-522, 1994.

Withrington PG. Ansari N. Croxton R. de Nucci G. Vane JR. The actions of endothelins-1 and -3 on the vascular and capular smooth muscle of the isolated blood perfused spleen of the dog. *Br. J. Pharmacol. 105*:490-494, 1992.

Wysolmerski JJ. Broadus AE. Zhou J. Fuchs E. Milstone LM. Philbrick WM. Overexpression of parathyroid hormone-related protein in the skin of transgenic mice interferes with hair follicle development. *Proc Nat Acad Sciences USA. 91*:1133-7, 1994.

Wysolmerski JJ. McCaughern-Carucci JF. Daifotis AG. Broadus AE. Philbrick WM. Overexpression of parathyroid hormone-related protein or parathyroid hormone in transgenic mice impairs branching morphogenesis during mammary gland development. *Development. 121*:3539-47, 1995.

Yamamoto I. Potts Jr JT. Segre GV. Circulating bovine lymphocytes contain receptors for parathyroid hormone. *J. Clin. Invest. 71*:404-407, 1983.

Yoshida T. Sakamoto H. Horiuchi T. Yamamoto S. Suematsu A. Oda H. Koshihara Y. Involvement of prostaglandin E(2) in interleukin-1alpha-induced parathyroid hormone-related peptide production in synovial fibroblasts of patients with rheumatoid arthritis. *J Clinical Endocrinol Metabol 86*:3272-8, 2001.

Yoshiike F. Koizumi T. Yoneyama A. Komatu M. Yamaguchi S. Hanaoka M. Kubo K. Eda S. Thymic squamous cell carcinoma producing parathyroid hormone-related protein and CYFRA 21-1. *Internal Med. 43*:493-5, 2004.

Yoshikawa T. Noguchi Y. Matsukawa H. Kondo J. Matsumoto A. Nakatani Y. Kitamura H. Ito T. Thymus carcinoid producing parathyroid hormone (PTH)-related protein: report of a case. *Surg Today. 24*:544-7, 1994.

Zeimer HJ. Greenaway TM. Slavin J. Hards DK. Zhou H. Doery JC. Hunter AN. Duffield A. Martin TJ. Grill V. Parathyroid-hormone-related protein in sarcoidosis. *Am J Pathol. 152*:17-21, 1998.

In: Novel Aspects of PTHrP Physiopathology
Editor: Claudio Luparello, pp. 191-233
ISBN: 978-1-60021-857-6

Chapter IX

MOLECULAR SIGNALING OF PTHrP IN TUMOR

Majed S. Alokail*
Department of Biochemistry, College of Science #5, King Saud University, PO Box 2455, Riyadh 11451, Kingdom of Saudi Arabia.

ABSTRACT

Parathyroid hormone-related peptide (PTHrP) a polyprotein discovered in 1987 and was originally identified as the factor responsible for the hypercalcemic paraneoplastic syndrome called humoral hypercalcemia of malignancy (HHM). PTHrP also plays crucial roles in various physiological systems and development associated with normal life. Both PTHrP and parathyroid hormone (PTH) signal through the same receptor, the PTH/PTHrP receptor (a class II G-protein-coupled receptor) (GPCR) know as PTH1R. In contrast with PTH, PTHrP is not normally present in the circulation, indicating that it acts in a paracrine/autocrine, rather than an endocrine manner. However, both endogenous and exogenous PTHrP also appear to have intracrine fashion through translocation into the nucleus or nucleolus and influence cellular events. Since PTHrP binding to PTH1R linked to different signal transduction pathways (cAMP/PKA and PLC/PKA cascades) can result in either mitogenic or antimitogenic responses, depending on the cellular system. It is not surprising that many cell specific mitogenic activity of PTHrP is partly dependent on the activation of the mitogen-activated protein kinases (MAPKs) pathway through protein kinase C (PKC) dependent manner. Activated MAPKs is a critical signal transduction event-mediated cell proliferation, cell migration and tumor progression. it has been shown recently that calcium-sensing receptor (CaR) and PTHrP are cross-talk by PKC, MEK, P38 MAPK, and JNK , which suggests that the mitogenic response is one major effect of PTHrP. Moreover, recent nuclear localization of PTHrP in number of tumor cells and its association with cellular survival and/or cellular proliferation has been extended the potential pathophysiological role of this extraordinary peptide and open exciting areas of investigation. This chapter will perform

* Correspondence concerning this article should be addressed to Dr. Majed S. Alokail Department of Biochemistry, College of Science #5, King Saud University, PO Box 2455, Riyadh 11451, Kingdom of Saudi Arabia. (e-mail: msalokail@yahoo.com).

a coherent overview on the concept of molecular targeting of PTHrP signaling, addressing the I) how does PTHrP binds to PTH1R in tumor cells; II) What are the mechanisms of PTH1R signaling in the cytoplasm and the nucleus; III) What are the consequences of nucleus signaling; and IV) How does PTHrP cross-talk with growth factors and nuclear receptors signaling. Understanding of PTHrP molecular signaling mechanisms will generate more effective anti-tumor therapeutic agents.

Introduction

Hypercalcaemia is a complication of malignancy which has been recognized since 1923 when Zondek *et al* reported the case in a 69-year-old man. The term "humoral hypercalcaemia of malignancy" (HHM) describes those patients in whom the blood calcium level is elevated due to production by the primary tumour of some substance which acts upon the skeleton to increase bone resorption. Bone metastases are a common cause of morbidity in breast cancer, and about 70% of women dying from the disease will have bone metastases (Coleman & Rubens, 1987). In 1936, Gutman *et al* reported extensive radiographic evidence for bone resorption in patients with multiple myeloma or breast cancer. In 1941 *Albright* described a patient in whom hypercalcaemia and hypophosphatemia were eradicated after the radiation of a single bone metastasis and removal of the primary renal carcinoma. He suggested that the tumour was secreting parathyroid hormone or parathyroid hormone like protein.

Since the 1950's and 60's many studies have confirmed that some cases of tumour-induced hypercalcaemia could be reversed by resection of the isolated malignancies, and that these tumours were often squamous or genitourinary malignancies. The humoral factors could induce hypercalcaemia through three distinct mechanisms; stimulation of osteoclastic bone resorption, increased calcium reabsorption from kidney and increased calcium absorption from the intestine (Rosol & Capen, 1988). It was suggested that the destruction of skeletal tissue in these patients occurred due to a secretory product from the primary malignancy (Insogna *et al*, 1989). HHM by definition occurs in patients with no metastases (yet) to bone. HHM is at least partially explained by the fact that these cancers produce a protein which has an action like that of parathyroid hormone (PTH), but which is chemically distinct from PTH. The condition of HHM is frequently associated with biochemical changes which include low plasma levels of phosphorus and increased nephrogenous renal production of cyclic 3'5'-adenosine monophosphate (cAMP) (Martin *et al.*, 1976; Stewart *et al.*, 1980).

Direct evidence for the existence of a distinct molecular form with PTH-like activity was obtained in the 1960s, when the first radioimmunoassays for PTH were developed (Berson and Yalow, 1966). Additional methods were developed, by the early of 1980s, to assay PTH-like activity using sensitive assays based on cAMP responses in clonal osteogenic sarcoma cells (Majeska *et al.*, 1980; Partridge *et al.*, 1980; Rodan *et al.*, 1983). These assays depend on the ability of PTH to activate adenylate cyclase, either in kidney or bone cell targets. Their use resulted eventually in the isolation of a PTH-like function from the conditioned medium of the lung cancer cell line, BEN (Rodda *et al.*, 1988). Considerable evidence rapidly accumulated that PTHrP was an important humoral mediator of paraneoplastic hypercalcaemia in patients with solid tumours such as squamous carcinoma of the lung (Martin & Suva, 1989).

The tumour extracts and plasma of patients with HHM showed definitive PTH-like activity (Broadus *et al*, 1985; Strewler *et al.*, 1983). A sensitive cytochemical assay for PTH was also used to show that tumour mRNA injected into Xenopus oocyte produced PTH-like activity which was inhibited by PTH antagonists but not by anti-PTH antisera. The same sensitive PTH assay was employed to detect increased circulating biological PTH-like activity in patients with HHM in the presence of low or undetectable immunoreactive PTH (Broadus *et al.*, 1985; Goltzman *et al.*, 1981; Gonzalez *et al.*, 1985; Ilardi & Faro, 1985; Riggs *et al.*, 1971).

These studies led to the realization that the tumours must be producing something that was capable of substituting for PTH in its action on major target tissues (Martin *et al.*, 1991; Rodda *et al.*, 1988; Rude *et al.*, 1981). Considerable evidence rapidly accumulated that PTHrP was an important humoral mediator of hypercalcaemia in patients with solid tumour such as squamous carcinoma of the lung (Martin, 1989), and the clinical similarities between HHM and primary hyperparathyroidism led to an intensive search for the common factor. This resulted in the purification, sequencing, cloning, expression, and synthesis of a PTH-related protein (PTHrP). The full length peptide contains 141 amino acids; eight of the first 13 amino acids residues are identical with PTH itself (Kemp *et al.*, 1987; Moseley *et al.*, 1987; Rosol *et al.*, 1987; Suva *et al.*, 1987).

Furthermore, many tissues synthesize PTHrP, including skin fibroblasts (Hayman *et al.*, 1989), smooth muscle when stretched (Nickols *et al.*, 1989; Winquist *et al.*, 1987) breast when stimulated by prolactin (Thiede, 1989), fetal parathyroid gland (Rodda *et al.*, 1988), the myometrium during pregnancy (Thiede *et al.*, 1990, 1991) and cartilage cells during chondrogenesis and mineralization (Karaplis *et al.*, 1992). The human lung cancer cell line (BEN), originally established from a patient with squamous cell carcinoma of the lung and hypercalcaemia (Ellison *et al.*, 1975), produces substantial amounts of PTHrP (Martin *et al.*, 1991). A protein of molecular weight 17000 to 18,000 Da was purified from BEN cells, and when applied in a sensitive biological assay employing the PTH-responsive UMR 106.01 osteogenic sarcoma cells caused an increase in cAMP (Moseley *et al.*, 1987). A similar protein has been purified from primary breast tumours (Burtis *et al.*, 1987). The structure of PTHrP and its activity have some similarity to those of PTH (Martin *et al.*, 1991). The N-terminal sequence of PTHrP retains 60% homology with that of PTH over the first 13 amino acids, and the PTH-like biological activity of PTHrP is contained within the first 34 amino acids (Moseley *et al.*, 1987; Danks *et al.*, 1989; Grill *et al.*, 1991; Orloff *et al.*, 1989).

In humans there are three mature peptide isoforms of 139, 141, and 173 amino acids translated from three splice forms of the mRNAs (Mangin *et al.*, 1990; Yasuda *et al.*, 1989). The expression of each one of them may be tissue-specific (Mangin *et al.*, 1988). Each form is rich in proteolytic sites and amidation signals (Mangin *et al.*, 1988; Thiede *et al.*, 1988; Suva *et al.*, 1987). Rat PTHrP is homologous with human PTHrP (1-141), and between these species, the amino acid sequences between 1 to 111 region differ by only two amino acids suggesting that conservation has a significant biological implication (Orloff *et al.*, 1989).

The human PTHrP gene is located on chromosome 12 (Mangin *et al.*, 1988, 1990; Suva *et al.*, 1989), whereas the PTH gene is located on chromosome 11 (Mannens *et al.*, 1987).

These two chromosomes are considered to be related in evolution and the PTHrP/PTH genes probably arose as a result of ancestral gene duplication (Martin *et al.*, 1991). The human PTHrP gene has been studied intensively by several groups (Mangin *et al.*, 1988, 1990, 1991; Suva *et al.*, 1989; Yasuda *et al.*, 1989), revealing that the gene is a single-copy containing eight exons. These exons span more than 15 kb of genomic DNA. The noncoding exons are 1A, 1B, 1C, and 2 (Burtis *et al.*, 1987; Mangin *et al.*, 1988; Suva *et al.*, 1989), and they can be fused together as a function of promoter usage and/or different splicing patterns to generate 5' untranslated regions. Exon 3 encodes the prepro-region of the peptide, except the dibasic endoproteolytic cleavage site, which is carried on exon 4. Exon 4 encodes the bulk of the PTHrP coding region, including the stop codon-splice donor sequence and 3' untranslated region. Exons 5 and 6 contain the sequences that encode the carboxy-terminal regions of the 173 and 141 amino-acid PTHrP isoforms respectively; each of these exons also has a stop codon (Mangin *et al.*, 1988, 1990; Suva *et al.*, 1987).

The 5'-flanking region of the PTHrP gene consists of four noncoding exons that are transcribed from at least three independent promoters, and these promoter elements are referred to as the upstream TATA, midregion GC and downstream TATA promoters (Mangen *et al.*, 1989; Yasuda *et al.*, 1989; Suva *et al.*, 1989). The downstream promoter structure includes a 45-base sequence; the upstream TATA promoter lies 2.7 kb 5' of the downstream promoter and the midregion GC promoter locates just 5' of exon 1C in a GC-rich region (Vasavada *et al.*, 1993). The GC-rich region of the PTHrP gene promoter in human tissue might be operated by some cytokines and/or growth factors (Brandt *et al.*, 1992). Moreover, the presence of GC and TATA boxes in the promoter regions advocates complex regulation of PTHrP expression. The 3′-untranslated regions of the various PTHrP mRNAs contain several copies of the AUUUA motif (AU-rich elements, ARE), involved in rapid degragation of mRNAs which is similar to the one in growth factor, proto-oncogene, and cytokine genes (Philbrick *et al.*, 1996; Sellers *et al.* (2004)). In addition, alternative splicing of the three isoforms of PTHrP results in unique 3′-untranslated regions with different half-lives. The human tissues express one or more of the alternatively spliced PTHrP mRNA isoforms and tissue-specific expression (Philbrick *et al.*, 1996; Gensure *et al.*, 2005).

The structure of the PTHrP gene in chicken, mouse and rat is less complicated than the human one, but they share a number of features in common implying a close evolutionary relationship (Moseley and Gillespie, 1995). The genes of these species encode for only one species of mature PTHrP, 139 amino acids in the mouse and 141 amino acids in the rat, as exons equivalent to human exons 7 and 8 are absent in these species (Moseley and Gillespie, 1995).

PTHrP in Cancer

HHM is a common paraneoplastic syndrome which complicates bone metastases from breast cancer in 10-20% of women before death (Coleman & Rubens, 1987). Of all the malignancies, mammary carcinomas have the highest incidence of tumour associated hypercalcaemia. This is partly due to the high rate of bone metastases in mammary carcinomas and local bone dissolution but it also occurs in the absence of bone metastasis due to the peripheral effects of the secreted PTHrP on bone (Gallacher *et al.*, 1990). The PTHrP production also increases renal tubular reabsorbtion of calcium and urinary cAMP levels (Gallacher *et al.*, 1990), therefore, high levels of PTHrP set a cycle in motion whereby elevated systemic levels of calcium resulting from its increased bone-resorptive and positive renal calcium-reabsorbing effects give rise to hypercalcemia, which in turn creates aggravating hypercalcemia by stimulating further release of PTHrP by the cancer cells (Chattopadhyay, 2006).

In addition, PTHrP is expressed in mammary carcinomas of various histological types. Danks *et al.*, (1989) found PTHrP in one of six mammary carcinomas, but recent reports found PTHrP in 60% of unselected breast cancer patients by immunohistological methods and by in situ hybridization (Southby *et al.*, 1990; Vargas *et al.*, 1992; Bundred *et al.*, 1996), and in 88% of breast tumours from patients with bone metastases compared with 52% of tumour without metastases (Bundred *et al.*, 1992). PTHrP was also detected previously by immunohistochemistry in breast tumours from nearly all investigated patients (Bucht *et al.*, 1998). PTHrP has been isolated from mammary tumours (Burtis *et al.*, 1987; Stewart *et al.*, 1987). PTHrP and PTH1R mRNA expression were identified in primary human breast tumour tissue which was surgically removed (Carron *et al.*, 1997). The comparison between PTHrP staining of the breast tumours and the radiological assessment of microcalcification in tumours showed a remarkable association, with 50% of PTHrP-positive breast cancers having microcalcification compared with 21% of PTHrP-negative tumours (Bundred *et al.*, 1996).

Furthermore, PTHrP stimulates osteoclastic bone resorption both in vitro and in vivo,and enhances renal tubular calcium reabsorption (Horiuchi *et al.* 1987, and Kemp *et al.* 1987). About 70 to 90% of metastatic lesions from breast tumour in bone express the PTHrP gene and produce the peptide (Vergas *et al.*, 1992). It is possible that the bone may activate or regulate PTHrP gene expression in metastatic breast carcinoma cells (Wysolmerski and Broadus, 1994). Transfection of MDA MB231 breast cancer cell line with the PTHrP gene enhanced secretion of PTHrP (Guise *et al.*, 1994). 92% of bone metastases secondary to breast cancer were shown to produce PTHrP (mRNA and protein) compared with 17% of metastases in non-bone sites such as liver, lung or soft tissue (Powell *et al.*, 1991). In another previous study, of 114 early breast cancer patients, 76% had detectable intact PTHrP 1-86, whereas, only 9 out of 27 (33%) of normal breast samples expressed PTHrP (Bundred *et al.*, 1996). Thus, tumour cells secreting potent osteoclast activating factors such as PTHrP seem to be a necessary prerequiste for the development of bone metastases (Arguello *et al.*, 1988).

The presence of multiple bioactive fragments of PTHrP were identified in vivo in studies on cancer patients using a cytochemical bioassy to demonstrate elevated plasma levels of PTH-like activity in the absence of detectable immunoreactive PTH (Goltzman *et al.*, 1981). Using a specific immunoassay (immunoradiometric assay, IRMA) to identified both N- and C-terminal moieties in the circulation of cancer patients Burtis and his group in 1990 found that both PTHrP-(1-36) and PTHrP-(37-74) epitopes could be detected, as well as the C-terminal-(109-138) fragment, but that PTHrP-(1-141) appeared to be absent from the circulation. Henderson *et al.* (1990) have reported also that a PTHrP species of small molecular weight corresponding to the amino terminal moiety (about 6-7KDa) and larger one (higher than 15KDa) were present in plasma of patients with breast adenocarcinoma and hypercalcaemia by using a radioimmunoassay based on an N-terminal antibody which had been raised against PTHrP-(1-34).

Moreover, in five breast cancer cell lines, the immunoreactive PTHrP 1-40 and 60-72 were detected in the conditioned medium (Tabuenca *et al.*, 1995), and the mid-region PTHrP 34-67 was detected using immunohistochemistry in 56% of epithelial cells of early breast cancer samples compared with 67% of primary breast cancer samples which had developed bone metastases (Bundred *et al.*, 1996). Based on the last data, the C-terminal fragments of PTHrP may be metabolized by the kidney. Proliferation studies on MCF7 and Hs578T breast cancer cell lines using ^{3}H thymidine incorporation, Birch *et al* (1995) found no effect of PTHrP-(1-34) or PTH-(1-34) to the Hs578T cells, but when MCF7 cells were treated with 100ng of PTHrP-(1-34) the level of intracellular cAMP and ^{3}H-thymidine uptake were significantly increased and no elevation were recorded at 10ng of the same peptide. In a mouse model of bone metastases, neutralizing antibodies to PTHrP-(1–34) inhibited the development of breast carcinoma metastases to bone of the human breast carcinoma cells MDA-MB-231, which produce moderate amounts of PTHrP (Thomas *et al.*, 1999). Conversely, in the same mouse model, overexpression of PTHrP by MCF-7 cells, which normally express low levels of PTHrP and do not cause osteolytic metastases, induced marked bone destruction associated with increased osteoclast formation compared with controls (Henderson *et al.*, 2001). These data suggest that tumor production of PTHrP is important for the establishment and progression of osteolytic bone metastases. However, Henderson *et al.*, (2001) reported that patients presenting with PTHrP-positive breast cancers have a more favorable outcome and have fewer metastases to bone and other sites. The PTHrP-mediated modulation of cell proliferation through apoptosis and cell cycle regulatory pathways in breast cancer is of both physiological and clinical relevance.

Aminoterminal Region of PTHrP

The first 34 N-terminal amino acids of PTHrP contain the PTH-like biological activity. This is similar to PTH in which the first 34 N-terminal amino acids are responsible for most of the biological activity. There is 70% sequence homology of the first 13 N-terminal amino acids of the PTHrP compared with PTH. These residues of the peptide are critical for most of the agonist effects of PTH on its classical target tissues (bone and kidney) in the regulation of calcium metabolism (Habener *et al.*, 1984). However, the PTHrP 14-36 region has almost no homology with the primary sequence of PTH (Kemp *et al.*, 1987). Orloff *et al* (1992) reported that the midregion and the C-terminal of PTHrP peptide did not bind specifically to several kinds of squamous carcinoma, Sqcc, cell lines and they suggested that the receptor binding domain of PTHrP may be located within the N-terminal of the PTHrP.

Nevertheless, studies carried out on synthesised hybrid peptides (PTH-1-14-PTHrP-15-34) found that this hybrid appears to have high affinity binding to LLC-PK1 cells compared to another Hybrid (PTHrP-1-14-PTH-15-34) which bound with much weaker affinity (Gardella *et al.*, 1995). The same group concluded that the amino acid in position 5 (Ile) in PTH contributes to the binding affinity in the first hybrid (PTH-1-14-PTHrP-15-34) and the amino acids in position 19 (Arg) and 21(Arg) in PTHrP are also contribute in the peptide-receptor interaction. Thus the way in which PTH and PTHrP bind to the PTH-receptor in LLC-PK1 cells may differ (Gardella, *et al.*, 1995). Moreover, Barden and Kemp (1996) reported that the arginine at position 19 and 20 on PTHrP have important roles in the binding.

The efficiency of PTHrP signal transduction may be affected by differences in species (Orloff *et al.*, 1991). The PTHrP-1-34 has a potent effect on renal cAMP production in isolated rat kidney preparations (Zhou *et al.*, 1989). N-terminal PTHrP is able to stimulate osteoclastic bone resorption in vitro and in vivo with similar potency to PTH (Evely *et al.*, 1991; Orloff *et al.*, 1989). N-terminal PTHrP imitates most effects of N-terminal PTH in kidney including increased tubular reabsorption of calcium and increased excretion of inorganic phosphate and cAMP (Rizzoli *et al.*, 1989; Carney *et al.*, 1991). Point mutation studies have revealed that the Ile^5-PTH-1-34 and His^5-PTH-1-34 bind to the PTH1R, stimulate cAMP accumulation, and release cytosolic free calcium in a clonal human embryonic kidney cell line (HEK293/C-21) (Behar *et al.*, 1996). In addition, Juppner *et al* (1994) found the PTH 7-34 fragment bound to opossum PTH1R receptor with high affinity, and this region is recognised to be important in the binding of PTH to its receptor (Nussbaum *et al.*, 1980). PTHrP 7-34 is well know as PTH1R antagonist, however, Asn^{10}-Leu^{11}-PTHrP-7-34 was reported to stimulates the adenylate cyclase activity in UMR 106-01 osteogenic sarcoma cells (Williams *et al.*, 1998).

MIDREGION OF PTHRP

The mid-region PTHrP is important for several reasons. First, it is highly conserved among species (Orloff & Stewart, 1995). Second, it is secreted by a variety of cell types (Soifer *et al.*, 1992). Finally, it is present in the circulation of patients with HHM syndrome in concentrations higher than those of any other PTHrP secretory form (Bucht *et al.*, 1992; Burtis *et al.*, 1994). The studies of Soifer *et al* (1992) described the existence of a midregion species of PTHrP that begins at alanine 38, which would be formed from any of the three isoforms of human PTHrP mRNA. However, the complete structure of the midregion peptide is unknown, but it appears to have a molecular mass of ~7,000 daltons by SDS-PAGE. This suggests that the midregion peptide contain 50-70 amino acids and this would place its carboxy terminus in the 80-108 regions of the predicted sequence (Soifer *et al.*, 1992).

The midregion peptide appears to be packaged into secretary granules both in rat insulinoma cells and in renal carcinoma cells, whereas, the amino-terminal PTHrP peptide appears predominantly in the Golgi apparatus (Soifer *et al.*, 1992). Based on the data summarized above, the midregion and the amino-terminal PTHrP fragments are packaged and secreted separately. Abbas *et al* (1989) found that the recombinant PTHrP-(1-84), PTHrP-(1-108) and PTHrP-(1-141) were capable of stimulating placental calcium transport, while synthetic PTHrP-(1-34) was inactive. The amidated midregion fragment of PTHrP-(67-86) amide was active in placentae derived from both normal and parathyroidectomized fetuses (Care *et al.*, 1990). It activated phospholipase C (PLC) and stimulated the cytosolic calcium responses in SqCC/Y1 (Orloff *et al*, 199). By performing radioreceptor assay (RRA) and affinity cross-linking studies, Inomata *et al* (1995) found the PTHrP (37-74) and PTHrP (109-141) show no binding to PTH/PTHrP receptors, but PTHrP (1-36) has very strong binding in several clonal cell lines. They also found that the PTHrP C-terminal and midregion caused no displacement of ^{125}I-PTH (1-84) peptide, suggesting that independent receptors for the mid-region peptide exist.

Furthermore, the mid-region PTHrP displays biological activity in placenta (Rodda *et al.*, 1988), and increases cytosolic calcium levels through a receptor coupled to the protein kinase C (PKC) but not to the protein kinase A (PKA) pathway in human squamous carcinoma line (YCC-SQ-1) and pancreatic β cell line (RIN 1046-38) (Orloff *et al.*, 1996; Wu *et al.*, 1996). The binding studies and calcium signalling pathway in the human embryonal kidney cells, C21, show no apparent interaction between the midregion or C-terminal PTHrP-67-94 and 107-139 (Pines *et al.*, 1996). In contrast, the radiolabelled PTHrP 67-86 did not bind to SqCC/Y1 cells, and did not compete for binding of ^{125}I-PTHrP-1-36^{Tyr} to PTH/PTHrP receptor in SaOS-2 osteosarcoma cells (Orloff *et al.*, 1996). These observations are important because they suggest that the mid-region of PTHrP has biological functions which probably occur via alternative, as yet unidentified, receptors that specifically recognised the PTHrP mid-region sequence.

Carboxy-Terminal Region

The mature PTHrP is highly conserved between chicken, human, mouse and rat up to amino acid 111 (Suva *et al.*, 1987; Mangin *et al.*, 1989; 1990; Yasuda *et al.*, 1989; Karaplis *et al.*, 1990). However, the sequence after 111 to the end of carboxy terminal, shows little inter-species homology (Moseley and Mathew, 1995). This suggests that the PTHrP amino acid residues up to 111 have biological functions, whereas, the remaining residues may be biologically irrelevant or may possibly have unique species-specific functions or may be involved in stabilizating the protein (Moseley and Gillespie, 1995). Seitz *et al* (1995) found that the C-terminal analogue of PTHrP (107-139) stimulated cAMP production in three osteoblast cell preparations, and they suggested that this region might interact with a receptor. The 107-139 peptide also inhibits the growth and DNA synthesis of human osteoblast-like cells. The antiproliferative effects of PTHrP 107-139 and 107-111 were found in UMR 106 cell line, and these effects of these C-terminal peptides may be independent of cAMP and mediated by PKC (Valin et al.., 1997). The same effect of PTHrP 107-111 was observed in human skin keratinocytes and BALB/MK-2 murine skin keratinocytes (Whitfield *et al.*, 1996).

On the other hand, in an in vivo study, when PTHrP 107-139 was injected for five consecutive days into adult male mice, the bone resorption was significantly decreased with a 70% decrease in osteoclast number and with 40% decrease in osteoblast number (Cornish *et al.*, 1997), and inhibited osteblast-like cell growth (Martinez *et al.*, 1997). Fenton *et al* (1991a,b) proposed that a carboxy terminal region of PTHrP that includes PTHrP-(107-111) (Thr-Arg-Ser-Ala-Trp) and the C-terminal region of PTHrP would inhibit bone resorption, and may also inhibit the activity of osteoclast cells (Dudley *et al.*, 1992). Figure 1.10 defines the biological active regions of PTHrP. In addition, Gagnon *et al* (1993) and Whitfield *et al* (1994) have shown that PTHrP-(107-111) stimulated membrane associated protein kinase C, but not adenylate cyclase in cultured ROS 17/2 rat cells and rat spleen lymphocytes in vivo and in vitro. Similar effects were seen at low concentrations of PTHrP-(107-111) in human skin keratinocytes and BALB/MK-2 murine skin keratinocytes (Whitfield *et al.*, 1996). PTHrP-107-111 was also reported to be antiproliferative for osteblast-like cells from adult human bone (Martinez *et al.*, 1997).

PTHrP Receptors

The PTH/PTHrP receptor (type 1 parathyroid hormone receptor, PTH1R) is a class II G-protein-coupled receptors (GPCRs) wich binds both PTH 1-34 and PTHrP 1-36 and transduces PTH and PTHrP signalling through adenylate cyclase-protein kinase A (AC-PKA) and phospholipase C-protein kinase C (PLC-PKC) (Abou-Samra *et al.*, 1992). PTH1R has been found to be express in different human tumors (Alokail. 2004; 2005; Alokail and Peddie. 2005) activation results in the generation of multiple second messengers including c'AMP and 1,4,5-inositol trisphosphate (IP_3) (Karpf *et al.*, 1987; Teitelbaum *et al.*, 1982), and changes in intracellular calcium (Abou-Samra *et al.*, 1992).

The transfected human receptor binds both PTH and PTHrP with equal affinity (Schipani *et al.*, 1993), and the binding affinity of PTHrP-1-34 in transfected HEK 293 cells (Blind *et al.*, 1995) was similar to that of PTH-1-34 in opossum kidney cells (Teitelbaum *et al.*, 1984). Orloff *et al* (1992) detected low affinity binding sites for PTHrP-1-36 in malignant squamous carcinoma cells (SqCC) but not in their nonmalignant counterpart HK (human epidermal keratinocytes). By [^{3}H] thymidine incorporation, Birch *et al* (1995) suggested that the both PTHrP-1-34 and PTH-1-34 mediate their effects through PTH1R in breast cancer cell lines MCF7 and Hs578T. These studies provided strong evidence that the PTH1R binds to both ligands, and initiates the signalling of PTH and PTHrP (Orloff *et al.*, 1995). However, a second receptor that binds PTH in vitro, the PTH2 receptor, is most closely related to the PTH1R (51% amino acid identity). PTH acts as an agonist at the human PTH2 receptor, but shows little or no agonism at the rat or fish homologs of this receptor. PTHrP shows no agonism at any of the known PTH2 receptors (Usdin *et al.*, 1995).

Direct comparison between transfected cloned opossum and rat PTH1R reveal some species differences (Segre *et al.*, 1979), and minor differences have also been shown between the properties of transfected cloned rat and human PTH1R (Karpf *et al.*, 1987). The receptors' amino acid sequences are highly homologous between species, and their lengths vary from 585 to 594 amino acids. Ten cysteine residues are located in the PTH1R, including two in the putative signal sequence, six in the amino-terminal extension and one in each of the first two extracellular loops. In addition, there are several charged side chain amino acid and proline residues within the receptor's membrane-spanning domains, and four potential glycosylation sites in the amino-terminal extension (Schipani *et al.*, 1993). Rat and mouse PTH1R are 99% homologous at the amino acid level whereas human and rat PTH1R are 91% homologous (Karpf *et al.*, 1987; Juppner *et al.*, 1988). The receptors' membrane-spanning helices are important for signal transduction across the cells' plasma membrane (Dohlman, *et al.*, 1991).

The physiochemical properties of the PTH1R have been characterized by affinity cross-linking with radioiodinated PTH ligands. The receptor is a glycoprotein with a molecular size of ~80,000 daltons; the peptide backbone accounts for ~59,000 daltons, and the remainder is due to asparagine-linked oligosaccharides (Abou-Samra *et al.*, 1992; Karpf *et al.*, 1988;

Juppner *et al.*, 1990, 1994, Nissenson *et al.*, 1993; Schipani *et al.*, 1993; Shigeno *et al.*, 1988b). The PTH1R is susceptible to cleavage by an endogenous proteolytic activity, and the site for this protease action is probably in the proximal portion of the C-terminal side (Nissenson *et al.*, 1993). The domains of the PTH1R involved in ligand-binding have been deduced by characterizing the interactions among several synthetic PTH and PTHrP fragments and analogs (Drake *et al.*, 1993). Receptors in which 45 amino acids were deleted from the amino-terminal region were unable to be expressed on cell surface to bind, or to activate adenylate cyclase (Segre *et al.*, 1993).

Moreover, mutating either cysteine residue in the first or second extracellular loop impaired binding (Segre *et al.*, 1993) while the point mutation of the third extracellular loop of the receptor led to impaired the binding to PTH. Replacement of the cysteine residues in the first and second extracellular loops also affected the receptor expression and PTH binding (Lee *et al.*, 1994), while treating plasma membranes with reducing agents indicated that the functional integrity of the PTH receptor requires intact cysteine bonds (Teitelbaum *et al.*, 1982). Deletion of the carboxy terminal portion of the first extracellular loop or most of the second extracellular loop diminished both PTH binding and cell surface expression (Lee *et al.*, 1994). Portions of the membrane spanning helices are also critical for PTH binding and receptor activation (Dohlman *et al.*, 1991). The regions of the receptor that lie between the third and the sixth membrane spanning helics are also important for binding and receptor activation (Segre *et al.*, 1993). The amino acids in the receptor amino terminal between 31 and 47 and in the loop 3 between 431 to 440 amino acids appear to have an essential role in the ligand-receptor interaction (Lee *et al.*, 1994). From these studies, it is clear that multiple regions in the receptor and all cysteines in the extracellular domain are engaged in ligand binding.

Ile^5-Bpa^{23}-PTHrP-1-36 is fully functional photoreactive analog of PTHrP was reported to cross-linked to 23-40 amino acids of the N-terminal extracellular domain of PTH1R in COS-7 cells, and using alanine scanning mutagenesis of this region revealed two residues, threonine 23 and glutamine 37, as being functionally involved in ligand binding (Mannstadt *et al.*, 1998). In order to identify the biomolecular interaction between hormone and receptor (the contact domain) interface, PTH-1-34 analog containing a photoderivatised lysine 13 was cross-linked to a 17-amino acid segment of the N-terminal receptor domain which is close to the first membrane-spanning helix (Zhou *et al.*, 1997). With the suggestion that PTH1R activation occurs via interaction between a discrete, N-terminal domain within the ligand and the receptor's juxtamembrane-domain, efforts have been made to synthesize minimum-length peptides capable of fully and efficiently activating the PTH1R. [Leu^{11}, d-Trp^{12}]PTHrP (7–34) and [Ile5, Trp^{23}]PTHrP(5–36) bind with high affinity, but are devoid of signaling activity (Carter *et al.*, 2001). Modification or substitution of valine 2 in PTH (1–34) or PTHrP (1–36) with a bulky amino acid or an amino acid derivative (Trp, Arg, or Bpa) also results in the generation of potent antagonists (Behar *et al.*, 2000).

In a series of generated clonal HEK-293 cell lines which expressed the PTH2 receptor, the BP-16 clone expressed an alternative subtype of the PTH1R recognised the ligand PTH-1-34, 7-34, and PTHrP-7-34, but not PTHrP-1-34 (Behar *et al.*, 1996), they found also that PTH-7-34 and PTHrP-7-34 are recognised by both the PTH2 and PTH1R subtypes. The lack of response to PTH by the rat PTH2 receptor, and the predominant localization of this receptor to the hypothalamus, which suggest a physiological role distinct from the regulation of calcium homeostasis. Further investigation led to the discovery of TIP39, a 39 amino acid peptide structurally related to PTH and PTHrP, which appears to be the natural ligand for this receptor (Usdin *et al.*, 1999). The PTH2 receptor agonist, TIP39, binds efficiently to the PTH1R, but does not activate it, and thus functions as a weak antagonist at this receptor. A chimeric peptide comprised of the N-terminal residues 1 through 20 of PTHrP and the C-terminal residues 23 through 39 of TIP39 (PTHrP(1–20)/TIP^{39}(23–39) binds to the PTH1R with higher affinity than does TIP39 and shows restored cAMP signaling activity (Jonsson *et al.*, 2001). However, this putative receptor has been characterized only partially and its cDNAs has not yet been isolated. A synthetic fragment of intact PTH, PTH(7–84), was recently shown to inhibit bone resorption (Slatopolsky *et al.*, 2000) possibly by impairing the differentiation of osteoclast precursors into mature bone-resorbing multinuclear cells (Divieti *et al.*, 2002). It remains to be determined, however, whether these actions of PTH (7–84) are mediated through the elusive C-PTH receptor. Biological roles distinct from those mediated through the PTH1R have also been described for C-terminal fragments of PTHrP. Some of these fragments may have, through a nuclear localization sequence within the fragment, intracrine roles and may act as transcriptional regulators while others appear to be secreted and interact with cell membrane receptors (Lam *et al.*, 1999a; Aarts *et al.*, 1999).

Role of G-Protein in PTH1R Activation

PTH1R belong to a family of G protein-linked receptors. Other members of this family are receptors for calcitonin (Lin *et al.*, 1991), growth hormone-releasing hormone (Mayo, 1992), glucagon (Jelinek *et al.*, 1993), glucagon-like peptide-I (Thorens, 1992), secretin (Ishihara *et al.*, 1991), and vasoactive intestinal peptide (Ishihara *et al.*, 1992). Because these receptors have no significant sequence identity (<12%) with the other G protein-linked receptors presented in data banks (Attwood *et al.*, 1991; Probst *et al.*, 1992), these receptors are classified as members of a distinct G protein-coupled receptor family. This family is highly homologous with many identical or conserved amino acids (Shigeno *et al.*, 1988a).

All G protein-linked receptors have relatively long amino-terminal, extracellular extensions, highly conserved cysteine residues in the amino-terminal and in each of the first two extracellular loops, and multiple potential asparagine-linked glycosylation sites (Shigeno *et al.*, 1988b; Abou-Samra *et al.*, 1992; Karpf *et al.*, 1988; Juppner *et al.*, 1990; Dohlman *et al.*, 1991). The last three membrane-spanning domains and the initial portion of their carboxyl-terminal intracellular region are especially highly conserved, the 16 amino acids 18 and the 17th of 18 in this region are identical between secretin and PTH1R and between calcitonin and PTH1R (Abou-Samra *et al.*, 1992; Attwood *et al.*, 1991; Dohlman *et al.*, 1991).

PTHrP activate multiple second messenger signalling pathways that are coupled by distinct G-proteins to the PTH1R (Abou Samra *et al.*, 1992). Binding of an agonist to its receptor activates the G-protein by releasing GDP, binding of GTP to the α-subunit, initiating the G-protein dissociation, and activation of α[GTP] and the $\beta\gamma$ dimer (Schwindinger *et al.*, 1998). Both dimers regulate signal effector molecules, such as adenylyl cyclase and β-isoforms of phospholipase C (Schwindinger *et al.*, 1998). Cell-specific expression of isoforms of adenylyl cyclase and phospholipase C that differ in their sensitivity to βγ-subunits and intracellular calcium can further modify hormone responses (Schwindinger *et al.*, 1998). The adenylate cyclase system is controlled by stimulatory (G_s) and inhibitory (G_i) proteins, whereas, PLC is linked to G_q (Hepler & Gilman, 1992).

PTH1R Signaling in Tumor

All three PTHrP isoforms are subjected to tissue-specific post-translational proteolysis on mono/multi basic (K/R) sites by members of the prohormone convertase family generating various daughter peptides all biologically active including amino-terminal PTHrP(1-36) interacting with the PTH1R, a mid-region PTHrP (38-94/95/101), and carboxy-terminal PTHrP (107-139) and (141-173) in humans, as well as combinations of theses peptides (Philbrick *et al.*, 1996; Talon *et al.*, 2005). To date, only the PTH1R has been cloned, and only pharmacological evidences support the existence of additional receptors recognizing the mid-region or carboxy-terminal PTHrP peptides. The perinatal letality of PTHrP or of the PTH1R knockout mice emphasizes the importance of this peptide system for normal life (Philbrick *et al.*, 1996). There are three potential biological roles have been assigned to PTHrP: (1) PTHrP is a regulator of transepithelial calcium transport in renal tubules and placenta and during lactation; (2) PTHrP is a potent myo-relaxant factor in vascular and non vascular smooth muscle; and (3) PTHrP is a regulator of cell differentiation, proliferation and death (Philbrick *et al.*, 1996). This latter property has been evidenced not only in normal cells and tissues but also in various tumor cells. The majority of the known biological properties of PTHrP are the consequences of its interaction with the PTH1R, which is coupled to adenylyl cyclase (AC) and/or phospholipase C (PLC) in a cell or tissue-specific manner, and subsequent protein kinase A (PKA)—and protein kinase C (PKC)-related signaling pathways (Clemens *et al.*, 2001; Gensure *et al.*, 2005).

The structure-function studies with PTH and PTHrP using truncated peptides have demonstrated that the first amino acids are essential for activation of adenylyl cyclase, and that the activation of PKC can be linked to a different domain of the molecule (Fujimori *et al.*, 1991). Nissenson *et al.*, (1993) showed that the activated receptor is more efficiently coupled to adenylate cyclase than to phospholipase C in transfected CHO cells. In ROS 17/2.8, PTH increase intracellular cAMP, via Gs, inhibits adenylyl cyclase via Gi, activates PLC, and leads to accumulation of IP3 and diacylglycerol (DAG) (Abou Samra *et al.*, 1992; Schneider *et al.*, 1994). IP3 increases intracellular free calcium by stimulating its release from the endoplasmic reticulum (Bringhurst *et al.*, 1992). In UMR-106 cells PTHrP and PTH increased the PLC activity and IP3 levels (Short *et al.*, 1991). Other studies demonstrated that PTH stimulated cAMP accumulation in human embryonal kidney cells, C21 (Schwindinger *et al.*, 1998). In COS-7 cells, both PTH and PTHrP stimulated with equal effect the cAMP response (Bergwitz *et al.*, 1998).

In SqCC and HK squamous cancer and normal epidermal keratinocytes cell lines, PTHrP stimulated an increase in intracellular calcium, but not cAMP (Orloff *et al.*, 1992). In SqCC/Y1, both PTH and PTHrP stimulate adenylate cyclase, indicating that these cells express the type I receptor and is capable of signalling through the adenylyl cyclase pathway

(Orloff *et al.*, 1995). These studies suggest the existence of an alternative receptor (type II) in the malignant cells. This type II PTH1R could arise from a different gene or through alternative processing of the type I receptor gene (Orloff *et al.*, 1995). The cloned full-length hPTH1R elicits both cAMP and IP3 responses when transiently transfected into monkey COS-1 cells, but the same receptor elicited only a cAMP responses when stably expressed in a human embryonic kidney cell line (HEK 293) (Schneider *et al.*, 1994). Using these cells, N-terminal PTH and PTHrP increased the accumulation of cAMP (Fukayama *et al.*, 1992), whereas, there was no cAMP stimulation or calcium signalling pathway initiated by any midregion or C-terminal PTH and PTHrP in C21 cells (Pines *et al.*, 1994, 1996).

The PTH1R structural requirements necessary for signal activation have been defined: the His^{223} in the human PTH1R or His^{220} in the opposum kidney PTH1R are necessary for receptor activation (Schipani *et al.*, 1995; 1997). Iida-Klein *et al* (1997) found that the receptor mutation in which the wild type (WT) rat receptor sequence EKKY (317-320 a.a.) of the second cytoplasmic loop was replaced with DSEL had little or no PLC stimulating ability in response to PTH when expressed in COS-7 cells. They suggested that the Lys-319 is critical for activating the PLC pathway, and that PTH was unable to produce inositol phosphates when the amino acids 317 to 320 were mutated in either HEK293 or LLC-PK1 cells.

The PTH1R was expressed in human embryonic kidney, HEK-293 cells, and ligand binding led to activation through PKA and PKC (Blind *et al.*, 1996). In addition, there were autophosphorylation sites at serine 491 (as a major site) in the cytoplasmic C-terminal tail of the receptor (Blind *et al.*, 1996), while serine 473 and/or 475 were the minor sites for PKA phosphorylation. The five threonine and serine residue of the third cytoplasmic loop of the PTH1R were not essential in receptor autophosphorylation (Blind *et al.*, 1996). In addition, a PKC-mediated receptor phosphorylation site(s) is located in the juxtamembrane portion of the C-terminal tail, and it may be located in the same region or may even overlap with the PKA sites (Blind *et al.*, 1996). The autophosphorylation sites are implicated in the regulation of receptor activation but their comperhinsive role had not been explained.

In addition, biological significance of alternative non-cAMP signaling pathways may relate to the diverse functions of the PTH1R in various tissues and its responsiveness to two different ligands. The effects of phospholipase C signaling have been investigated using a PTH1R mutant, which stimulates cAMP formation normally but does not lead to inositol trisphosphate formation (Iida-Klen *et al.*, 1997). Mutant mice exclusively expressing this mutant receptor have delayed ossification and enhanced chondrocyte proliferation. This finding suggests that the normal function of phospholipase C signaling by the PTH1R receptor is to slow proliferation and promote differentiation of chondrocytes in the growth plate and to thereby oppose the primary, cAMP-mediated, actions of the receptor (Guo *et al.*, 2002). Further studies selectively ablating each putative signaling pathway in the various target tissues will be required to determine how each signaling cascade contributes to the individual cellular responses induced by the PTH1R receptor.

Furthermore, PTHrP has been shown to be an auto/paracrine cell growth regulator in proximal tubular cells proliferation of either animal or human origin (Esbrit and Egido, 2000; Talon *et al.*, 2005). In this cell type, PTHrP stimulates proliferation through the PTH1R via a mechanism which seems to involve both PKA and PKC signaling pathways (Esbrit and

Egido, 2000). In 1990, Burton *et al.*, Raised the possibility that PTHrP, in addition to its role in inducing HHM, might involve in the growth regulation of RCC. Indeed, in this early study, PTHrP antiserum almost totally inhibited the growth in vitro of a human renal cell carcinoma, CRCC, cell line (SKRC-1), known to secrete PTHrP, and growth was significantly inhibited by PTH (3-34) NH_2, a competitive PTH1R antagonist. Until our recent works (Massfelder *et al.*, 2004; Talon *et al.*, 2005), there were no other reports to study further such property of PTHrP in human RCC. Massfelder *et al* (2004) have recently shown that inhibiting PTHrP with antibodies or antagonizing the PTH1R, dramatically blunts the growth of three VHL-deficient human CRCC cell lines (786-0, UOK-126 and UOK-128 cell lines) in vitro by promoting cell apoptosis. In nude mice implanted subcutaneously with 786-0 tumors, anti-PTHrP treatment using a specific PTHrP-neutralizing antibody directed against amino-terminal PTHrP induced complete regression of the implanted tumors in 70% of mice by inducing cell death. While the treatment with a specific PTH1R antagonist induced no tumor regression, it completely blocked tumor growth also through induction of tumor cell apotosis. These results raise an argument about the auto/paracrine nature of PTHrP-induced CRCC cell death. Interestingly, another significant finding in these studies was the increased microvessel density in CRCC tumors grown in nude mice in response to PTH1R system inhibition. In the same study, they also demonstrated that the pVHL negatively regulates PTHrP expression specifically at the post-transcriptional level by decreasing PTHrP mRNA stability. These studies identify PTHrP as a critical growth factor for VHL-deficient CRCC.

Akino *et al.* (2000) have observed an increased microvessel density in CCRC tumors grown in nude mice in response to PTH1R system inhibition. This latter observation strongly suggests that PTHrP is an anti-angiogenic factor in CCRC. In support of this, PTHrP has been shown to behave as an angiogenic or anti-angiogenic factor, depending on the cell or tissue-type (Akino *et al.*, 2000; Bakre *et al.*, 2002). As a rule, vascularization leads to a phase of rapid growth of a given tumor, a pre-requisite for the development of invasive processes. However, it has been proposed that in CCRC tumors with poor prognosis, decreased microvessel density is associated with the development of large vessels, which facilitate metastatic spread (MacLenna *et al.*, 1995; Delahunt *et al.*, 1997). Thus, the angiogenic effect, i.e. increased microvessel density, in response to the anti- PTH1R manoeuvres might be beneficial therapeutically, together with the induction of tumor apoptosis. This is an interesting new field of research and efforts should be put to understand the significance of the tumor vascular supply in terms of tumor metastatic spread and patient survival.

Current information suggests that PTH and PTHrP interact with the PTH1R (Type I) through multiple sites and that these are dispersed throughout the extracellular surface of the receptor (Offermanns *et al.*, 1996). Affinity cross-linking studies demonstrated that a PTH-1-34 analog containing a photoderivatised lysine 13 crosslinked to a 17-amino acid segment of the amino terminal extracellular receptor domain (Zhou *et al.*, 1997). In HEK293/C-21 cells, the 173 to 189 amino acids domain of the N-terminal extracellular PTH1R domain were identified as the contact region with the lysine in the PTH agonist [^{125}I-all-R-K13]. To further define PTHrP-receptor interaction, Mannstadt *et al* (1998) found a photoreactive analog of PTHrP (Ile^5-Bpa^{23}-PTHrP-1-36^{Tyr}) bound covalently and specifically to the PTH1R in COS-7 cells; (they suggested that this analog cross-linked to amino acids 23-40 of the PTH1R). They identified that the Thr^{33} and Gln^{37} on the receptor were involved functionally in ligand binding.

PTHrP 14-38 and PTHrP 14-34 analogs have been shown to interact with PTH1R receptors in ROS cells (Abou-Samra *et al.*, 1989), and PTH 14-34 and PTHrP 14-34 were found to be equipotent in binding to the PTH1R receptors in both bovine and renal cortical plasma membranes (Caulfield *et al.*, 1990). A series of experiments using PTH/PTHrP-PTH2 chimeras found that with amino-terminal of the PTH1R spliced to the PTH2 receptor, PTH bound and fully activated the receptor, but there was no detectable interaction of PTHrP with this receptor (Clark *et al.*, 1998). Transfer of the PTH2 receptor amino terminus to the PTH1R eliminated the PTHrP binding and significantly decreased activation of the receptor by the PTHrP but retained binding and activation by PTH, replacing of the PTH2 receptor amino-terminal by the amino-terminal of the PTH1R did not effect on ^{125}I-PTHrP binding or ability to stimulate adenylate cyclase. In addition, a mutation study carried out in the transmembrane domain on 3 and 7 (TM3 & TM7) in the PTH2 receptor showed that PTHrP was able to bind and activate the receptor. Both PTH2 and PTH1R receptors have residues important for activation, and residues (His^{180} and Arg^{190}) may form part of the receptor activation mechanism (Turner *et al.*, 1998). Dissociation of receptor binding and receptor activation was also observed in a previous study in which mutation of Arg^{233} in the second transmembrane domain and Gln 451 in the seventh transmembrane domain of the PTH1R resulted in disruption of receptor signalling (Gardella *et al.*, 1996a).

In contrast, deletion of amino acids 62-106 of the PTH1R revealed that these residues are involved in receptor function, and substitution of the PTH2 receptor third extracellular loop (429-441a.a.) with the corresponding loop of the PTH1R decreased the PTHrP affinity 5-fold, but had no effect on PTH binding (Clark *et al.*, 1998). They established that the Gln440 and Arg394 on the PTH1R play a crucial role in the transduction process, and that the third extracellular loop of PTH2 and PTH1R receptors have similar interaction with PTH. These receptor chimeras show the involvement of the amino-terminal and third extracellular loop of PTH1R in PTHrP interaction. Specific amino acids within the two peptides were also defined. The native phenylalanine at position 23 in the PTH was shown to be involved in the PTH ligand binding specificity to the PTH2 receptor (Gardella *et al.*, 1996b).

MARK PATHWAY AND PTHRP SIGNALING

The PTHrP gene contains nucleotide sequence motifs common in members of the immediate-early gene family, as well as other hallmark features which include induction by growth factors, serum or cycloheximide and relatively short-lived mRNA (Martin *et al.*, 1997; Allinson *et al.*, 1992). While PTHrP acts as a hormone when produced in excess by various tumors, in lactating women and during fetal development, it is now clear that PTHrP is an important local regulator of several tissue-specific functions. Thus, PTHrP appears now as a key player of cellular differentiation, growth and death. There is a growing body of evidence, especially in bone cells, epithelial cells, smooth muscle cells, skin cells and chondrocytes, that supports such notion (Fiaschi-Taesch *et al.*, 2003). The growth factor-like properties of PTHrP are the consequences not only of its interaction with the PTH1R and subsequent signal transduction cascades but also of its nuclear translocation. Similarly, PTHrP promotes or suppresses apoptosis in various settings depending on cell type and context (Amling *et al.*, 1997; Hastings *et al.*, 2003). PTHrP inhibits apoptosis in chondrocytes through Bcl-2 expression (Amling *et al.*, 1997), but stimulates apoptosis in type II pneumocytes through a mechanism involving PLC cascade and caspase 3 activity. As evoked in the precedent chapter, nuclear translocation of PTHrP represents an additional mechanism by which PTHrP modulates a number of cellular functions related to growth and survival. Thus, expression of PTHrP peptides containing the bNLS prolongs survival of chondrocytes under conditions that promote cell apoptosis (serum starvation) and stimulates proliferation of vascular smooth muscle cells, while PTHrP forms lacking the nuclear targeting sequence negate these effects (Henderson *et al.*, 1995). In addition, to add complexity in a single cell type, PTHrP may inhibit or stimulate proliferation depending on whether it acts through the auto/paracrine pathway or through the intracrine pathway, respectively. Such a paradoxical effect of PTHrP on cell proliferation has been demonstrated initially in vascular smooth muscle cells, IEC-6 intestinal epithelial cells and in PC-3 prostate cancer cells (Massfelder *et al.*, 1997; Ye *et al.*, 2001; Tovar Sepulveda and Falzon, 2002).

PTHrP is frequently expressed or overexpressed in various neoplasms in humans and animals regardless of calcemia. PTHrP has been shown to stimulate adhesion, migration, proliferation and/or apoptosis in breast, prostate and lung cancers in vitro and in vivo in immunodeficient mouse models. These effects are the consequence of either interaction of PTHrP with the PTH1R and subsequent signaling cascade or nuclear translocation of PTHrP, or both (Luparello *et al.*, 2001; Dougherty *et al.*, 1999; Hastings *et al.*, 2001). Interestingly, evidence of altered regulation of PTHrP mRNAs in cancer cells was demonstrated in breast, lung and squamous carcinomas (Bouizar *et al.*, 1999; Sellers *et al.*, 2004). Although transcripts for PTHrP (1-139) and/or (1-141) are more common than PTHrP (1-173) transcript in benign tissues, malignant tissues tend to be enriched in PTHrP (1-173) mRNA. The significance of such dysregulation is still largely unknown but could be related to tumor progression, at least in some cancers. This is undoubtedly a new domain to investigate in the PTHrP-cancer field to uncover the role of PTHrP not only in tumor progression but also in the development of HHM (Sourbier and Massfelder, 2005).

PTHrP is now well recognised as an important factor in the development of osteolytic BM from breast cancer. The mechanisms involved remain to be fully resolved but studies by Guise and colleagues provide evidence that production of PTHrP forms part of a vicious cycle involving osteoclast activation followed by the release of mitogenic growth factors such as IGF-1 from the bone matrix (Guise, 2000). In this model, PTHrP exerts its actions by binding to receptors present on osteoblasts, which in response secrete factors leading to osteoclast activation. The presence or absence of the PTH1R on the tumour cells themselves is unlikely to exert a major influence in such a process. On the other hand, PTH1R expression may give metastatic breast cancer cells a selective advantage that allows them to colonise and expand in secondary sites by permitting autocrine PTHRP signalling. In this study, the expression of PTH1R was maintained in breast cancer BM. These data suggest that PTH1R expression occurs more frequently and at a higher level in BM compared to the primary cancer and tumour cells overexpressing the PTH1R have a selective survival or growth advantage in BM. Alternatively, tumour cells may upregulate PTH1R expression as a result of their exposure to the bone microenvironment. Distinguishing between these possibilities is a goal for future studies. Aklilu *et al* (2000) have shown that the proliferation of MCF7 cells overexpressing the PTH1R is sustained in part by PTHrP acting in an autocrine manner. They observed that PTHrP gene expression is promoted via the Ras-signal-regulated kinase (ERK) pathway (Aklilu *et al.*, 2000).

Mitogen-activated protein kinase (MAPK) cascade is also called the extracellular signal-regulated kinase (ERK) cascade and has been found to be involved in cell adhesion, proliferation, differentiation, viability, and apoptosis (Zhu and Assoian. 1995). Many extracellular growth factors signal through GTPase Ras/MAPK pathways to activate gene expression (Xiao *et al.*, 2002). Another GTPase of the Ras superfamily, Rap1, is activated by PKA phosphorylation in human neutrophils (Altschuler *et al.*, 1995) and activates the MAPK pathway (Stork and Schmitt. 2002). Activation of the MAPK cascade involves phosphorylation of MAPKKK (Raf-1), MAPKK, and MAPK (ERK). Active MAPK subsequently phosphorylates transcription factors, other downstream kinases, and substrates leading to biologic activity (Hagemann and Blank. 2001). The MAPKs are a family of serine/threonine kinases involved in the transduction of externally derived signals regulating cell growth, division, differentiation, and apoptosis (Aklilu *et al.*, 2000). Mammalian cells contain at least three major classes of MAPK, ERK1/2, c-Jun N-terminal kinase/stress-activated protein kinases, and p38/HOG1 MAPKs. MAPK activity is regulated by a series of parallel protein phosphorylation cascades, each comprised of three kinases that successively phosphorylate and activate the downstream component. In the ERK1/2 cascade, the proximal kinases, cRaf-1 and B-Raf, phosphorylate and activate MAPK kinase 1 and 2 (MEK1 and MEK2). MEK1 and -2 are dual-function threonine/tyrosine kinases that, in turn, phosphorylate and activate ERK1/2. Once activated, MAPKs phosphorylate a variety of membrane, cytoplasmic, and cytoskeletal substrates. Activated MAPKs also translocate to the nucleus, where they phosphorylate and activate nuclear transcription factors involved in DNA synthesis and cell division (Pearson *et al.*, 2001).

Many cellular effects of PTHrP signaling though the MAPK pathway have been reported in several tissues (Chan *et al.*, 2001; Shimo *et al.*, 2006) In addition, it has been shown that transactivation of the ubiquitously expressed epidermal growth factor receptor (EGFR) contribute to PTH1R-mediated ERK1/2 activation (Ahmed *et al.*, 2003), and this activation taken place by balance exists between G_s- and G_q-mediated signaling pathways and EGFR transactivation in ERK1/2 activation. However, it still remains unclear whether activation of ERK1/2 occurs via trafficking-dependent or -independent mechanisms (Syme *et al.*, 2005). Bisello and his group have shown previously that modifications of residue 1 in the biologically active N-terminal fragment of PTHrP result in ligands (PTHrP-(2–36) and Bpa^1-PTHrP-(1–36) that are unable to stimulate G_q/protein lipase C/protein kinase C-mediated signaling but still cause cAMP accumulation as a result of G_s signaling (Bisello *et al.*, 2002). Certainly, several studies have suggested that G_s/cAMP/PKA-mediated signaling inhibits ERK1/2 activity and results in reduced cell proliferation (Swarthout *et al.*, 2001; Massfelder *et al.*, 1997). These data indicate that G_q-mediated signaling and/or receptor trafficking is necessary for activating ERK1/2. In addition, cross-talk between EGFR and PTH1R have been confirmed in HEK-293 cells through predominant mechanism of PTH1R-mediated activation of ERK1/2 and both G_q signaling and PTH1R trafficking contribute to the activation of ERK1 and ERK2 through the transactivation of EGFR (Syme *et al.*, 2005). Their observation based on a PTHrP-based analog ([p-benzoylphenylalanine[1], Ile[5], Arg[11,13], Tyr[36]] PTHrP-(1–36) NH_2), which selectively activates the G_s/cAMP pathway without inducing PTH1R endocytosis, unsuccessful to stimulate ERK1/2 activity. ERK1/2 phosphorylation occurred following internalization of a PTH1R mutant induced by PTH-(7–34) in the absence of G protein signaling. These data show that PTH1R trafficking and G_q (but not G_s) signaling independently contribute to ERK1/2 activation, mainly through transactivation of the EGFR (Syme *et al.*, 2005) They suggested that parallel pathways exist with G_q-mediated and trafficking-dependent components. Thus, the cross-talk mechanism involves ERK1/2 phosphorylation and PTH1R signaling by mitogenic activity of PTHrP is seems to be still complex and tissue specific.

An additional explanation for the apparent increased mitogenic responsiveness of cells expressing the PTH1R derives from the results of previous analysis of ERK signalling. PTHrP found indirectly influences signalling through the ERK pathway; while PTHrP had little effect on its own, it increased the resulting activation of ERK when cells were stimulated by EGF and IGF-1. The mechanisms involved remain to be established, although it is interesting to note that ATP, which also signals via a GPCR, potentiated EGF signalling in MCF-7 cells (Wagstaff *et al.*, 2000). Since the ERK pathway appears critical for optimal proliferation in MCF-7 cells (Hermanto *et al.*, 2000), the potentiation of its activation by PTH1R may be significant and could provide a further explanation for the enhanced mitogenesis in cells overexpressing the PTH1R.

p38 MAPK is a stress-activated kinase that was originally identified as the target of pyridinylimidazole compounds found to suppress inflammatory cytokine release and cell death following cellular stress (Nebreda and Porras. 2000). The data revealed that high $(Ca^{2+})_o$-induced PTHrP release was satisfied in the presence of a specific inhibitor of p38α and -β subtypes called SB-203580. they also indicated that high $[Ca^{2+}]_o$ induced the phosphorylation of p38 MAPK. When p38 MAPK activated by phosphorylation, p38 MAPK will activates ATF-2, which then acts as a transcription factor for various target genes. The fast activation of ATF-2 observed in our studies in H-500 cells in response to high $(Ca^{2+})_o$ may be due to other intracellular signaling pathways that also activate ATF-2. Recently, p38 MAPK was shown to be involved in the Smad-independent induction of PTHrP release from MDA-MB-231 breast cancer cells by transforming growth factor-β (Kakonen *et al.*, 2002). They suggested that TGF-β stimulates PTHrP release through both Smad-dependent and MAP kinase signaling pathways. The combined inhibition of p38 MAP kinase and Smad signaling eliminated TGF-β stimulation of PTHrP release as successfully as the overexpression of dominant-negative TGF-β type II receptor.

Furthermore, the phosphorylation of p38 MAP kinase increase TGF-β increased in a time-dependent fashion consistent with appropriate MAP kinase activation which is supporting the role of p38 MAP kinase in TGF-β-induced PTHrP release (Kakonen *et al.*, 2002). These data indicate that the effects of TGF-β on MAP kinase pathways are mediated through the TGF-β receptor. These data suggested that MDA-MB-231 breast cancer cells use both Smad and MAP kinase pathways to regulate PTHrP production. Another investigation revealed that MAP kinase involved in other indicators of the metastatic phenotype in MDA-MB-231 cells. In matrix invasion, the activated p38 MAP kinase is essential by breast cancer cells such as MDA-MB-231 (Huang *et al.*, 2000). Likewise, both p38 MAP kinase and Smad pathways are activated by activin, a member of TGF-β gene family in the human breast cancer T47D cell line (Cocolakis *et al.*, 2001). In addition, there are widespread cross-talk examples in leteratures between the Smad pathway and the ERK, JNK, and p38 MAP kinase pathways that might participate in the TGF-β signaling to increase PTHrP upstream of p38 kinase as well as regulating PTHrP production upstream of MEK kinase (Mulder *et al.*, 2000). For instance, p38 kinase activated by TAK1 through MKK6 or MKK3 and JNK via MKK4. Since MKK4 can also activate p38, TGF-β-activated kinase 1 (TAK1) could activate p38 via MKK4. Smads also have direct effect in target gene expression in TGF-β- activated cells and it can integrate multiple signaling pathways (Verschueren *et al.*, 1999). Engel *et al* (1999) have observed interdependence between Smad and JNK pathways in TGF-β-mediated transcription, and transcriptional cross-talk between Smad, ERK1/2, and p38 MAP kinase pathways in TGF-β induction of the aggrecan gene have also been reported (Watanabe *et al.*, 2001).

Käkönen (2002) proposed the following mechanism by which TGF-β promotes breast cancer osteolysis. Metastatic breast cancer cells in the bone microenvironment secrete PTHrP, which stimulates osteoclastic bone resorption by increasing osteoblastic expression of RANK ligand (Thomas *et al.*, 1999). TGF-β, released in active form from the mineralized bone matrix as a consequence of osteoclastic bone resorption, activates the TGF-β receptors on tumor cells, which signal via both Smad and MAP kinase pathways. TGF-β signaling further stimulates tumor production of PTHrP. In HEK-293 cells that cross-talk between EGFR and PTH1R represents the predominant mechanism of PTH1R-mediated activation of ERK1/2. Another group demonstrated that in HEK-293 cells PTH1R endocytosis occurs exclusively via β-arrestin- and dynamin-dependent mechanisms. PTH1R trafficking affects neither acute cAMP signaling nor desensitization and resensitization of G_s signals. In contrast, we show that both G_q signaling and PTH1R trafficking contribute to the activation of ERK1 and ERK2 through the transactivation of EGFR (Syme *et al.*, 2005).

Furthermore, Shimo *et al* (2006) have reported in very recent data that the PTHrP activated certain MAPK signaling pathways through PTH1R in cancer cells. There results have indicated that PTHrP induced activation of ERK MAPK in MDA231 breast cancer cells. Moreover, PTHrP induces connective tissue growth factor (CCN2) which is a mediator of local angiogenesis induced by breast cancer. The PTHrP induction of CCN2 taken places throughout PKC and ERK1/2 p38 MAPK pathways. Additionally, a few number of studies found that MAPK regulation by PKA requires members of the Src family (Schmitt *et al.*, 2002), and Src might have a role in cross-talk between MAPK and PKA pathways to induce the CCN2 transcription by PTHrP in breast cancer cell line (Shimo *et al.*, 2006).

As we mentioned above, the extracellular ERK cascade also known as MAPK cascade has been found to be involved in cell adhesion, proliferation, differentiation, viability, and apoptosis. Activation of many genes by xtracellular growth factors signal through GTPase Ras/MAPK pathways (Xiao *et al.*, 2002) and Rap1 of the Ras superfamily is activated by PKA phosphorylation in human neutrophils (Altschuler *et al.*, 1995). Further activation of the MAPK cascade involves phosphorylation of MAPKKK (Raf-1), MAPKK, and MAPK (ERK) subsequently phosphorylates transcription factors, other downstream kinases, and substrates leading to biologic activity (Haqemann and Blank. 2001). In MG-63 osteosarcoma cells,

PTHrP induction of osteoblast differentiation in via multiple signaling pathways including PKA, PKC, and MAPK (Carpio *et al.*, 2001), and PTHrP regulation of osteblast specific gene expression, cellular proliferation, and differentiation through both the cAMP-activated PKA and MAPK pathway (Xiao *et al.*, 2002). Because the PTH1R promoter lacks elements that respond to mediators of the MAPK pathway, the inhibition of the MAPK pathway did not alter basal levels or the PTHrP-mediated down-regulation of the PTH1R. However, there are other puzzling factors like growth factor expression that may act as indirect mediators of MAPK pathway. PTH1R is sensitive to growth factor regulation since there was no alteration in the response of the PTH1R to MAPK inhibition (Chen *et al.*, 2004).

CaR and PTHrP Signaling

Calcium-sensing receptor (CaR) is a member of the GPCR family that uses $G\alpha_{q/11}$ for coupling to its major signaling pathway, PI-PLC. The CaR is a mediator of calcium-induced inhibition of the release of PTH in the parathyroid gland and has been shown to have a variety of functions, including the regulation of the cell cycle, peptide release, and apoptosis in other systems (Tfelt-Hansen *et al.*, 2002). Because the CaR is a member of the GPCR family that uses $G\alpha_{q/11}$ for coupling to its major signaling pathway, PI-PLC, they investigated whether PTHrP release could be induced by activation of other GPCRs coupled to $G\alpha_{q/11}$The role of the CaR in the regulation of PTHrP release has been also reported in a prostate cancer cell line, PC-3 and human embryonic kidney (HEK)) cells stably transfected with the CaR (HEK-CaR), whereas nontransfected HEK cells, which lack endogenous CaR expression, showed no such effect (Sanders *et al.*, 2001; MacLeod *et al.*, 2003).

Moreover, Tfelt-Hansen *et al* (2003) have confirmed that regulation of PTHrP release by the CaR involves in activation of PKC as well as ERK1/2, p38 MAPK, and JNK pathways and high $[Ca^{2+}]_o$-induced activation of the stress-activated protein kinase (SEK1) is PKC independent (Tfelt-Hansen *et al.*, 2003). This specific induction of PTHrP release by the CaR has important PTHrP pathophysiological implications in HHM, in which the PTHrP under the dominant role of the CaR (Grill *et al.*, 1991). In addtion, Tfelt-Hansen *et al* (2003) group have shown that the CaR mediated PTHrP release by PKC as well as by PKC-independent activation of ERK1/2, p38 MAPK and its downstream activating transcription factor (ATF)-2 cascade, and the SEK-1, in which the high $[Ca^{2+}]_o$ upregulates the PTHrP expression at transcriptional level. PKC has been reported to regulate PTHrP release in the NCI-H727 nonsmall lung cancer cell and in alveolar epithelial cells (Brandt *et al.*, 1991; Hastings *et al.*, 1994). It has recently been confirmed that Ras/MEK/ERK pathway involved in the production of PTHrP from cardiac myocytes likely acting at the transcriptional level (Ho *et al.*, 1998). The CaR acts via Ras/PKC/MEK pathway to induce PTHrP release at the transcriptional level since this pathway represents a classical signaling cascade. The occurrence of nuclear translocation of ERK1/2 in response to prolonged activation suggests that high $[Ca^{2+}]_o$-induced activation of ERK acts at the transcriptional level to increase PTHrP release (Tfelt-Hansen *et al.*, 2003).

PTHrP expression and release have been shown to be regulated by a variety of nuclear and membrane-bound receptor ligands. These various forms of regulation are mostly at the transcriptional level and are often exerted in a cell type-specific fashion. The postreceptor mechanisms by which the CaR stimulates PTHrP release involve activation of PKC, MEK, JNK, and p38 MAPK pathways. Regulation of PTHrP release by PKC has been reported in the NCI-H727 nonsmall lung cancer cell and in alveolar epithelial cells (Brandt *et al.*, 1991; Hastings *et al.*, 1994). Tfelt-Hansen *et al.*, (2004) observed that CaR-mediated induction of PTHrP release is potentiated by a PKC activator and blunted by a PKC inhibitor. Activation of PKC participates in the activation of the ERK1/2 cascade in some cells systems (Hastings *et al.*, 1994). A Ras/MEK/ERK pathway has recently been associated in PTHrP release from cardiac myocytes likely acting at the transcriptional level (Ho *et al.*, 1998). Because the Ras/PKC/MEK pathway represents a classical signaling cascade, it is therefore conceivable that the CaR acts via this pathway to induce PTHrP release at the transcriptional level. In case of ERK activation periods, the potential determinant is the balance between activating kinases and inactivating phosphatases. In contrast, the occurrence of nuclear translocation of ERK1/2 in response to prolonged activation suggests that high $[Ca^{2+}]_o$-induced activation of ERK acts at the transcriptional level to increase PTHrP release (Tfelt-Hansen *et al.*, 2004). The effect of sustained activation of ERK1/2 has been demonstrated in Swiss 3T3 fibroblasts, where it led to translocation of activated ERK and was associated with proliferation (Murphy *et al.*, 2002). Because the CaR induces PTHrP release, it is possible that the mitogenic and antiapoptotic effects of elevated Ca^{2+} could be indirect and mediated via PTHrP (Tfelt-Hansen *et al.*, 2004).

Furtheromre, several studies have indicatec that PTHrP signaling transiently stimulates mRNA expression of immediate-early genes, including c-fos (MAPK-independent), fra-2, and interleukin-6 (IL-6) (MAPK-dependent) (Chen *et al.*, 2004). The cAMP-dependent protein kinase A and MAPK pathways with minor extent of the protein kinase C pathway involved in Regulation of IL-6, and a promoter region containing an activator protein-1 site was important for PTHrP-induced IL-6 gene transcription. Phosphorylation of the transcription factor cAMP-response element-binding protein (CREB) cAMP-response element-binding protein was also essential but not adequate for PTHrP-mediated IL-6 promoter activity. PTHrP increasing phosphorylated ERK in undifferentiated MC4 cells but decreasing phosphorylated ERK in differentiated cells. Chen *et al* (2004) observation indicate that inactivation of the MAPK pathway shows differential regulation of PTHrP-stimulated activator protein-1 members, blocks PTHrP-stimulated IL-6, and synergistically down-regulates certain osteoblastic markers associated with differentiation. Collectively, these data indicate that the MAPK pathway plays a selective but potential role in the actions of PTHrP (Chen *et al.*, 2004).

In addition, IL-6 is a pro-resorptive cytokine suggesting that the MAPK pathway may be important in the catabolic actions of PTHrP; in contrast, it has been reported that fra-2 associated with increased bone formation, and modification of PTHrP actions by the MAPK pathway with anabolic or catabolic actions of PTHrP. It was found that regions containing activator protein-1 (AP-1) and NFκB influence the basal activity of the IL-6 promoter with opposite effects, and the region containing the AP-1 site played a potential role for PTHr action (Chen *et al.*, 2004). Additionally, the specific promotion of AP-1 activity by PTHrP was not dependent on MAPK activity. It has been reported that regulation of IL-6 gene transcription in other cell systems involve at least four different transcription factors, NF-κB, AP-1, CCAAT/enhancer-binding protein β(C/EBP-β), and CREB (Baccam *et al.*, 2003), and there role varies between different cell types and may also vary within the same cells depending on the stimulus (Zhang *et al.*, 2001). Altogether, these findings identifies PTHrP-responsive genes that are impacted by the MAPK pathway demonstrating that there are genes up-regulated by PTHrP (*fra*-2 and IL-6) and down-regulated by PTHrP bone sialoprotein (BSP)) and genes whose PTHrP mediation is not dependent on the MAPK pathway (c-*fos* and PTH-1R), and the regulation of IL-6 involves the PKA and MAPK pathway (Chen *et al.*, 2004). on the other hand, these results show that a GPCR can regulate PTHrP production via the p38 MAPK pathway in a pathophysiological setting. Future studies required to clarify of the p38 and MEK kinases in regulation of PTHrP signaling and the possible cross-talk between the MAP kinase and GPCR signaling pathways.

Nuclear Targeting

The full-length PTHrP has also been associated with an intracrine role that is dependent on nuclear localization sequence (NLS) which is absent in the PTH molecule, and PTHrP NLS composed of multibasic amino acids in the 88-91 and 89-106 region of the peptide. Following post-translation processing of PTHrP results in the NLS (88-101) remaining within midregion PTHrP-38-101 (Henderson *et al.*, 1995; 1997; Massfelder *et al.*, 1997). Midregion PTHrP-38-101 contains an NLS similar to those found in steroid hormone receptors, growth factors and transcription factors (Wu TL *et al.*, 1996) and several studies have found that NLS is required for various cells growth (Henderson *et al.*, 1995, Massfelder *et al.*, 1995, Tovar Sepulveda *et al.*, 2002). As well, NLS- dependent nuclear protein import can be mediated by several nuclear import receptors (importins) and the nuclear import receptor for PTHrP is called importins beta which has been mapped to PTHrP-67-94 and when importins beta binding inhibited when PTHrP is phosphorylated at Thr 85 by cyclin-dependent kinase (Lam *et al.*, 1999b).

In addition, cell type specific expression of PTHrP mRNA isoforms occurred between the various cell lines (Sellers *et al.*, 2004). The peptide may interact with key proteins involved in cell cycle regulation and/or with nucleic acids via an intracrine pathway independent of its classical nuclear localization sequence (Lehrer *et al.*, 2004). This novel pathway could mediate the effects of PTHrP on tumor progression. One of the particularily of the PTHrP gene is the presence in the 3′ region of an untranslated exon (VII, VIII and IX) specific for each PTHrP isoform. These exons are AU-rich and contain multiple AUUUA sequence, known to be involved in rapid mRNA degradation ((Mitchell and Tollervey. 2001), but more recent data also suggest that these regions might be involved in the binding of mRNA-stabilizing proteins (Bevilacqua *et al.*, 2003). It will be interesting in the next future to identify PTHrP mRNA-stabilizing proteins, if any that are targets of the VHL/HIF system, and to determine whether the other targets of this system share common mRNA stabilizing proteins. Informations triggered from these studies could lead to the development of new thearpeutic options based on the blockade of these regulatory proteins.

The growth properties of PTHrP are the consequence of its interaction with the PTH1R and subsequent intracellular pathways activation and recent data argue for a possible involvement of PTHrP nuclear translocation. In CRCC cells, we localized PTHrP and the

PTH1R to both the cytosol and nucleolar compartments (Massfelder *et al.*, 1997). Nuclear/nucleolar localization of PTHrP not only has been described in various cell types including normal and tumoral cells, but also has been associated with cell survival and/or proliferation (Massfelder *et al.*, 1997). On the other hand, the molecular targets for PTHrP in the nucleus have not yet been identified. Although the PTH1R has also been seen in the nuclear/nucleolar compartment in a number of tissues (Watson *et al.*, 2000), and its role in the nucleus, as well as its possible interaction with nuclear PTHrP is incompletely understood. This leads to the fundamental question of what are the molecular events activated by PTHrP leading to such a substantial effect of PTHrP on human CRCC tumor growth. Indeed, since anti-PTH1R treatments have shown complete human CRCC tumor regression in the xenograft mouse model, the answer to that question should bring new insight into the mechanism of tumor resistance, not only intrinsic but also in response to therapies. In contrast, It remains to be determined whether these actions of PTH (7–84) are mediated through the elusive C-PTH receptor. Biological roles distinct from those mediated through the PTH1R have also been described for C-terminal fragments of PTHrP. Some of these fragments may have, through a nuclear localization sequence within the fragment, intracrine roles and may act as transcriptional regulators while others appear to be secreted and interact with cell membrane receptors (Lam *et al.*, 1999a; Aarts *et al.*, 1999).

Important findings accumulated over the last decade have demonstrated that, in addition to this classical auto/paracrine pathway, PTHrP acts through what is called the intracrine pathway involving the translocation of the native protein into the nuclear compartment (Fiasch-Taesch and stewart, 2003). Indeed, PTHrP has been shown to contain in its mid-region 88–107, a bipartite nuclear/nucleolar localization signal (bNLS) similar to sequences found in viral andmammalian proteins (Fiasch-Taesch and stewart, 2003). Nuclear/nucleolar localization of PTHrP has been demonstrated to regulate cell death and proliferation (Clemens *et al.*, 2001; Fiasch-Taesch and stewart, 2003). In contrast, although a role for PTHrP in the regulation of gene transcription and/or nuclear organization is suggested by these results, the molecular mechanism as well as the molecular targets of nuclear PTHrP remain unknown. Since, the PTH1R has also been detected in the nucleus in cells of various tissues, the possibility exists that an active PTH1R system functions in the nuclear compartment.

PTHrP has a nuclear localization signal and has been reported to enhance proliferation of PC3 prostate cancer cells in an intracrine fashion. PTHrP can also protect MCF-7 breast cancer cells against serum starvation-induced apoptosis via acting in an intracrine manner (Tovar Sepulveda *et al.*, 2002). PTHrP can be accomplished via protein that is endocytosed from the cell exterior, even in cells that do not express the PTH/PTHrP receptor (Massfelder *et al.*, 1997; Aarts *et al.*, 1999), and lternative translation start sites may bypass the PTHrP N-terminal signal sequence and result in a peptide that cannot enter the endoplasmic reticular space to be secreted, but, having the NLS sequence, can travel directly to the nucleus (Massfelder *et al.*, 1997). Moreover, breast cancer MCF-7 cells overexpressing mutant PTHrP, showed unequivocally that deleting either multibasic cluster (88–91 or 102–106) or both (88–91 + 102–106) in the NLS of PTHrP negated its ability to protect against apoptosis. Mutant PTHrP was also ineffective in preventing against valinomycin-induced nuclear degradation. These findings indicate that an intact NLS is required for the PTHrP-mediated protective effects against apoptosis and suggest that this action requires that PTHrP enter the nucleus (Tovar Sepulveda *et al.*, 2002), and the protective effects of PTHrP on apoptosis and survival have been noted in prostate cancer cells (Dougherty *et al.*, 1999). In very recent investigation, the effect of midregion PTHrP (38-94/95/101) containing NLS-87-106 have shown to increase the growth of MCF-7 and MDA-MB231 breast cancer cells through independent pathway of PTH1R. They also observed that an increase in intracellular calcium mobilisation in breast cancer cells stimulated with both PTHrP-(67-101) and PTHrP-(67-86), and ERK independent growth response mediated by PTHrP-(67-101) (Kumari *et al.*, 2006). However, studies using midregion PTHrP-67-94 or PTHrP-(67-86) lacking the full length of NLS have shown anti-growth and anti-invasive roles in breast cancer cells. The post-translational, nuclear targeting and growth focus in the dependence of PTHrP on nuclear targeting as growth-promoter and PTHrP-containing NLS-88-101 as mitogenic inducer (Luparello *et al.*, 1997, 2001, Kumari *et al.*, 2006). Inhibition of several breast cancer cell lines (MDA-MB231, BC3A, Hs578T, 8701BC) growth and invasion has been indicated PTHrP-38-94 peptide with shorter NLS sequence (87-94) which revealed anti-mitogenic results (Luparello *et al.*, 2001). Collectively, these data indicated that NLS-containing midregion PTHrP peptide is dependent on both internalisation and nuclear translocation to induce growth in breast cancer cells and the findings highlight the importance of PTHrP midregion.

The mechanisms underlying the ability of PTHrP to protect against apoptosis may be mediated via the Bcl-2 family of proteins. The proapoptotic protein Bax binds to the antiapoptotic Bcl-2 and Bcl-x_L through interaction of their BH3 domains, forming heterodimers (Zha *et al.*, 1996). The balance of homodimers of Bcl-2 and Bcl-x_L to Bcl-2/Bax and Bcl-x_L/Bax heterodimers influences cell fate (Sedlak *et al.*,1995). In addition, cells overexpressing wild-type PTHrP were enriched in G_2 + M stage of the cell cycle compared with cells overexpressing NLS-mutated PTHrP, indicating an intracrine role for PTHrP in cell cycle regulation. Wild-type PTHrP also protected MCF-7 cells from serum starvation-induced apoptosis. Cells overexpressing wild-type PTHrP showed significantly greater cell survival than cells overexpressing NLS-mutated PTHrP. The ratios of the apoptosis-regulating proteins Bcl-2 to Bax and Bcl-x_L to Bax were higher in cells overexpressing wild-type, but not NLS-mutated, PTHrP compared with control cells. These findings suggest that the proliferative effects of PTHrP in breast cancer cells are mediated through regulation of the cell cycle and apoptosis, and that controlling PTHrP production in breast cancer may be therapeutically useful (Tovar Sepulveda *et al.*, 2002). Deletion of either one or both of these multibasic clusters within the NLS also abolished the proliferative effects of PTHrP in MCF-7 cells, normal rat small intestinal crypt cell-derived IEC-6 cells, vascular smooth muscle cells, and COS-1 cells (Tovar Sepulveda *et al.*, 2002; Ye *et al.*, 2001; Massfelder *et al.*, 1997; Henderson *et al.*, 1995).

CONCLUSION

PTHrP emerge as a multifunctional protein with pleiotropic effects on tumor cells through simultaneously secreted with multitarget to the cytosolic and nucleus. Many findings accumulated to date indicate that although PTHrP was discovered as an hypercalcemic factor one of its primary role might be to regulate cell differentiation, proliferation and death at pathological levels including cancer. Since PTHrP discovery, data have accumulated in the last 17 years argumenting favorably a role for PTHrP as a bioactive factor participating to tumor initiation, growth and invasion in various carcinomas. However, conflicting results have been reported in the literature in vitro, in vivo studies as well as in clinical studies. Therefore, while recent advances have contributed to a better understanding of PTHrP pathophysiology, concluding remarks are difficult to set up. The new nuclear functions and recent identified cytoplasmic PTHrP signaling further extend the potential pathophysiological role of this extraordinary peptide and open exciting areas of investigation.

REFERENCES

Aarts M. M. Rix, A/ Guo, J. Bringhurst, R. & Henderson, J. E. (1999). The nucleolar targeting signal (NTS) of parathyroid hormone related protein mediates endocytosis and nucleolar translocation, *Journal of Bone and Mineral Research, 14*, 1493–1503.

Abbas, S. K. Pickard, D. W. Illingworth, D. Storer, J. Purdie, D. W. Moniz, C. Dixit, M. Caple, I. W. Ebeling, P. R. Rodda, C. P. Martin, T. J. & Care, D, A. (1990). Measurement of parathyroid hormone-related protein in extracts of fetal parathyroid glands and placental membranes. *Journal of Endocrinology, 124*, 319-325.

Abou-samra, A. Goldsmith, P. K. Xie, L. Y. Juppner, H. Spiegel, A. M. & Segre, G. V. (1994). Down-regulation of parathyroid hormone/parathyroid hormone-related peptide receptor immunoreactivity and PTH binding in opossum kidney cells by PTH and dexamethasone. *Endocrinology. 135*, 2588-2594.

Abou-samra, A. Juppner, H. Force, T. Freeman, M. W. Kong, X. Schipani, E. Urena, P. Richards, J. Bonventre, J. V. Potts, J. T. J. R. Kronenberg, H. M. & Segre, G. V. (1992). Expression cloning of a common receptor for parathyroid hormone and parathyroid hormone-related peptide from rat osteoblast-like cells: A single receptor stimulates intracel lular accumulation of both cAMP and inositol trisphosphates and increases intracellular free calcium. *Proceeding National Acadamy of Sciences. USA, 89*, 2732-2736.

Abou-Samra, A-B, Uneno, S. Juppner, H. Keutmann, H. Potts, J.T. Segre, G. V. & Nussbaum, S. R. (1989). Non-homologous sequences of parathyroid hormone and the parathyroid hormone-related peptide bind to a common receptor on ROS 17/2.8 cell. *Endocrinology. 125*, 2215-2217.

Ahmed, I. Gesty-Palmer, D. Drezner, M. K. & Luttrell, L. M. (2003). Transactivation of the epidermal growth factor receptor mediates parathyroid hormone and prostaglandin F2 alpha-stimulated mitogen-activated protein kinase activation in cultured transgenic murine osteoblasts. *Mol. Endocrinol, 17*, 1607–1621.

Akino, K. Ohtsuru, A. Kanda, K. Yasuda, A. Yamamoto, T. Akino, Y. Naito, S. Kurokawa, M. Iwahori, N. Yamashita, S. (2000). Parathyroid hormone-related peptide is a potent angiogenic factor, *Endocrinology, 141*, 4313–4316.

Aklilu, F. Gladu, J. Goltzman, D. & Rabbani, S. A. (2000). Role of mitogen-activated protein kinases in the induction of parathyroid hormone-related peptide. *Cancer Res, 60*, 1753-1760.

Albright, F. (1941). Case records of the Massachusetts general hospital (case 27401). *New England Journal of Medicine, 225*, 789-791.

Allinson, E. T. & Drucker, D. J. (1992). Parathyroid hormone-like peptide shares features with members of the early response gene family: rapid induction by serum, growth factors, and cycloheximide, *Cancer Res, 52*, 3103–3109.

Alokail, M. S. (2005). Influence of parathyroid hormone-related peptide gene in colon cancer cell line growth. *Saudi Med J, 26*, 714-717.

Alokail, M. S. (2004). Potential regulation of PTH/PTHrP receptor expression in choriocarcinoma cells. *Saudi Med J, 25*, 615-620.

Alokail, M. S. & Peddie, M. J. (2005). Characterisation of ligand binding to the parathyroid hormone/parathyroid hormone-related peptide receptor in MCF7 breast cancer cells and SaOS-2 osteosarcoma cells. *Cell Biochem Funct.*

Altschuler, D. L. Peterson, S. N. Ostrowski, M. C. & Lapetina, E. G. (1995). Cyclic AMP-dependent activation of Rap1b. *J. Biol. Chem, 270*, 10373–10376.

Amling, M. Neff, L. Tanaka, S. Inoue, D. Kuida, K. Weir, E. Philbrick, W. M. Broadus, A. E. & Baron, R. (1997). Bcl-2 Lies downstream of parathyroid hormone-related peptide in a signaling pathway that regulates chondrocyte maturation during skeletal development. *Journal of Cellular Biology, 136*, 136-205.

Ardawi, M. S. Nasrat, H. A. & Ba'aqueel, H. S. (1997). Calcium-regulating hormones and parathyroid hormone-related peptide in normal human pregnancy and postpartum: a longitudinal study. *European Journal of Endocrinology, 137*, 402-409.

Arguello, F. Baggs, R. B. & Frantz, C. N. (1988). A murine model of experimental metstasis to bone and bone marrow. *Cancer Research, 48*, 6876-6881.

Asa, S. L. Henderson, J. Goldzman, D. & Drucker, D. J. (1990). Parathyroid hormone-like peptide in normal and neoplastic human endocrine tissues. *Journal of Clinical Endocrinology and Metabolism, 38,* 1112-1118.

Attwood, T. K. Eliopoulos, E. E. & Findlay, J. B. (1991). Multiple sequence alignment of protein families showing low sequence homology: a methodological approach using database patternmatching discriminators of G-protein-linked receptors. *Gene, 98*, 153-159.

Baccam, M. Woo, S. Vinson, C. & Bishop, G. A. (2003). CD40-mediated transcriptional regulation of the IL-6 gene in B lymphocytes: involvement of NF-kappa B, AP-1, and C/EBP. *J. Immunol, 170*, 3099–3108.

Bakre, M. M. Zhu, Y. Yin, H. Burton, D. W. Terkeltaub, R. & Deftos, L. J. (2002). Parathyroid hormone-related peptide is a naturally occuring, protein kinase A-dependent angiogenesis inhibitor, *Nat. Med, 8*, 995–1003.

Barden, A. J. & Kemp, B. E. (1996). Evidence that the PTH receptor binding site on PTHrP-1-34 can hinge at Arg19/Arg20. *Biochemical and Biophysical Research Communications, 220*, 431-436.

Behar, V. Nakamoto, C. Greenberg, Z. Bisello, A. Suva, L. J. Rosenblatt, M. & Chorev, M. (1996). Histidine at position 5 is the specificity "switch" between two parathyroid hormone receptor subtypes. *Endocrinology, 137*, 4217-4224.

Bergwitz, C. Klein, P. Kohno, H. Forman, S. R. Lee, Rubin, D. & Juppner, H. (1998). Identification, functional characterization, and developmental expression of two nonallelic parathyroid hormone (PTH)/PTH-related peptide receptor isoforms in xenopus laevis (daudin). *Endocrinology, 139*, 723-732.

Berson, S. A. & Yalow, R. S. (1966). Parathyroid hormone in plasma in adenomatous hyperparathyroidism, uremia and bronchogenic sarcoma. *Science, 154*, 907-909.

Bevilacqua, A. Ceriani, M. Capaccioli, S. & Nicolin, A. (2003). Post-transcriptional regulation of gene expression by degradation of messenger RNAs, *J. Cell Physiol, 195*, 356–372.

Birch, M. A. Carron, J. A. Scott, M. Fraser, W. D. & Gallagher, J. A. (1995). Parathyroid hormone (PTH) / PTH-related protein (PTHrP) receptor expression and mitogenec responses in human breast cancer cell lines. *British Journal of Cancer, 72*, 90-95.

Bisello, A. Chorev, M. Rosenblatt, M. Monticelli, L. Mierke, D. F. & Ferrari, S. L. (2002). Selective ligand-induced stabilization of active and desensitized parathyroid hormone type 1 receptor conformations. *J. Biol. Chem, 277*, 38524–38530.

Blind, E. Bambino, T. Huang, Z. Bliziotes, M. & Nissenson, R. A. (1996). Phosphorylation of the cytoplasmic tail of the PTH/PTHrP receptor. *Journal of Bone and Mineral Research, 11*, 578-586.

Blind, E. Bambino, T. & Nissenson, A. (1995). Agonist-Stimulated phosphrylation of the G protein-coupled receptor for parathyroid hormone (PTH) and PTH-related protein. *Endocrinology, 136*, 4271-4277.

Blind, E. Raue, F. Knappe. V. Schroth, J. & Ziegler, R. (1993). Cyclic AMP formation in rat bone and kidney cells is stimulated by parathyroid hormone-related peptide PTHrP(1-34) and PTH (1-34). *Experimental and Clinical Endocrinology, 101*, 150-155.

Bouizar, Z. Spyratos, F. & De vernejoul, M. C. (1999). The parathyroid hormone-related protein (PTHrP) gene: use of downstream TATA promotor and PTHrP 1-139 coding pathways in primary breast cancers vary with the occurrence of bone metastasis. *Journal of Bone & Mineral Research, 14*, 406–414.

Brandt, D. W. Bruns, M. E. Bruns, D. E. Ferguson, J. E. Burton, D. W. & Deftos, L. J. (1992). The parathyroid hormone-related protein (PTHrP) gene preferentially utilizes a GC-rich promoter and the PTHrP-1-139 coding pathway in normal human amnion. *Biochemical and Biophysical Research Communications, 189*, 938-943.

Brandt, D. W. Pandol, S.J. & Deftos, L. J. (1991). Calcium-stimulated parathyroid hormone-like protein secretion: potentiation through a protein kinase-C pathway. *Endocrinology, 128*, 2999–3004.

Bringhurst, F. R. Juppner, H. Guo, J. Urena, G. P. Potts, J. T. Jr. Kronenberg, H. M. Abou-Samra, A. B. & Segre, G. V. (1992). Cloned, stably-expressed parathyroid hormone

(PTH)/PTH-related peptide receptors activate multiple messenger signals and biological responses in LLC-PK, kidney cells. *Endocrinology, 132*, 2090-2098.

Broadus, A. E. Goltzman, D. Webb, A. C. & Kronenberg, H. M. (1985). Messenger ribonucleic acid from tumors associated with humoral hypercalcemia of malignancy directs the synthesis of a secretory parathyroid hormone-like peptide. *Endocrinology, 117*, 1661-1666.

Bucht, E. Eklund, A. Toss, G. Lewensohn, R. Granberg, B. Sjostedt, U. Eddeland, R. & Torring, O. (1992). Parathyroid-hormone related peptide, measured by a midmolecule radioimmunoassay, in various hypercalcaemic and normocalcaemic conditions. *Acta Endocrinol (Capenh), 127*, 294-300.

Bundred, N. J. Ratcliffe, W. A. Walker, R. A. Coley, S. Morrison, J. M. & Walker, J. G. (1991). Parathyroid hormone-related protein and hypercalcemia in breast cancer. *British Medical Journal, 303*, 1506-1509.

Bundred, N. J. Walls, J. & Ratcliffe, W. A. (1996).Parathyroid hormone-related protein, bone metastases and hypercalcaemia of malignancy. *Annual Royal College of Surgents, England, 78*, 354:358.

Burtis, W. J. Wu, T. Bunch, C. Wysolmerski, J. J. Insogna, K. L. Weir, E. C. Broadus, A. E. & Stewart, A. F. (1987). Identification of a novel 17,000-dalton parathyroid hormone-like adenylate cyclase-stimulating protein from a tumor associated with humoral hypercalcemia of malignancy. *The Journal of Biological Chemistry, 262*, 7151-7156.

Burton, P. B. Moniz, C. & Knight, D. E. (1990). Parathyroid hormone related peptide can function as an autocrine growth factor in human renal cell carcinoma, *Biochem. Biophys. Res. Commun, 167*, 1134–1138.

Carney, S. L. Ray, C. Ebeling, P. R. Martin, T. J. & Gillies, A. H. B. (1991). Synthetic human parathyroid hormone-related protein and rat renal electrolyte transport. *Mineral Electrolyte Metabolism, 17*, 41-45.

Carpenter, T. O. Ellis, B. K. Insogna, K. L. Philbrick, W. M. Sterpka, J. & Shimkets, R. (2005). Fibroblast growth factor 7: an inhibitor of phosphate transport derived from oncogenic osteomalacia-causing tumors. *J Clin Endocrinol Metab, 90*, 1012-1020.

Carron, J. A. Fraser, W. D. & Gallagher, J. A. (1997). PTHrP and the PTH/PTHrP receptor are co-expressed in human breast and colon tumours. *British Journal of Cancer, 76*, 1095-1098.

Carter, P. H. Carter, P. H. Petroni, B. D. Gensure, R. C. Schipani, E. Potts, J. T. Jr. & Gardella, T. J. (2001). Selective and nonselective inverse agonists for constitutively active type-1 parathyroid hormone receptors: evidence for altered receptor conformations, *Endocrinology, 142*, 1534–1545.

Caulfield, M. P. McKee, R. L. Goldman, M. E. Duong, L. T. Fisher, J. E. Gay, C. T. DeHaven, P. A. Levy, J. J. Roubini, E. Nutt, R.F. Chorev, M. & Rosenblatt, M. (1990). The bovine renal parathyroid hormone (PTH) receptor has equal affinity for two different amino acid sequences: the receptor binding domains of PTH and PTH-related protein are located within the 14-34 region. *Endocrinology, 127*, 83-87.

Chan, G. K. Chan, G. K. Deckelbaum, R. A. Bolivar, I. Goltzman, D. & Karaplis, A. C. (2001). PTHrP inhibits adipocyte differentiation by down-regulating PPAR gamma activity via a MAPK-dependent pathway, *Endocrinology, 142*, 4900–4909.

Chen, C. Koh, A. J. Datta, N. S. Zhang, j. Keller, E. T. Xiao, G. Franceschi, R. T. D'Silva, N. J. & McCauley. L. K. (2004). Impact of the Mitogen-activated Protein Kinase Pathway on Parathyroid Hormone-related Protein Actions in Osteoblasts. *J. Biol. Chem., 279*, 29121-29129.

Chattopadhyay, N. (2006). Effects of calcium-sensing receptor on the secretion of parathyroid hormone-related peptide and its impact on humoral hypercalcemia of malignancy. *Am J Physiol Endocrinol Metab, 290*, E761-E770.

Chen, X. Macica, C. M. Dreyer, B. E. Hammond, V. E. Hens, J. R. Philbrick, W. M. & Broadus A. E. (2006). Initial characterization of PTH-related protein gene-driven lacZ expression in the mouse. *Journal of Bone & Mineral Research. 21*, 113-123.

Chorev, M. Goldman, M. E. McKee, R. L. Roubini, E. Levy, J. J. Gay, C. T. Reagan, J. E. Fisher, J. E. Caporate, L. H., Golub, E. E. Caulfield, M. P. Nutt, R. F. & Rosenblatt, M. (1990). Modifecations of position 12 in parathyroid hormone and parathyroid hormone related protein: toward the design of highly potent antagonists. *Biochemistry, 29*, 1580-1586.

Clark, J. A. Bonner, T. I. Kim, A. S. & Usdin, T. B. (1998). Multiple regions of ligand discrimination revealed by analysis of chimeric parathyroid hormone 2 (PTH2) and PTH/PTHrP-related peptide (PTHrP) receptor. *Molecular Endocrinology, 12*, 193-206.

Clemens, T. L. Cormier, S. Eichinger, A. Endlich, K. Fiaschi-Taesch, N. Fischer, E. Friedman, P. A. Karaplis, A. C. Massfelder, T. Rossert, J. Schluter, K. D. Silve, C. Stewart, A. F. Takane, K. & Helwig, J. J. (2001). Parathyroid hormone-related protein and its receptors: nuclear functions and roles in the renal and cardiovascular systems, the placental trophoblasts and the pancreatic islets, *Br. J. Pharmacol, 134*, 1113-1136.

Clines G. A. & Guise, T. A. (2005). Hypercalcaemia of malignancy and basic research on mechanisms responsible for osteolytic and osteoblastic metastasis to bone. *Endocrine-Related Cancer, 12*, 549-583.

Coleman, R. E. & Rubens, R. D. (1987). The clinical course of bone metastases from breast cancer. *British Journal of Cancer, 55*, 61-66.

Cornish, J. Callon, K. E. Nicholson, G. C. & Reid, I. R. (1997). Parathyroid hormone-related protein-(107-139) inhibits bone resorption in vitro. *Endocrinology, 138*, 1299-1304.

Danks, J. A. Ebeling, P. R. Hayman, J. Chou, S. T. Moseley, J. M. Dunlop, J. Kemp, B. E. & Martin, T. J. (1989). Parathyroid hormone-related protein: immunohistochemical localization in Cancers and in normal Skin. *Journal of Bone and Mineral Research, 4*, 273-278.

Delahunt, P.B. Bethwaite, P. B. & Thornton, A. (1997), Prognostic significance of microscopic vascularity for clear cell renal cell carcinoma, *Br. J. Urol, 80*, 401–404.

Divieti, P. John, M. R. Juppner, H. & Bringhurst, F. R. (2002). Human PTH-(7–84) inhibits bone resorption in vitro via actions independent of the type 1 PTH/PTHrP receptor, *Endocrinology, 143*, 171–176.

Dohlman, H. G. Thorner, J. Caron, M. G. & Leftkowitz, R. J. (1991). Model system for the study of seven-transmembrane-segment responses. *Annual Review of Biochemistry, 60*, 653-688.

Dougherty, K. M. Blomme, E. A. Koh, A. J. Henderson, J. E. Pienta, K. J. Rosol, T. J. & McCauley, L. K. (1999). Parathyroid hormone-related protein as a growth regulator of prostate carcinoma. *Cancer Res, 59*, 6015–6022.

Drake, M. T. Gardella, T. Abou-Samra, A-B. & Segre, G. V. (1993). Mutational analysis of the rat PTH/PTHrP receptor: structural determinants for activation of the stimulatory G protein. *Journal of Bone and Mineral Research, 8*, S128.

Dudley. A. King. K. Mathias. J. Burnier. J. P. Burdick. D. Horton. M. & Hammonds, R. G. (1992). Effect of human parathyroid-hormone related peptide-107-139 on osteoclast formation and bone-resorption Invitro. *Journal of Bone and Mineral Research, 7*, S309.

Ellison, M. Woodhouse, D. Hillyard, C. J. Dowsett, M. Coombes, R. C. & Gilby, E. D. (1975). Immunoreactive calcitonin production by human lung cancer cells in culture. *British Journal of Cancer, 32*, 373-379.

Engel, M. E. McDonnell, M. A. Law, B. K. & M oses, H. L. (1999). Interdependent SMAD and JNK signaling in transforming growth factor-beta-mediated transcription. *J. Biol. Chem, 274*, 37413-37420.

Esbrit, P. & Egido, J. (2000). The emerging role of parathyroid hormone-related protein as a renal regulating factor, *Nephrol. Dial. Transplant, 15*, 1109–1111.

FalzonM, & Du P. (2000). Enhanced growth of MCF-7 breast cancer cells overexpressing parathyroid hormone-related peptide. *Endocrinology, 141*, 1882-1892.

Fenton, A. J. Kemp, B. E. Hammonds, R. G. Mitchelhill, K. Moseley, J. M. Martin, T. J. & Nicholson, G. N. (1991a) A potent inhibitor of osteoclastic bone resorption within a highly conserved pentapeptide region of parathyroid hormone related protein: PTHrP-[107-111]. *Endocrinology, 129*, 3424-3426.

Fenton, A. J. Kemp, B. E. Kent, G. N. Moseley, J. M. Zheng, J. M. Rowe, D. J. Dritta, J. M. Martin, T. J. & Nicholson, G. N. (1991b). Carboxy terminal peptide from the parathyroid hormone related protein inhibits bone resorption by osteclasts. *Endocrinology, 129*, 1762-1768.

Fiaschi-Taesch, N. M. & Stewart, A. F. (2003). Minireview: parathyroid hormone-related protein as an intracrine factor-trafficking mechanisms and functional consequences, *Endocrinology, 144*, 407–411.

Fujimori, A. Cheng, S. L. Avioli, L. V. & Civitelli, R. (1992). Structure-function relationship of parathyroid hormone: activation of phospholipase C, protein kinase-A and -C in osteosarcoma cells. *Endocrinology, 130*, 29-36.

Fukayama, S. Tashjian, A. H. Jr. & Bringhurst, F. R. (1992). Mechanisms of desensitization to parathyroid hormone in human osteoblast-like SaOS-2. *Endocrinology, 131*, 1757-1769.

Gagnon, L. Jouishomme, H. Whitefield, J. P. MacLeans, S. Neugebauer, W. Willick, G. Rixon, R. H. & Chakravarthy, B. (1993). Protein kinase C activating domains of parathyroid hormone-related protein. *Journal of Bone and Mineral Research, 8*, 497-503.

Gallacher, S. J. Fraser, W. D. Patel, U. Logue, F. C. Soukop, M. Boyle, I. T. & Ralston, S. H. (1990). Breast cancer-associated hypercalcemia: a reassessment of renal calcium and phosphate handling. *Annual Clinical Biochemistry, 27*, 551-556.

Gardella, T. J. Luck, M. D. Wilson, A. K. Keutmann, H. T. Nussbaum, S. R. Segre, G. V. Potts, J. T. Jr. & Kronenberg, H. M. (1995). Parathyroid hormone (PTH)-PTH-related peptide hybrid peptides reveal functional interactions between the 1-14 and 15-34 domains of the ligand. *The Jouranl of Biological Chemistry, 270*, 6584-6588.

Gardella, T. J. Luck, M. D. Fan, M. H. & Lee. C. (1996). Transmembrane residues of the parathyroid hormone (PTH) and PTH-related peptide receptor that specifically affected binding and signalling by agonist ligands. *The Jouranl of Biological Chemistry, 271*, 12820-12825.

Gardella, T. J. Juppner, H. Wilson, A. K. Keutmann, H. T. Abou-samra, A. Segre, G. V. Bringhurst, F. R. Potts, J. T. JR., Nussbaum, S. R. & Kronenberg, H. M. (1994). Determinants of [Arg2]PTH-(1-34) binding and signaling in the transmembrane region of the parathyroid hormone receptor. *Endocrinology, 135*, 1186-1194.

Gensure, R. C. T.J. Gardella T. J. & Juppner, H. (2005). Parathyroid hormone and parathyroid hormone-related peptide, and their receptors, *Biophys. Res. Commun., 328*, 666–678.

Goltzman, D. Stewart, A. F. & Broadus, A. E. (1981). Malignancy-associated hypercalcemia evaluation with a cytochemical bioassay for parathyroid hormone. *Journal of Clinical Endocrinology and Metabolism, 52*, 899-905.

Gonzalez, R. D. Barrientos, A. Larrodera, L. Ruilope, L. M. Leiva, O. & Barobia, V. (1985). Squamous cell carcinoma of the renal pelvis associated with hypercalcemia and the presence of parathyroid hormone-like substances in the tumor. *Journal of Urology, 133*, 1029-1034.

Grill, V. Ho, P. Body, J. J. Johanson, N. Lee, S. C. Kukreja, C. Moseley, N. M. & Martin, T. J. (1991). Parathyroid hormone-related protein: elevated levels in both humoral hypercalcemia of malignancy and hypercalcemia complicating metastatic breast cancer. *Journal of Clinical Endocrinology and Metabolism, 73*, 1309-1315.

Guise, T. A. (2000). Molecular mechanisms of osteolytic bone metastases. *Cancer, 88*, 2892-2898.

Guo, J. Liu, B-Y. & Bringhurst, R. (1997). Mechanism of homologus and heterologous desensitization of PTH/PTHrP receptor signaling in LLC-PK1 cells. *American Journal of Physiology, 273*, E383-E393.

Guo, J. Guo, J. Chung, U. I. Kondo, H. Bringhurst, F. R. & Kronenberg, H. M. (2002). The PTH/PTHrP receptor can delay chondrocyte hypertrophy in vivo without activating phospholipase C, *Dev. Cell, 3*, 183–194.

Gutman, A. B. Tyson, T. L. & Gutman, E. B. (1936). Serum calcium, inorganic phosphorus and phosphatase activity in hyperparathyroidism, Paget's disease, multiple myeloma and neoplastic disease of the bone. *Archive of Internal Medicine, 57*, 379-413.

Habener, J. F. Rosenblatt, M. & Potts, J. T. Jr. (1984). Parathyroid hormone: biochemical aspects of biosynthesis, secretion, action, and metabolism. *Physiology Review, 64*, 985-1035.

Hagemann, C. & Blank, J.L. (2001). The ups and downs of MEK kinase interactions. *Cell. Signal, 13*, 863–875.

Hastings, R. H. Burton, D. W. Quintana, R. A. Biederman, E. Gujral, A. & Deftos, L. J. (2001). Parathyroid hormone-related protein regulates the growth of orthotopic human lung tumors in athymic mice, *Cancer, 92*, 1402–1410.

Hastings, R. H. Duong, H. Burton, D. W. & Deftos, L. J. (1994). Alveolar epithelial cells express and secrete parathyroid hormone-related protein. *Am J Respir Cell Mol Biol, 11*, 701–706,

Hastings, R. H. Quintana, R. A. Sandoval, R. Rascon, Y. Burton, D. W. & Deftos, L. J. (2003). Proapoptotic effects of parathyroid hormone-related protein in type II pneumocytes, *Am. J. Respir. Cell Mol. Biol, 29*, 733–742.

Hayman, J. A. Danks, J. A. Ebeling, P. R. Moseley, J. M. Kemp, B .E. & Martin, T. J. (1989). Expression of parathyroid hormone-related protein in normal skin and in tumors of skin and skin appendages. *Journal of Pathology, 158*, 293-296.

Henderson, J. E. Amizuka, N. Warshawsky, H. Biasotto, D. Lanske, B. M. K. Goltzman, D. & Karaplis, A. (1995). Nucleolar localization of parathyroid hormone-related peptide enhances survival of chondrocytes under conditions that promote apoptotic cell death. *Molecular & Cellular Biology, 15*, 4064-4075.

Henderson, M. A, Danks, J. A. Moseley, J. M. Slavin, J. L. Harris, T. L. McKinlay, M. R. Hopper, J. L. & Martin, T. J. (2001). Parathyroid hormone-related protein production by breast cancers, improved survival, and reduced bone metastases. *J Natl Cancer Inst, 93*, 234–237.

Henderson, J. E. Kremer, R. Rhim, J. S. & Glotzman, D. (1992). Identification and functional characterisation of adenylate cyclase-linked receptors for parathyroid hormone-related peptides on immortalised human keratinocytes. *Endocrinology, 130*, 449-457.

Henderson, J. E. Shustik, C. Kremer, R. Rabbani, S. A. Hendy, G. N. & Goltzman, D. (1990). Circulating concentrations of parathyroid hormone-related peptide in malignancy and hyperparathyroidism. *Journal of Bone and Mineral Research, 5*, 105-113.

Hepler, J. R. & Gilman, A. G. (1992). G-proteins. *Trends in Biochemical Sciences, 17*, 383-387.

Hermanto, U. Zong, C. S. Wang, L. H. (2000). Inhibition of mitogen-activated protein kinase kinase selectively inhibits cell proliferation in human breast cancer cells displaying enhanced insulin-like gr owth factor I-mediated mitogen-activated protein kinase activation. *Cell Growth Differ, 11*, 655-664.

Ho, P. D. Zechner, D.K. He, H. Dillmann, W.H. Glembotski, C. C. & McDonough P. M. (1998). The Raf-MEK-ERK cascade represents a common pathway for alteration of intracellular calcium by Ras and protein kinase C in cardiac myocytes. *J Biol Chem, 273*, 21730–21735.

Huang, S. New, L. Pan, Z. Han, J. & Nemerow, G. R. (2000). Urokinase plasminogen activator/urokinase-specific surface receptor expression and matrix invasion by breast cancer cells requires constitutive p38alpha mitogen-activated protein kinase activity. *J. Biol. Chem, 275*, 12266-12272.

Iida-Klein, A. Guo, J. Takemura, M. Drakes, M. T. Jr, J. T. P. Abou-Samra, A. Bringhurst. F. R. & Segre, G. V. (1997). Mutations in the second cytoplasmic loop of the rat parathyroid hormone (PTH)/PTH-related protein receptor result in selective loss of PTH-stimulated phospholipase C activity. *The Journal of Biological Chemistry, 272*, 6882-6889.

Ilardi, C. F. & Faro, J. C. (1985). Localization of parathyroid hormone-like substance in squamous cell carcinomas. *Archives Pathology and Laboratory Medicine, 109*, 752-755.

Inomata, N. Akiyama, M. Kubota, N. & Juppner, H. (1995). Characterization of a novel parathyroid hormone (PTH) receptor with specificity for the carboxy-terminal region of PTH-1-86. *Endocrinology, 136*, 4732-4740.

Insogna, K. L. (1989). Humoral hypercalcemia of malignancy: the role of parathyroid hormone-related protein. *Endocrinology and Metabolism Clinics of North America, 18*, 779-794.

Ishihara, T. Shigemoto, R. Mori, K. Takahashi, K. & Hagata, S. (1992). Functional expression and tissue distribution of a novel receptor for vasoactive intestinal polypeptide. *Neuron, 8*, 811-819.

Ishihara, T. Nakamura, S. Kaziro, Y. Takahashi, T. Takahashi, K. & Nagata, S. (1991). Molecular cloning and expression of a cDNA encoding the secretin receptor. *Embryology Journal, 7*, 1635-1641.

Jelinek, L. J. Lok, S. & Rosenberg, G. B. (1993). Expression cloning and signaling properties of the rat glucagon receptor. *Science, 259*, 1614-1616.

Jonsson, K. B. Jonsson, K. B. John, M. R. Gensure, R. C. Gardella, T. J. & Juppner, H. (2001). Tuberoinfundibular peptide 39 binds to the parathyroid hormone (PTH)/PTH-related peptide receptor, but functions as an antagonist, *Endocrinology,142*, 704–709.

Joun, H. Lanske, B. Karperien, M. Qian, F. Defize, L. & Abou-Samra, A. (1997). Tissue-specific transcription start sites and alternative splicing of the parathyroid hormone (PTH/PTH-related peptide (PTHrP) receptor gene: a new PTH/PTHrP receptor splice varient that lacks the signal peptide. *Endocrinology. 138*, 1742-1749.

Juppner, H. Abou-Samra, A. B. Uneno, S. Gu, W-X. Potts, J. T. JR., & Segre, G. V. (1988). The parathyroid hormone-like peptide associated with humoral hypercalcemia of malignancy and parathyroid hormone bind to the same receptor on the plasma membrane of ROS 17/2.8 cells. *The Journal of Biological Chemistry, 263*, 8557-8560.

Juppner, H. Schipani, E. Bringhurst, F. R. MCClure, I. Keutmann, H. T. Potts, J. T. Jr. Kronenberg, H. M. Abou-Samra, A. B. Segre, G. V. & Gardella, T. J. (1994). The extracellular amino-terminal region of the parathyroid hormone (PTH)/PTH-related peptide receptor determines the binding affinity for carboxyl-terminal fragments of PTH-(1-34). *Endocrinology, 134*, 879-884.

Käkönen, S. M. Selander, K. S. Chirgwin, J. M. J. Yin, J. J. , Burns, S. Rankin, W. A. Grubbs, B. G. Dallas, M. Cui, Y. &. Guise. T. A. (2002). Transforming Growth Factor-beta Stimulates Parathyroid Hormone-related Protein and Osteolytic Metastases via Smad and Mitogen-activated Protein Kinase Signaling Pathways. *J. Biol. Chem, 277*, 24571-24578.

Karaplis, A. C. Tybulewicz, V. Mulligan, R. C. & Kronenberg, H. M. (1992). Distripution of parathyroid hormone-related peptide gene leads to multiple skeletal abnormalities and perinatal mortality. *Journal of Bone and Mineral Research, 7*, S93.

Karpf, D. B. Arnaud, C. D. King, K. Duffy, D. King, K. L. Winer, J. & Nissenson, R. A. (1987). The canine renal parathyroid hormone receptor is a glycoprotein: characterization and partial purification. *Biochemistry, 26*, 7825-7833.

Kemp, B. E. Moseley, J. M. Rodda, C. P. Ebeling, P. R. Wettenhall, R. E. H. Stapleton, D. Diefenbach-Jagger, H. Ure, F. Michelangeli, V. P. Simmons, H. A. Raisz, L. G. &

Martin, T. J. (1987). Parathyroid hormone-related protein of malignancy: Active synthetic fragments. *Science, 238*, 1568-1570.

Kronenberg, H. Lee, K. Lanske, B. & Segre, G. V. (1997). Parathyroid hormone-related protein and Indian hedgehog control the pace of cartilage differentiation. *Journal of Endocrinology, 154*, S39-S45.

Kumari, R. Robertson, J. F. & Watson, S. A. (2006). Nuclear targeting of a midregion PTHrP fragment is necessary for stimulating growth in breast cancer cells. *Int J Cancer, 119*, 49-59.

Lam, M.C.H., Olsen, S. L., Rankin, W. A., Ho, P. W. M., Martin, T. J., Gillespie, M. T. & Moseley, J. M. (1997). PTHrP and cell division: expression and localization of PTHrP in a keratinocyte cell line (HaCat) during the cell cycle. *Journal of Cellular Physiology, 173*, 433-446.

Lam, M. H. Briggs, L. J. Hu, W. Martin, T. J. Gillespie, M. T. & Jans, D. A. (1999a). Importin beta recognizes parathyroid hormone-related protein with high affinity and mediates its nuclear import in the absence of importin alpha, *J. Biol. Chem, 274*, 7391–7398.

Lam, M. H, House, C. M. Tiganis, T. Mitchelhill, K. I. Sarcevic, B. Cures, A. Ramsay, R. Kemp, B. E. Martin, T. J. & Gillespie, M. T. (1999b). Phosphorylation at the cyclin-dependent kinases site (Thr85) of parathyroid hormone-related protein negatively regulates its nuclear localization. *J Biol Chem, 274*, 18559-18566.

Lee, C. Gardella, T. J. Abou-Samra, A. Nussbaum, S. R. Segre, G. V. Potts, J. T. Jr. Kronenberg, H. M. & Juppner, H. (1994). Role of the extracellular regions of the parathyroid hormone (PTH)/PTH-related peptide receptor in hormone binding. *Endocrinology, 135*, 1488-1495.

Lefebvre, M. F. Guillot, C. Crepin, M. & Saez, S. (1995). Influence of tumor derived fibroblasts and 1,25-dihydroxyvitamin D_3 on growth of breast cancer cell lines. *Breast Cancer Research and Treatment, 33*, 189-197.

Lehrer, S. Diamond, E. J. Mamkine, B. Stone, N. N. & Stock, R. G. (2004). Serum interleukin-8 is elevated in men with prostate cancer and bone metastasis. *Technol Cancer Res Treat, 3*, 411.

Lin, H. Y. Harris, T. L. & Flannery, M. S. (1991). Expression cloning of adenylate cyclase-coupled calcitonin receptor. *Science, 254*, 1022-1024.

Luparello, C. Birch, M. A. Gallagher, J. A. & Burtis, W. (1997). Clonal heterogeneity of the growth and invasive response of a human breast carcinoma cell line to parathyroid hormone-related peptide fragments. *Carcinogenesis, 18*, 23-29.

Luparello, C. Burtis, W. Raue, F. Birch, M. A. & Gallagher, J. A. (1995). Parathyroid hormone-related peptide and 8701-BC breast cancer cell growth and invasion in vitro: evidence for growth-inhibiting and invasion-promoting effects. *Molecular and Cellular. Endocrinology, 111*, 225-232.

Luparello, C. Ginty, A. F. Gallagher, J. A. Pucci-Minafra, I. & Minafra, S. (1993). Transforming growth factor-β1, β2, β3, urokinase and parathyroid hormone-related peptide expression in 8701-BC breast cancer cells and clones. *Differentiation, 55*, 73-80.

Luparello, C. Romanotto, R. Tipa, A. Sirchia, R. Olmo, N & Lopez de Silanes, I Turnay, J. Lizarbe, M. A. & Stewart, A. F. (2001). Midregion parthyroid hormone-related protein inhibits growth and invasion in vitro and tumorigenesis in vivo of human breast cancer cells. *Journal of Bone and Mineral Research, 16*, 2173–2181.

MacLennan, G. T. & Bostwick, D. G. (1995). Microvessel density in renal cell carcinoma: lack of prognostic significance, *Urology, 46*, 27–30.

MacLeod, R. J. Chattopadhyay, N. & Brown, E. M. (2003). PTHrP stimulated by the calcium-sensing receptor requires MAP kinase activation. *Am J Physiol Endocrinol Metab, 284*, E435–E442.

Maioli, E, & Fortino, V. (2004). The complexity of parathyroid hormone-related protein signalling. *Cell Mol Life Sci, 61*, 257-262.

Majeska, R. J. Rodan, S. B. & Rodan, G. A. (1980). Parathyroid hormone-responsive clonal cell lines from rat osteosarcoma *Endocrinology, 107*, 1494-1503.

Mangin, M. Ikeda, K. Dreyer, B. E. & Broadus, A. E. (1989). Isolation and characterization of the human parathyroid hormone-like peptide gene. *Proceeding National Acadamy of Sciences, 86*, 2408-24124.

Mangin, M. Ikeda, K. Dreyer, B. E. & Broadus, A. E. (1990). Identification of an upstream promoter of the human parathyroid hormone-related peptide (PTHrP) gene. *Molecular Endocrinology, 4*, 851-858.

Mangin, M. Webb, A. C. Dreyer, B. E. Posillico, J. T. Ikeda, K. Weir, E. C. Stewart, A. F. Bander, N. H. Milstone, L. Barton, D. E. Francke, U. & Broadus, A.E. (1988). Identification of a cDNA encoding a parathyroid hormone-like-peptide from a human tumor associated with humoral hypercalcemia of malignancy. *Proceeding National Academy of Science U.S.A, 85*, 597-601.

Mannstadt, M., Luck, M., Gardella, T. J. Juppner, H. (1998). Evidence for a ligand interaction site at the amino-terminus of the parathyroid hormone/parathyroid hormone-related protein receptor from cross-linking and mutational studies. *The Journal of Biological Chemistry, 273*, 16890-16896.

Mannens, M. Slater, R. M. Heyting, C. Guerts Van Kessek, A. Goedde-salz, B. Frants, R. R. Van-Ommen, G. J. B. & Pearson, P. L. (1987). Regional localization of DNA probed on the short arm of chromosome 11 using anirdia-Wilms' tumor associated deletions. *Human Genetics, 75*, 180-187.

Martin, T. J. Allan, E. H. Caple, I. W. Care, A. D. Danks, J. A. Diefenbach-Jagger, H. Ebeling, P. R. Gillespie, M. T. Hammonds, G. Heath, J. A. Hudson, P. J. Kemp, B. E. Kubota, M. Kukeja, S. C. Moseley, J. M. N. G. K. W. Raisz, L. G. Rodda, C. P. Simmons, H. A., Suva, L. J. Wettenhall, R. E. H. & Wood. W. I. (1989). Parathyroid hormone-related protein: Isolation, molecular cloning, and mechanism of action. *Recent Progress in Hormone Research, 45*, 467-506.

Martin, T. J. Ingleton, P. M. Underwood, J. C. E. Melick. R. A. Michelangeli, V. P. & Hunt, N. H. (1976). Parathyroid hormone-responsive adenylate cyclase in induced transplantable osteogenic rat sarcoma. *Nature, 260*, 436-438.

Martin, T. J. Moseley, J. M. & Gillespe, M. T. (1991). Parathyroid hormone-related protein: Biochemistry and Molecular Biology. *Critical Review in Biochemistry and Molecular Biology, 26*, 377-395.

Martin, T. J. & Suva, L. J. (1988). Parathyroid hormone-related protein: a novel gene product. *Bailliere Clinical Endocrinology and Metabolism, 2*, 1003-1029.

Martin, T. J. & Suva, L. J. (1989). Parathyroid hormone-related protein in hypercalcaemia of malignancy. *Clinical Endocrinology, 31*, 631-647.

Martinez, M. E. Garcia-Ocana, A. Sanchez, M. Medina, S. Del Campo, T. Valin, A. Sanchez-Cabezudo, M. J. & Esbrit, P. (1997). C-terminal parathyroid hormone-related protein inhibits proliferation and differentiation of human osteoblast-like cells. *Journal of Bone and Mineral Research, 12*, 778-785.

Massfelder, T. Dann, P. Wu, T. L. Vasavada, R. Helwig, J-J. & Stewart, A. F. (1997). Opposing mitogenic and anti-mitogenic actions of parathyroid hormone-related protein in vascular smooth muscle cells: a critical role for nuclear targeting. *Proc Natl Acad Sci USA, 94*, 13630–13635.

Massfelder, T. Lang, H. Schordan, E. Lindner, V. Rothhut, S. & Welsch, S. (2004). Parathyroid hormone-related protein is an essential growth factor for human clear cell renal carcinoma and a target for the von Hippel-Lindau tumor suppressor gene, *Cancer Res, 64*, 180–188.

Mayo, K. E. (1992). Molecular cloning and expression of a pituitary-specific receptor for growth hormone-releasing hormone. *Molecular Endocrinology, 6*, 1734-1744.

Mitchell P. & Tollervey, D. (2001). mRNA turnover, *Curr. Opin. Cell. Biol, 13*, 320–325.

Moseley, J. M. & Gillespie, M. T. (1995). Parathyroid hormone-related protein. *Critical Reviews in Clinical Laboratory Sciences, 32*, 299-343.

Moseley, J. M. Kubota, M. Diefenbach-Jagger, H. Wettenhall, R. E. H. Kemp, B. E. Suva, L. J. Rodda, C. P. Ebeling, P. R. Hudson, P. J. Zajac, J. D. & Martin, T. J. (1987). Parathyroid hormone-related protein purified from a human lung cancer cell line. *Proceeding National Academy of Science, 84*, 5048-5052.

Mulder, K. M. (2000). Role of Ras and Mapks in TGFbeta signaling. *Cytokine Growth Factor Rev, 11*, 23-35.

Nebreda, A. R. & Porras, A. (2000). p38 MAP kinases: beyond the stress response. *Trends Biochem Sci, 25*, 257–260.

Nickols, G. A. Nan, A. D. Nickols, M. A. Dipette, J. & Asimakis, G. K. (1989). Hypotension and cardiac stmulation due to the parathyroid hormone and parathyroid hormone-related protein, humoral hypercalcemia of malignancy. *Endocrinology, 125*, 834-841.

Nissenson, R. A. Huang, Z. Blind, E. & Shoback, D. (1993). Structure and function of the receptor for parathyroid hormone-related protein. *Receptor, 3*, 193-202.

Nussbaum, S. Rosenblatt, M. & Potts, J. T. Jr. (1980). Parathyroid hormone-renal receptor interactions. *The Journal of Biological Chemistry, 255*, 10183-10187.

Offermanns, S. Iida-Klein, A. Segre, G. V. & Simon, M. I. (1996) G alpha q family members couple parathyroid hormone (PTH)/PTH-related peptide and calcitonin receptors to phospholipase C in COS-7 cells. *Mol Endocrinol, 10*, 566-474.

Orloff, J. J. Ganz, M. B. Ribaudo, a. e. Burtis, W. J. Reiss, M. Milstone, L. M. & Stewart, A. F. (1992). Analysis of PTHRP binding and signal transduction mechanisms in benign and malignant squamous cells. *American Journal of Physiological, 262*, E599-E607.

Orloff, J. J. Wu, T. L. Heath, H. W. Brady, T. G. Brines, M. L. & Stewart, A. F. (1989a) Characterization of canine renal receptors for the parathyroid hormone-like protein associated with humoral hypercalcemia of malignancy. *The Journal of Biological Chemistry, 64*, 6097-6103.

Orloff, J. J. Wu, T. L. & Stewart, A. E. (1989b). Parathyroid hormone-like proteins: biochemical responses and receptor interactions. *Endocrine Review, 10*, 476-495.

Paget, S. (1889). The distribution of secondary growths in cancer of the breast. *Lancet, I*, 571-573.

Partridge, N. C. Frampton, R. J. Eisman, J. A. Michelangeli, V. P. Elms, E. Bradley, T. R. & Martin, T. J. (1980). Receptor for 1,25$(OH)_2$- vitamin D_3 enriched in cloned osteoblast-like rat osteogenic sarcoma cells. *FEBS Lett, 115*, 139-142.

Pearson, G. Robinson, F. Beers Gibson, T. Xu, B-E. Karandikar, M. Berman, K. & Cobb, M. H. (2001). Mitogen-activated protein (MAP) kinase pathways: regulation and physiologic functions. *Endocr Rev, 22*, 153–183.

Philbrick, W. M. Wysolmerki, J. J. Galbraith, S. Holt, E. Orloff, J. J. Yang, K. H. Vasavada, R. C. Weir, E. C. Broadus, A. E. & Stewart, A. F. (1996). Defining the roles of parathyroid hormone-related peptide in normal physiology. *Physiological Reviews, 76*, 127-173.

Pines, M. Adams, A. E. Stueckle, S. Bessalle, R. Rashti-Behar, V. Chorev, M. Rosenblatt, M. & Suva, L. J. (1994). Generation and characterization of human kidney cell lines stably expressing recombinant human PTH/PTHrP receptor: lack of interaction with a c-terminal human PTH peptide. *Endocrinology, 135*, 1713-1716.

Pines, M. Fukayama, K. C. Costas, K. Meurer, E. Goldsmith, P. K. Xu, X. Muallem, S. Behar, V. Chorev, M. Rosenblatt, M. Tashjian, Jr. A. H. & Suva, L. J. (1996). Inositol 1-,4-,5-triphosphate-dependent Ca^{2+} signaling by the recombinant PTH/PTHrP receptor stably expressed in a human kidney cell line. *Bone, 18*, 381-389.

Powell, G. J. Southby, J. Danks, J. A., Stillwell, R. G. Heyman, J. A. Henderson, M. A., Bennett, R. C. & Martin, T. J. (1991). Localization of parathyroid hormone-related protein in breast cancer metastases: increase in incidence in bone compared with other sites. *Cancer Research, 51*, 3059-3061.

Riggs, B. L. Arnaud, C. D. Reynolds, J. C. & Smith, L. H. (1971). Immunological differentiation of primary hyperparathyroidsm from hyperparathyroidism due to non-parathyroid cancer. *Journal Clinical Investigation, 50*, 2079-2083.

Rihani-Bisharat, S. Maor, G. & Lewinson, D. (1998). In vivo anabolic effects of parathyroid hormone (PTH) 28-48 and N- terminal fragments of PTH and PTH-related protein on neonatal mouse bones. *Endocrinology, 139*, 974-981.

Rizzoli, R. Sappino, A. P. Aubert, M. L. & Bonjour, J.-P. (1990). Effect of cAMP-stimulators on parathyroid hormone-related protein (PTHrP) release by a cultural lung squamous cell carcinoma (BEN cells). *Calcification Tissue International, 46*, A58.

Rizzoli, R. & Bonjour, J. P. (1989). High extracellular calcium increases the production of a parathyroid hormone-like activity by culture leydig tumor cells associated with humoral hypercalcaemia. *Journal of Bone and Mineral Research, 4*, 839-844.

Rodda, C. P. Kubota, M. Heath, J. A. Ebeling, P. R. Moseley, J. M. Care, A. D. Caple, I. W., & Martin, T. J. (1988). Evidence for a novel parathyroid hormone-related peptide (PTHrP) in fetal lamb Parathyroid gland and sheep placenta. *Journal of Endocrinology, 117*, 261-271.

Rodan, S. B. Insogna, K. L. Vignery, A. M. C. Stewart, A. F. Broadus, A. E. D'Souza, S. Bertolini, D. R. Mundy, G. R. & Rodan, G. A. (1983). Factors associated with humoral hypercalcemia of malignancy stimulate adenylate cyclase in osteoblastic cells, *Journal of Clinical Investigation, 72*, 1511-1515.

Rodan, S. B. Noda, M. Wesolowski, G. Rosenblatt, M. & Rodan, G. A. (1988). Comparison of postreceptor effects of 1-34 human hypercalcemia factor and 1-34 human parathyroid hormone in rat osteosarcoma cells. *Journal of Clinical Investigatio, 81*, 924-927.

Rosol, T. J. Capen, C. C. & Horst, R. L. (1988). Effects of infusion of human parathyroid hormone-related protein-(1-40) in nude mice: histomorphometric and biochemical investigations. *Journal of Bone and Mineral Research, 3*, 699-706.

Rosol, T. J. Capen, C. C. & Brooks, C. L. (1987). Bone and kidney adenylate cyclase-stimulating activity produced by a hypercalcemia canine adenocarcinoma line (CAC-8) maintained in nude mice. *Cancer Research, 47*, 690-695.

Rude, R. K. Sharp, C. F. Fredericks, R. S. Oldham, S. B. Elbaum, N. Link, J. Irvin, L. & Singer, F. R. (1981). Urinary and nephrogenous adenosine 3'5'-monophosphate in the hypercalcaemia of malignancy. *Journal of Clinical Investigation, 52*, 765-771.

Sanders. J. L. Chattopadhyay. N. Kifor. O. Yamaguchi, T. & Brown, E. M. (2001). Ca(2+)-sensing receptor expression and PTHrP secretion in PC-3 human prostate cancer cells. *American Journal Physiology and Endocrinology metabolism, 281*, E1267–E1274.

Schipani, E. Karga, H. Karaplis, A. C. Potts, JR. J. T. Kronenberg, H. M. Segre, G. V. Abou-Samra, A. B. & Juppner, H. (1993). Identical complementary deoxyribonucliec acids (cDNA) encode a human renal and bone parathyroid hormone (PTH)/PTH-related peptide receptor. *Endocrinology, 132*, 2157-2165.

Schmitt, J. M. & Stork, P. J. (2002). PKA phosphorylation of Src mediates cAMP's inhibition of cell growth via Rap1. *Mol Cell, 9*, 85-94.

Schneider, H. Feyen, J. H. M. & Seuwen, K. (1994). A c-terminally truncated human parathyroid-hormone receptor is functional and activates multiple G-proteins. *FEBS Letters, 351*, 281-285.

Schwindinger, W. F. Fredericks. J., Watkins, L. Robinson, H. Bathon, J. M. Pines, M. Suva, L. J. & Levine, M. (1998). Coupling of the PTH/PTHrP receptor to multiple G-proteins; Direct demonstration of receptor activation of G_s, $G_{q/11}$, and $G_{i\ (1)}$ by [α-^{32}P]GTP-γ-azidoanilide photoaffinity labeling. *Endocrine, 8*, 201-209.

Sedlak, T. W. Oltvai, Z. N. Wang, K. Boise, L. H. Thompson, C. B. & Korsmeyer, S. J. (1995). Multiple Bcl-2 family members demonstrate selective dimerizations with Bax. *Proceeding National Academy of Science USA, 92*, 7834–7838.

Segre, G. V. Rosenblatt, M. Reiner, B. L. Mahaffey, J. E. & Potts, J. T. Jr. (1979). Characterization of parathyroid hormone receptors in canine renal critical plasma membranes using a radioiodinated sulfin-free hormone analogue: correlation of binding with adenylate cyclase activity. *Journal of Biological Chemistry, 254*, 6980-6986.

Seitz, P. K. Zhang, R-W. Simmons, D. J. & Cooper, C. W. (1995). Effects of c-terminal parathyroid hormone-related peptide on osteoblasts. *Mineral and Electrolytes Metabolism, 21*, 180-183.

Sellers, R.S., Luchin, A. I., Richard, V., Brena, R. M. Lima D. & Rosol, T. J. (2004). Alternative splicing of parathyroid hormone-related protein mRNA: expression and stability. *Journal of Molecular Endocrinology, 33*, 227–241.

Shigeno, C. Hiraki, Y. Westerberg, D. P. Potts, J. T. Jr. & Serge, G. V. (1988a). Photoaffinity labeling of parathyroid hormone receptors in clonal rat osteosarcoma cells. *The Journal of Biological Chemistry, 263*, 3864-3871.

Shigeno, C. Hiraki, Y. Westerberg, D. P. Potts, J. T. Jr. & Serge, G. V. (1988b). Parathyroid hormone receptors are plasma membrane glycoproteins with asparagine-link oligosaccharides. *Journal of Biological Chemistry, 263*, 3872-3878.

Shimo, T. Kubota, S. Yoshioka, N. Ibaragi, S. Isowa, S. Eguchi, T. Sasaki, A. & Takigawa, M. (2006). Pathogenic role of connective tissue growth factor (CTGF/CCN2) in osteolytic metastasis of breast cancer. *Journal of Bone and Mineral Research, 7*, 45-59.

Short, A. D. Brown, B. L. & Dobson, P. R. M. (1991). The effect of retinoic acid on parathyroid hormone- and parathyroid hormone-related peptide-induced intracellular calcium in a rat osteosarcoma cell line, UMR 106. *Journal of Endocrinology, 129*. 75-81.

Slatopolsky, E. Finch, J. Clay, P. Martin, D. Sicard, G. Singer, G. Gao, P. Cantor, T. & Dusso, A. (2000). A novel mechanism for skeletal resistance in uremia, *Kidney International, 58*, 753–761.

Soifer, N. E. Dee, K. E. Insogna, K. L. Burtis, W. J. Matovcik, L. M. Wu, T. L. Milstone, L. M. Broadus, A. E. Philbrick, W. M. Stewart, A. F. (1992) Parathyroid hormone-related protein. Evidence for secretion of a novel mid-region fragment by three different cell types. *Journal Biological Chemistry, 267*, 18236-18243.

Sourbier, C. & Thierry Massfelder, T. (2006). Parathyroid hormone-related protein in human renal cell carcinoma. *Cancer Letter. 240*, 170-82.

Southby, J. Kissin, M. W. Danks, J. A. Hayman, J. A. Moseley, J. M. Henderson, M. A. Bennet, R. C. & Martin, T. J. (1990). Immunohistochemical localization of parathyroid hormone-related protein in human breast cancer. *Cancer Research, 50*, 7710-7716.

Stewart, A. F. Horst, R. Deftos, L. J. Cadman, E. C. Lang, R. & Broadus, A. E. (1980). Biochemical evaluation of patients with cancer-associated hypercalcemia. Evidence for humoral and non-humoral groups. *New England Journal of Medicine, 303*, 1377-1381.

Stork, P. J. S. & Schmitt, J. M. (2002). Crosstalk between cAMP and MAP kinase signaling in the regulation of cell proliferation.*Trends Cellular Biology, 12*, 258–266.

Strewler, G. J. Williams, R. D. & Nissenson, R. A. (1983). Human renal carcinoma cells produce hypercalcemia in the nude mouse and a novel protein recognized by parathyroid hormone receptors. *Journal of Clinical Investigation, 71*. 769-774.

Suva, L. J. Mather, K. A., Gillespie, M. T. Webb, G. C. Ng, K. W. Winslow, G. A. Wood, W. I. Martin, T. J. & Hudson, P. J. (1989). Structure of the 5' flanking region of the gene encoding human parathyroid hormone-related peptide (PTHrP). *Gene, 77*, 95-105.

Suva, L. J. Winslow, G. A. Wettenhall, R. E. H. Hammonds, R. G. Moseley, J. M. Diefenbach-Jagger, H. Rodda, C. P. Kemp, B. E. Rodriguez, H. Chen, E. Y. Hudson, P. J. Martin, T. J. & Wood, W. I. (1987). A parathyroid hormone-related protein implicated in malignant hypercalcemia: Cloning and expression. *Science, 237*, 893-896.

Swarthout, J.T. Doggett, T. A. Lemker, J. L. & Partridge, N. C. (2001). Stimulation of extracellular signal-regulated kinases and proliferation in rat osteoblastic cells by parathyroid hormone is protein kinase C-dependent. *J. Biol. Chem, 276*, 7586–7592.

Syme, C. A. Friedman, P. A. & Bisello, A. (2005). Parathyroid Hormone Receptor Trafficking Contributes to the Activation of Extracellular Signal-regulated Kinases but Is Not Required for Regulation of cAMP Signaling. *J. Biol. Chem, 2*80, 11281-11288.

Tabuenca, A. Mohan, S. Garberoglio, C. A. Borgen, P. I. Rosol, T. & Linkhart, T. A. (1995). Parathyroid hormone-related protein: primary osteolytic factor produced by breast tumor cell in vitro. *World Journal of Surgery. 19*, 292-298.

Takasu, H. & Bringhurst, F. R. (1998). Type-1 parathyroid hormone (PTH)/PTH-related peptide (PTHrP) receptors activate phospholipase C in response to carboxyl-turncated analogs of PTH (1-34). *Endocrinology, 139*, 4293-4299.

Talon, I. Lindner, V. Sourbier, C. Schordan, E. Rothhut, S. I. Talon, V. Lindner, C. Sourbier, E. Schordan, S. Rothhut & Lang, H. Helwig, J. J. Massfelder, T. (2005). Anti-tumor effect of parathyroid hormone-related protein neutralizing antibody in human renal cell carcinoma in vitro and in vivo, *Carcinogenesis, 27*, 73-83.

Tovar Sepulveda, V. A. & Falzon, M. (2002). Parathyroid hormone-related protein enhances PC-3 prostate cancer cell growth via both autocrine/paracrine and intracrine pathways, *Regul. Pept, 105*, 109–120.

Teitelbaum, A. P. Nissenson, R. A. & Arnaud, C. D. (1982). Coupling of the canine renal parathyroid hormone receptor to adenylate cyclase: modulation by guanyl ucleotides and N-ethylmaleimide. Endocrinology, 11, 1524-1533.

Tfelt-Hansen, J. Chattopadhyay, N. Yano, S. Kanuparthi, D. Rooney, P. Schwarz, P. & Brown. E. M. (2004). Calcium-Sensing Receptor Induces Proliferation through p38 Mitogen-Activated Protein Kinase and Phosphatidylinositol 3-Kinase But Not Extracellularly Regulated Kinase in a Model of Humoral Hypercalcemia of Malignancy. *Endocrinology, 145*, 1211-1217.

Tfelt-Hansen, J. Yano, S. Brown, E. M. & Chattopadhyay, N. (2.002), The role of the calcium-sensing receptor in human pathophysiology. *Curr Med Chem, 2*, 175–193.

Tfelt-Hansen, J. MacLeod R. J, Chattopadhyay, N. Yano, S. Quinn, S. Ren, X. Terwilliger, E. F. Schwarz, P. & Brown, E. M. (2003). Calcium-sensing receptor stimulates PTHrP release by pathways dependent on PKC, p38 MAPK, JNK, and ERK1/2 in H-500 cells. *Am J Physiol Endocrinol Metab, 285*, E329-E337.

Thiede, M. A. (1989). The mRNA encoding a parathyroid hormone-like protein is produced in mammary tissue in response to elevation inserum prolactin. *Molecular Endocrinology, 3*, 1443-1048.

Thiede, M. A. Daifotis, A. G. & Weir, E. C. (1990). Intraauterine occupancy controls expression of the parathyroid hormone-related peptide gene in preterm rat myometrium. *Proceeding of National Academy of Science, USA,* 87, 6969-6973.

Thiede, M. A. Harm, S. C. McKee, R. L. Grasser, W. A. Duong, L. T. & Leach, R. M. Jr. (1991). Expression of the parathyroid hormone-related protein gene in the avian oviduct: potential role as a local modulator of vascular smooth muscle tension and shell gland motility during the egg-lying cycle. *Endocrinology, 129*, 1958-1966.

Thomas, R. J. Guise, T. A. Yin, J .J. Elliott, J. Horwood, N.J. Martin, T. J. & Gillespie, M. T. (1999). Breast cancer cells interact with osteoblasts to support osteoclast formation. *Endocrinology, 140*, 4451–4458.

Thorens, B. (1992). Expression cloning of a pancreatic B cell receptor for the gluco-incretin hormone, glucagon-like peptide 1. *Proceeding of National Academy of Sciences USA, 89*, 8641-8645.

Turner, P. R. Mefford, S. Bambion, T. & Nissenson, R. A. (1998). Transmembrane Residues Together with the amino terminus limit the response of the parathyroid hormone (PTH) 2 receptor to PTH-related peptide. *Journal of Biological Chemistry, 273*, 3830-3837.

Usdin, T. B. Gruber, C. & Bonner, T. I. (1995). Identification and functional expression of a receptor selectively recognising parathyroid hormone, the PTH2 receptor. *Journal of Biological Chemistry, 270*, 15455-15458.

Usdin, T. B. Hoare, S. R. Wang, T. Mezey, E. Kowalak, J. A. (1999). TIP39: a new neuropeptide and PTH2-receptor agonist from hypothalamus, *Nat. Neurosci, 2*, 941–943.

Valin, A. Garcia-Ocana, A. DeMiguel, F. Sarasa, J. L. & Esbrit, P. (1997). Antiproliferative effect of the C-terminal fragments of parathyroid hormone-related protein, PTHrP-107-111 and 107-139 on osteoblastic osteosarcoma cells. *Journal of Cellular Physiology, 170*, 209-215.

Vargas, S. J. Gillespie, M. T. Powell, G. J. Southby, J. Danks, J. A. Moseley, J. M. & Martin, T. J. (1992). Localization of parathyroid hormone-related protein mRNA expression and metastatic lesions by in situ hybridization. *Journal of Bone and Mineral Research, 7*, 971-980.

Vasavada. R. C. Wysolmerski. J. J. Broadus. A. E. & Philbrick. W. M. (1993). Identification and characterization of a GC-rich promoter of the human parathyroid hormone-related peptide gene. *Molecular Endocrinology. 7*, 273-282.

Verschueren, K. & Huylebroeck, D. (1999). Remarkable versatility of Smad proteins in the nucleus of transforming growth factor-beta activated cells. *Cytokine Growth Factor Rev, 10*, 187-199.

Wada, T. Qian, X. & Greene, M. I. (1990). Intermolecular Association of the P185^{neu} protein and EGF receptor modulates EGF receptor function. *Cell, 61*, 1339-1347.

Wagstaff, S. C. Bowler, W. B. Gallagher, J. A. Hipskind, R. A (2000) Extracellular ATP activates multiple signalling pathways and potentiates growth factor-induced c-fos gene expression in MCF-7 breast cancer cells. *Carcinogenesis, 21*, 2175-81.

Watanabe, H. de Caestecker, M. P. & Yamada, Y. (2001). Transcriptional cross-talk between Smad, ERK1/2, and p38 mitogen-activated protein kinase pathways regulates transforming growth factor-beta-induced aggrecan gene expression in chondrogenic ATDC5 cells. *J. Biol. Chem, 276*, 14466-14473.

Watson, P. H. Fraher, L. J. Hendy, G. N. Chung, U. I. Kisiel M. & Natale B. V. (2000). Nuclear localization of the type 1 PTH/PTHrP receptor in rat tissues, *J. Bone Miner. Res, 15*, 1033–1044.

Wettschureck, N. Lee, E. Libutti, S. K. Offermanns, S. Robey, P. G. Spiegel, A. M. (1995). G alpha q family members couple parathyroid hormone (PTH)/PTH-related peptide and calcitonin receptors to phospholipase C in COS-7 cells, *Mol. Endocrinol, 10*, 566–574.

Whitfield, J. F. Isaacs, R. J. Chakravarthy. B. R. Durkin. J. P. Morley. P. Neugebauer. W. Williams. R. E. Willick. G. Rixon. R. H. (1994). C-terminal fragments of parathyroid hormone-related protein, PTHrP-(107-111) and PTHrP-(107-139), and the n-terminal

PTHrP-(1-40) fragment stimulate membrane-associated protein-kinase-c activity in rat spleen Lymphocytes. *Journal of Cellular Physiology. 158*, 518-522.

Whitfield, J. F. Isaacs, R.I. Jouishomme, H. MacLean, S. Chakravarthy, B. R. Morley, P. Barisoni, D. Regalia, E. & Armato, U. (1996). C-terminal fragment of parathyroid hormone-related protein, PTHrP-(107-111), stimulates membrane-associated protein kinase C activity and modulates the proliferation of human and murine skin keratinocytes. *Journal of Cellular Physiology, 166*, 1-11.

Williams, E. D. Major, B. J. Martin, T. J. Moseley, J. M. & Leaver, D. D. (1998) Effect of antagonism of the parathyroid hormone (PTH/PTH-related protein receptor on decidualization in rat uterus. *Journal of Reproduction and Fertility, 112*, 59-67.

Winquist, R. J. Baskin, E. P. & Vlasuk, G. P. (1987). Synthetic tumor-derived human hypercalcemic factor exhibits parathyroid hormone-like vasorelaxation in renal arteries. *Biochemical Biophysical Research Communication, 149*, 227-232.

Wu, T. L. Vasavada, R. C. Yang, K. H. Massfelder, T. Ganz, M. Abbas, S. K. Care, A. D. & Stewart, A. F. (1996). Stractural and physiologic characteriztion of the mid-region secretory species of parathyroid hormone-related protein. *Journal of Biological Chemistry, 271*, 24371-24381.

Wysolmerski, J. J. & Broadus, A. E. (1994). Hypercalcemia of malignancy: the central role of parathyroid hormone-related protein. *Annual Review of Medicine, 45*, 189-200.

Yasuda, T. Banville, D. Hendy, G. N. & Goltzman, D. (1989). Characterization of the human parathyroid hormone-like peptide gene; Functional and evolutionary aspects. *The Journal of Biological Chemistry, 264*, 7720-7725.

Yasuda, Y. Benville, D. Rabbani, S. A. Hendy, G. N. & Goltzman, D. (1989). Rat parathyroid hormone-like peptide: comparison with the human homologue and expression in malignant and normal tissue. *Molecular endocrinology, 3*, 518-525.

Ye, Y. Falzon, M. Seitz, P. K. & Cooper, C. W. (2001). Overexpression of parathyroid hormone-related protein promotes cell growth in the rat intestinal cell line IEC-6, *Regul. Pept, 99*, 169–174.

Zha, H. Aime-Sempe, C. Sato, T. & Reed, J. C. (1996). Proapoptotic protein Bax heterodimerizes with Bcl-2 and homodimerizes with Bax via a novel domain (BH3) distinct from BH1 and BH2. *J Biol Chem, 271*, 7440–7444.

Zhang, J., Johnston, G. Stebler, B. & Keller, E. T. (2001). Hydrogen peroxide activates NFkappaB and the interleukin-6 promoter through NFkappaB-inducing kinase. *Antioxid. Redox. Signal, 3*, 493–504.

Zhou, A. T. Bessalle, R. Bisello, A. Nakamoto, C. Rosenblatt, M. Suva, L. & Chorev, M. (1997). Direct mapping of an agonist-binding domain within the parathyroid hormone/parathyroid hormone-related protein receptor by photoaffinity crosslinking. *Proceeding of National Academy of Science.USA, 94*, 3644-3649.

Zhou, H. Leaver, D. D. Moseley, J. M. Kemp, B. Ebeling, P. R. & Martis, T. J. (1989). Actions of parathyroid hormone-related protein on the rat kidney in vivo. *Journal of Endocrinology, 122,* 229-135.

Zhu, X. & Assoian, R. K. (1995). Integrin-dependent activation of MAP kinase: a link to shape-dependent cell proliferation. *Mol. Biol. Cell, 6*, 273–282.

Zondek, H. Petow, H. & Siebert, W. (1923). Die bedeutung der calciumbestimmung im blute fur die diagnose der niereninsuffizienz. Z. *Klin. Med, 99*, 129-138.

Zumkeller. W. & Schofield. P. (1995). Growth factors, cytokines and soluble forms of receptor molecules in cancer patients. *Anticancer Research, 15*, 344-348.

Xiao, G. Jiang, D. Gopalakrishnan, R. & Franceschi, R. T. (2002). Fibroblast growth factor 2 induction of the osteocalcin gene requires MAPK activity and phosphorylation of the osteoblast transcription factor, Cbfa1/Runx2. *J. Biol. Chem, 277*, 36181–36187.

In: Novel Aspects of PTHrP Physiopathology
Editor: Claudio Luparello, pp. 235-270
ISBN: 978-1-60021-857-6

Chapter X

MECHANISMS INVOLVED IN THE REGULATION OF PTHRP EXPRESSION

Jürgen Dittmer*

Clinic for Gynecology, University of Halle, 06120 Halle (Saale), Germany.

ABSTRACT

PTHrP (parathyroid hormone-related protein) is a protein with many biological functions. Expressed by a high percentage of epithelial cancers, it is also thought to contribute to tumor development and progression. This chapter addresses the mechanisms by which PTHrP gene expression is regulated in normal and tumor cells. PTHrP expression is mainly controlled on the transcriptional level involving three different promoters, P1, P2 and P3. The best analyzed promoter, the proximal P3 promoter, displays binding site for Ets, Sp-like and Smad transcription factors through which a number of stimulatory factors, such as HTLV-I Tax, TGFβ and phorbol ester, exert their effects on PTHrP transcription. Ligands of receptor tyrosine kinases, G-protein coupled receptors and protein kinase C often employ the Ras/Raf/MEK-1/ERK1/2 pathway to stimulate P3-dependent PTHrP transcription probably via Ets1 or Ets2. Ligands of nuclear receptors rather inhibit PTHrP expression. The nuclear receptor ligand vitamin D interacts with sequences in the P1 promoter suggesting a role for the P1 promoter in steroid-dependent suppression of PTHrP transcription. The list of factors that interfere with PTHrP expression is long. Some factors, such as angiotensin II, gastrin or N-methyl-D-aspartic acid, act as cell-specific PTHrP regulators supporting the notion that PTHrP modulates highly diverse, but specific biological activities.

* Correspondence concerning this article should be addressed to: Jürgen Dittmer, Clinic for Gynecology, University of Halle, Ernst-Grube-Str. 40, 06120 Halle (Saale), Germany. E-mail: juergen.dittmer@medizin.uni-halle.de; Tel: +49-(0)345-557-1338; Fax: +49-(0)345-557-5261.

Introduction

PTHrP, discovered as a factor that induces hypercalcaemia of malignancy, is expressed and secreted by many cells [1]. It plays a role in a variety of important biological processes, such as bone and breast development [2-4]. PTHrP interferes with cellular activities, including proliferation, migration and apoptosis [5], and modulates gene expression [6,7]. The diverse activities of the PTHrP protein are based on its complex nature featuring three functional domains able to exert their effects independently of each other. Epithelial cancer that often overexpress PTHrP may benefit from PTHrP. Increased mitogenic and migratory abilities of cancer cells as well as their resistance to apoptotic agents have been associated with PTHrP expression. PTHrP may also facilitate growth of metastatic cells in bone due to its osteoclast-stimulatory activity [8]. Knowing the mechanisms underlying PTHrP regulation may help to find new targets for therapeutic interventions to control PTHrP production. PTHrP expression is primarily regulated on the transcriptional level. Three promoters, P1, P2 and P3, have been identified to control transcription of the human PTHrP gene [9-12]. The existence of three promoters predicts that the regulation of the PTHrP gene is rather complex. This chapter intends to provide an overview of the current knowledge on the regulatory mechanisms that drive PTHrP gene expression in mammalian cells.

Organization of the PTHrP Gene

The human PTHrP gene encompasses nine exons spanning 15 kbp of DNA (Figure 1) [10,12,13]. Exons 1-4 (also known as exons Ia, Ib, Ic and II) contain sequences that are not translated. Exon 5 (or exon III) encodes the prepro-sequence of PTHrP. Exon 6 (or exon IV) codes for most of the coding region. The other exons 7, 8, 9 (or exon V, VII and VII) harbor sequences for different 3'-termini [14]. Depending on which 3'-terminus exon 6 is spliced to, the PTHrP protein will either be 139, 141 or 173 amino acids long. Different splicing events are also observed at the 5'-terminus. The splicing pattern at the 5'-terminus is dictated by the promoter that controls PTHrP transcription. P1 generates transcripts that at their 5'-termini contain the sequences of exons 1, 2 and 3 or exon 1 and 3 only, but never exon 4. P2-derived RNAs harbor the sequence of exon 3, but not 4, and P3-guided transcription leads to transcripts carrying the sequence of exon 4, but not 3, at its 5'-terminus. Independent of the promoter that induced its production, each transcript contains the sequences of exon 5 and 6 which code for the full length PTHrP protein. The distal promoter P1 and the proximal promoter P3 feature TATA-boxes for the assembly of the transcription initiation complex. In contrast, the P2 promoter located inbetween P1 and P3 harbors a GC-rich transcriptional start site (note that the P3 promoter was called P2 before the GC-rich promoter was detected) [10]. As PTHrP RNAs carry a "promoter mark" identifying their origin, the importance of the three different promoters in PTHrP-producing cells can be determined. Studies showed that promoter usage was very different depending on the PTHrP-producing cell type that was analyzed. E.g., MT-2 T-cell leukemia cells initiated most of their PTHrP transcription from the P3 promoter, whereas OsA-CL osteosarcoma cells used preferentially the upstream promoters [15]. In contrast, lung fibroblast produced PTHrP through the P2 and P3 promoters

[16]. A comprehensive study on promoter usage in breast, renal, lung and parathyroid tumors revealed that, in epithelial cancer cells, the P3 promoter is preferentially used to drive PTHrP transcription [17]. Studying lung cancer, Ganderton et al. confirmed the importance of the P3 promoter for PTHrP expression, but also found the P1 and P2 promoter to substantially contribute to PTHrP transcription [16].

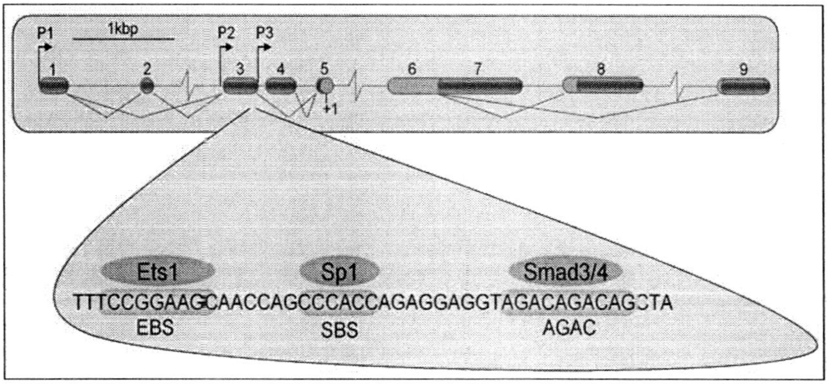

Figure 1. Organization of the human PTHrP gene. Boxes represent exons. Coding regions are striped. The translational start site is indicated by +1. Splicing events are denoted below the map by dashes lines. A blown-up map of a characterized regulatory control region within the P3 promoter is shown below. Examples of transcription factors that can bind to this control region are indicated. AGAC = binding motif for Smad proteins, EBS = Ets binding site, SBS = binding site for Sp-like factors.

Regulation of PTHrP Expression by DNA Methylation

One effective way to control gene transcription is by DNA methylation. DNA methylation takes place on cytosines of CG dinucleotides, so-called CpG sites [18]. Many CpG sites together can form a CpG island that, if located in a sensitive area within a promoter, may have an impact on gene expression. Methylated CpG islands are recognized by MeCP (methyl CpG binding protein) which is able to further recruit co-repressors and HDACs (histone deacetylases) to the modified DNA. This leads to chromatin compaction and will eventually result in blockage of gene transcription. Importantly, methyl CpG are epigenetic marks that can be maintained through mitotic cell division as a result of the action of an enzyme, termed DNMT1 (DNA methyltransferase 1). DNMT1 copies the methylation pattern of the parental strand onto the daughter strand. Epigenetic changes in gene expression play an important role in carcinogenesis. Hypo- and hypermethylation of DNA have been found to take place during carcinogenesis causing inactivation of critical tumor suppressor genes or activation of proto-oncogenes [19,20]. In the PTHrP gene, a CpG island has be detected upstream of exon 4 [21,22]. It encompasses the sequences of promoter 3 and most of promoter 2. The importance of this CpG island for PTHrP expression has been analyzed by using renal and lung cancer cells and tissues. In all cases, this CpG island was found to be unmethylated irrespective of whether the cells produce PTHrP or not [16,21]. Surprisingly, four isolated CpG sites between -2030 and -1500 relative to the translational start site were identified to have an impact on PTHrP expression in renal carcinoma [21]. When these CpG sites were methylated, the renal carcinoma cells did not produce PTHrP, whereas, when unmethylated, cells were PTHrP-positive. In the PTHrP-negative cells, PTHrP expression could be restored by feeding cells with the DNMT1 inhibitor azacytidine. This suggested that, when methylated, these four CpG sites blocked PTHrP transcription in renal cancer cells. This simple on- and off- mechanism, however, does not apply to the regulation of PTHrP expression in lung cancer cells and fibroblasts. In these cells, methylation pattern of the four CpG sites did not correlate with PTHrP expression [16]. This suggests cell-type specific factors to be involved in the epigenetic control of the PTHrP gene transcription.

HTLV-I TAX$_1$, ETS1 AND SP1

All three different promoters can contribute to PTHrP transcription. The activities of these promoters can be regulated by a variety of stimulating and inhibitory factors. The best analyzed promoter is the proximal P3 promoter. Its counterpart in rodents, the P2 promoter, shows close structurally and functionally homologies suggesting that regulation of this major PTHrP promoter is conserved across mammalian species.

In the first promoter assay performed to gain insights into the regulation of the PTHrP gene a large upstream PTHrP gene fragment containing the P2 and P3 promoters was analyzed for its responsiveness to the HTLV-I (human T-cell leukemia virus-I)-Tax (Tax$_1$) protein [23]. HTLV-I is the agent that causes adult T-cell leukemia (ATL), a disease often associated with hypercalcaemia of malignancy and high serum PTHrP levels [24]. Tax$_1$, a unique viral 40kD trans-activating protein, is encoded by the so-called pX region of the HTLV-I genome. When Tax$_1$ was co-transfected with the PTHrP P2/P3 containing DNA fragment, a strong increase in promoter activity was observed [23]. Further analysis showed that Tax$_1$ acts primarily on the P3 promoter [15]. This notion was supported by the finding that, in Tax$_1$-producing MT-2 T-cell leukemia cells, the P3 promoter is the most active PTHrP promoter. As Tax$_1$ is unable to bind to DNA by itself and, therefore, needs to tether to transcription factors to activate transcription, we searched for Tax$_1$-binding factors that interact with the P3 promoter. One of these Tax$_1$-binding factors was found to be Ets1 [15,25]. Ets1 is primarily expressed in haematopoietic cells where it controls T-cell apoptosis, B-cell differentiation and the development of natural killer cells [26-28]. In epithelial cancer, Ets1 is primarily expressed by more advanced tumors and plays a role in the acquisition of invasiveness and in the onset of neo-angiogenesis [29]. Increased expression of Ets1 has been found to be predictive for unfavorable prognosis in a number of cancer, including breast cancer [30]. Ets1 is the founding member of a family of transcription factors, the ETS protein family. Its members share a unique DNA binding domain, the ETS domain which recognizes a GGAA/T core motif [31]. The P3 promoter harbors two overlapping Ets binding sites (EBS I and II) approximately 70bp upstream of its transcriptional start site (Figure 1) [15]. EBSI (CCGGAAGC) was found to be functionally active, allowing Ets1 to activate the PTHrP P3 promoter. EBSI was also required for Tax$_1$-induced promoter activity. It could be shown that Tax$_1$ and Ets1 use this element to cooperatively activate the P3 promoter [25]. On its own, Ets1 is a weak activator. To fully unleash its transcriptional activity, it relies on other transcription factors [29]. One factor that supports Ets1-dependent activation of the P3 promoter was found to be Sp1 [32]. Sp1 is a ubiquitiously expressed transcription factor, which is known to be a common partner for Ets1 in the regulation of Ets-responsive genes. In the P3 promoter, Sp1 recognizes the G-rich sequence on the complementary strand of a CCCACC motif downstream of EBSI. Not only was this motif important for the synergistic effect of Ets1 and Sp1 on the P3 promoter in Ets1- and Sp1-deficient *Drosophila* Schneider cells, but it was also required for maintaining basal P3 promoter activity in Sp1- and Ets1-positive Jurkat T-cell leukemia cells. Mutations in the Sp1 binding site also affected P3 promoter activation of Tax_1 [25]. By immunoprecipitation assays it was shown that Tax_1 forms a ternary complex with Ets1 and Sp1 that likely strengthen the Ets1/Sp1 cooperative effect [25]. The Ets1/Sp1 composite element of the P3 promoter resembles a sequence within the TRE-2 (Tax-responsive element 2) of the HTLV-I promoter, the HTLV-I LTR (long terminal repeat) [33]. This homologous sequence within the TRE-2 also recruits Ets1, Sp1 and Tax_1 and allows these three transcriptional activators to functionally interact [34]. In Tax_1-producing MT-2 leukemia cells, PTHrP transcription can be further increased by interleukin-2 (IL-2), prostaglandin E1 or cAMP [35,36]. The mechanism(s) by which these agents upregulate PTHrP expression has not yet been analyzed.

PROTEIN KINASE C AND RAS

More than half of all breast cancers express PTHrP [37]. The P3 promoter strongly contributes to the PTHrP production in breast cancer cells [17]. E.g., in MDA-MB-231 breast cancer cells, approximately 25% of the PTHrP transcripts derives from P3-dependent transcription which increases to 55-75% upon treatment with TGFβ (transforming growth factor β) [38]. In phorbol ester-treated MCF-7 breast cancer cells, the P3 promoter gives rise to approximately 50% of the PTHrP RNA that is produced [39]. Promoter studies showed that, for basal and stimulated P3 activity in MDA-MB-231 and MCF-7 cells, the Ets binding site EBSI is important [38,39]. Similar data were found when the P3 promoter was analyzed in the breast cancer cell line NS2T2A1 [40]. P3 promoter activity could be stimulated in these breast cancer cells by ectopic expression of Ets1 and/or its close relative Ets2 which depended upon EBSI. In MDA-MB-231 and MCF-7 cells, these stimulatory effects of Ets1 and Ets2 were supported by members of the protein kinase C (PKC) family. PKCs are kinases that upon activation bind to phospholipids of membranes, thereby rendering the catalytic domain of the kinase accessible for substrates [41]. Most PKC subtypes can be activated by diacylglycerol or by its mimetic phorbol ester. Some subtypes, such as PKCα, are involved in carcinogenesis [42]. PKCα regulates Ets1 expression and activity in cancer cells and can phosphorylate the Ets1 protein [43,44]. In MCF-7 breast cancer cells that lack PKCα, addition of a constitutively active form of PKCα was required to allow Ets1 to transactivate the PTHrP P3 promoter [44]. In contrast, in MDA-MB-231 cells whose endogenous PKCα enzyme is permanently activated, the ability of Ets1 to activate the P3 promoter did not rely on the presence of exogenous PKCα. This suggests that PKCα is indispensable for Ets1 to drive P3-dependent transcription in breast cancer cells.

Although MCF-7 cells lack both Ets1 and PKCα, phorbol ester was shown to strongly increase transcription from the P3 promoter in an EBSI-dependent fashion [39]. Further analysis demonstrated that Ets2 was the major regulator of the P3 promoter in this case. Phorbol ester was able to upregulate Ets2 expression and to increase the potency of Ets2 to activate the P3 promoter. This Ets2-supporting effect of phorbol ester could be mimicked by an activated form of PKCε and was sensitive to PD98059, an inhibitor of MEK-1 (MAPK/ERK1/2 kinase-1). This suggested the involvement of PKCε and the Ras/Raf/MEK-1/ERK1/2 (extracellular signal regulated kinase 1/2) pathway. Ras is able to superactivate Ets1 and Ets2 by inducing the phosphorylation of a single threonine at the N-termini of these Ets proteins via ERK1/2 [45]. Subsequently, mutation of this threonine to alanine was shown to abrogate the Ets2/phorbol ester and the Ets2/PKCε cooperative effects. Since PKCε can activate ERK1/2 by stimulating Raf [46], the signaling cascade that leads to Ets2-dependent P3 promoter activation in response to phorbol ester is likely to be phorbol ester/PKCε/Raf/MEK-1/ERK1/2/Ets2 (Figure 2).

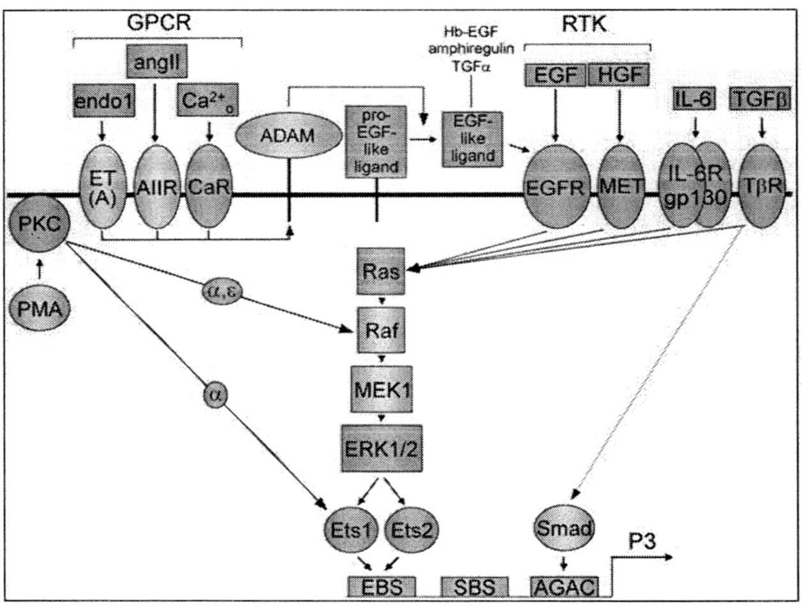

Figure 2. The central role of the Ras/Raf/MEK-1/ERK1/2 pathway in the regulation of PTHrP expression. A number of GPCR and RTK ligands as well as IL-6 and to some extent also TGFβ act via the Ras/Raf/MEK-1/ERK1/2 pathway on PTHrP expression. For some of these ligands, it has been shown that they also activate Ets1/Ets2-dependent transcription from the P3 promoter. This suggests that most, if not all of these stimulators exert their effects on PTHrP transcription through Ets proteins. Proteins that are known to contribute to carcinogenesis are marked in yellow. Ligands are indicated in green, DNA binding elements are indicated in pink. Abbreviations: AIIR = angiotensin II receptor, AGAC = binding motif for Smad proteins, angII = angiotensin II, endo1 = endothelin-1, ET = endothelin receptor, PMA = phorbol ester, SBS = binding site for Sp-like factors, all other abbreviations are explained in the text.

Phorbol ester and the Ras/Raf/MEK-1/ERK1/2 signaling pathway were also shown to affect PTHrP expression in other cells. Ras was demonstrated to upregulate PTHrP expression in Leydig H-500 tumor cells, in Fisher 3T3, NRK 49F kidney and embryo fibroblasts as well as in various prostate cell lines [47-52]. Conversely, Ras and MEK-1 inhibitors were found to inhibit PTHrP expression in MDA-MB-231 breast cancer and MG-63 osteosarcoma cells [53,54]. Phorbol ester upregulated PTHrP expression also in NCI-H727 lung carcinoid cells, Saos-2/B-10 osteosarcoma cells, BEN lung carcinoma cells, T-leukemia cells, umbilical vein endothelial and mammary epithelial cells [39,55-59].

Promoter assays using keratinocytes and T-leukemia cells support the view that phorbol ester and the Ras/Raf/MEK-1/ERK1/2 pathway act on PTHrP expression predominantly by stimulating transcription from the P3 promoter. First, dominant negative forms of Ras and Raf blocked transcription from the P3 promoter in keratinocytes [60]. Second, Ets1 cooperated with MEK-1 to increase promoter activity in T-leukemia cells [57]. Third, the Ets1/MEK-1 cooperation mimicked the combined effect of phorbol ester and ionomycin on the P3 promoter. It should be noted, however, that P3 may not be the only PTHrP target of phorbol ester. In fact, in MCF-7 cells, phorbol ester also affected the levels of P1 and P2-derived PTHrP transcripts [39].

TRANSFORMING GROWTH FACTOR β

The P3 promoter also mediates the stimulatory effect of TGFβ (transforming growth factor β) on PTHrP expression in MDA-MB-231 breast cancer cells [38]. TGFβ is important for PTHrP production in breast cancer cells that have metastasized to bone. As an osteolytic factor PTHrP induces the degradation of the TGFβ-rich bone matrix, leading to activation of TGFβ that further fuels PTHrP secretion [61]. This vicious cycle promotes osteolysis and allows tumor cells to grow in the dense bony environment. TGFβ-induced transcription from the PTHrP P3-promoter not only requires the Ets/Sp1 composite element, but also depends on an AGAC motif located downstream of the Sp1 binding site (Figures 1 and 2) [38]. The AGAC motif was found to recruit TGFβ effectors Smad3/4 to the promoter. This places Smad3/4 in close contact with the Ets1 protein and allows these transcription factors to synergistically activate the P3 promoter. A cooperation between Smad3 and Ets1 has also been found to be involved in TGFβ-induced tenascin-C and CCN2 (connective tissue growth factor) regulation in fibroblasts [62,63] suggesting that the interaction between these transcription factors is of general importance for TGFβ-regulated transcription. There is also evidence that p38 MAP kinase contributes to the TGFβ effect on the PTHrP P3 promoter [53]. Activated by TGFβ, p38 may help to shuttle the Smad proteins from the cytoplasm to the nucleus [64]. In addition, TGFβ also increases the expression of Ets1 which may further enhance PTHrP P3 promoter activity [64].

TGFβ affects PTHrP expression not only in MDA-MB-231 cells. A number of other cancerous and non-cancerous cell lines show increased PTHrP expression in response to TGFβ. These include SCC2/88 and COLO16 squamous carcinoma cells, HOC21 ovarian cancer cells, prostate carcinoma cells and Walker carcinosarcoma 256 cells [65-70]. For untransformed cells, an upregulating effect of TGFβ on PTHrP has been shown for prostate and breast epithelial cells, granulosa cells, keratinocytes, kidney cells, endometrial stromal cells and chondrocytes [71-79]. TGFβ2 plays also an important role in PTHrP-regulatory action on hypertrophic differentiation of chondrocytes. Here it mediates the stimulatory effect of sonic hedgehog (Shh) on PTHrP expression in the perichondrium of embryonic metatarsal bones [80]. It seems that, in chondrocytes, the PTHrP P2 promoter is the most active promoter to drive PTHrP expression and to mediate the TGFβ response [79]. This suggests that, depending on the cell type, the mechanism by which TGFβ stimulates PTHrP expression may vary.

TGFβ does not only affect the transcription of PTHrP, but it seems also to interfere with the stability of the PTHrP transcripts. Such an effect has been shown to contribute to the TGFβ-dependent upregulation of PTHrP expression in SCC2/88 squamous carcinoma cells and Walker carcinosarcoma 256 cells [70,81]. TGFβ may even preferentially stabilize certain isoforms of PTHrP. In SCC2/88 cells, TGFβ has been found to primarily stabilize the PTHrP (1-141) isoform [81], whereas, in chondrocytes, TGFβ seems to specifically upregulate the level of the PTHrP (1-173) protein [79]. To add to the complexity of TGFβ-dependent PTHrP regulation, TGFβ has also been shown to be able to downregulate PTHrP expression in canine prostate stromal cells and murine MCT chondrocytes [81,82].

Receptor Tyrosine Kinases

Receptor tyrosine kinases (RTKs) are membrane-bound kinases that are involved in carcinogenesis [83]. When activated, RTKs stimulate important signaling cascades, such as the Ras/Raf/MEK-1/ERK1/2 pathway. The activation of a number of RTKs, including EGFR (epidermal growth factor receptor), c-MET RTK, insulin receptor and insulin-like growth factor I (IGF-I) receptor, results in an increase in PTHrP production in cancerous and non-cancerous cells [49,56,60,84-94]. The MET RTK is critically involved in invasive growth of epithelial cells during embryonal development [95] and the invasiveness of cancer cells [96]. It has been shown that activation of MET RTK by hepatocyte growth factor/scatter factor (HGF/SF) stimulates Ets1-dependent transcription via the Ras/Raf/MEK-1/ERK1/2 pathway [97]. Ras was also found to mediate the upregulating effect of Trp-MET, a constitutively active form of MET, on PTHrP [49]. This suggests that Ets1 is involved in MET-induced PTHrP synthesis. In support of this notion, Trp-MET was demonstrated to upregulate the PTHrP P3 promoter activity through the Ets binding site (R.K. Lindemann, J. Dittmer, unpublished results).

Like MET RTK, EGFR often plays a role in carcinogenesis [98]. EGFR can be activated by epidermal growth factor (EGF) or EGF-like ligands, such as Hb-EGF (heparin-binding EGF), amphiregulin and TGFα (transforming growth factor α) [99]. Activation of EGFR leads to a number of intracellular events, including the stimulation of the Ras/Raf/MEK-1/ERK1/2 pathway and activation of AKT [100]. Most studies addressing the importance of the EGFR-dependent pathway for PTHrP expression used EGF. EGF was found to stimulate PTHrP in a number of cell types, including prostatic and mammary epithelial cells [56,87,92], keratinocytes [88,101] and various cancer cells [84-86,91]. Nuclear run-on experiments suggested that, in NCI H520 lung squamous cancer cells, the EGF effect on PTHrP is mediated via the P1 promoter [84]. In contrast, in HaCaT keratinocytes, the P2 and P3 promoters were shown to be responsible for the increased expression of PTHrP in response to EGF [88]. A couple of studies addressed the effect of EGF-like ligands on PTHrP expression [60,89,102]. In one study, EGF-like ligand TGFα was shown to upregulate PTHrP expression in BEN-57 lung cancer cells [89]. Another study identified amphiregulin to be responsible for the constitutively activation of the EGR receptor in primary keratinocytes leading to elevated PTHrP expression [60]. Inhibition of EGFR in these cells negatively affected not only PTHrP expression but also P3-dependent transcription. Similar effects on P3 activity was achieved by overexpression of dominant negative forms of Ras or Raf or by mutation of the Ets binding site. This suggested that, in keratinocytes, EGFR mediates its effect on PTHrP expression by activating the Ras/Raf/MEK-1/ERK1/2 pathway which then increases P3 promoter activity through the Ets binding site (Figure 2). Both Ets1 and Ets2 were able to activate the P3 promoter implying that Ets1 or Ets2 may be the downstream targets of the Ras/Raf/MEK-1/ERK1/2 pathway also in keratinocytes.

G-Protein-Coupled Receptors

EGF-like ligands are synthesized as pro-ligands that needs to be converted into their active forms to allow interaction with the EGF receptor. This ligand shedding is mediated by metalloproteases of the ADAM (a disintegrin and metalloprotease) family. Activation of ADAM proteases can occur via GPCRs (G-protein-coupled receptors). This cross-talk between GPCRs and EGFR allows GPCR ligands to regulate PTHrP expression through EGFR signaling (Figure 2). One of the GPCR ligands that has been shown to interfere with PTHrP expression is extracellular calcium ($Ca^{2+}{}_o$). $Ca^{2+}{}_o$ was shown to stimulate PTHrP synthesis and secretion by a number a cell types, including breast cancer cells, H-500 Leydig cells, normal and neoplastic glia cells, HEK293CaR embryonic kidney cells and CH-8 chondrocytes [102-110]. The $Ca^{2+}{}_o$ effect could be mimicked by polyvalent cations (calcimimetics), such as spermine or neomycin. $Ca^{2+}{}_o$ and calcimimetics act as agonists for the calcium sensing receptor (CaR). This G protein-coupled receptor is primarily expressed in cells of the parathyroid gland where it maintains calcium homeostasis by controlling parathyroid hormone production, but is also found in other cell types [111]. Various pathways lie downstream of CaR. One of these pathways is the Ras/Raf/MEK1/ERK1/2 signaling cascade. This cascade appears to be predominantly used by CaR to stimulate PTHrP expression. In rat H-500 Leydig cancer cells and in human PC-3 prostate carcinoma cells, stimulation of endogenous CaR led to phosphorylation of ERK1/2 along with an increase in PTHrP expression [106,107]. Likewise, overexpression of CaR in CaR-deficient HEK293 embryonic kidney cells and treatment with extracellular calcium induced both the activation of ERK1/2 and production of PTHrP [102]. There is evidence that the EGF receptor is involved in this process. In H-500 Leydig and HEK293 cells, EGFR kinase inhibitor AG1478, an EGFR or Hb-EGF neutralizing antibody abrogated $Ca^{2+}{}_o$-induced ERK1/2 phosphorylation and PTHrP expression [102,107]. Hence, CaR may upregulate PTHrP expression by stimulating EGF-ligand shedding leading to activation of EGFR and, consequently, stimulation of the Ras/Raf/MEK-1/ERK1/2 pathway (Figure 2). Besides ERK1/2, CaR is also able to activate the MAP kinases p38 and JNK as well as protein kinase C [107]. Not in all cases did $Ca^{2+}{}_o$ upregulate PTHrP expression. In 8701-BC breast cancer cells, extracellular calcium suppressed the transcript levels of all three PTHrP promoters [112].

The ability of $Ca^{2+}{}_{o}$ to upregulate PTHrP expression may be relevant in the light of the fact that PTHrP can mobilize calcium from the bone and increase calcium concentration in the blood. In hypercalcaemic tumor patients, elevated extracellular calcium levels may further fuel PTHrP secretion by the tumor cells. Also, tumor cells that metastasized to bone may use the bone-borne calcium to increase secretion of PTHrP and, subsequently, to promote osteolysis. Such a putative $Ca^{2+}{}_{o}$/PTHrP vicious cycle may combine with the TGFβ/PTHrP vicious cycle to further accelerate bone degradation. In support of this hypothesis, TGFβ and calcium have been shown to act in tandem to increase PTHrP expression in MDA-MB-231 cells [103]. The same cell line has been shown to utilize the TGFβ/PTHrP vicious cycle to facilitate its growth in the bone [61].

Besides CaR, other GPCRs are able to communicate with EGFR [113]. Among these are angiotensin type I and endothelin A receptor. Ligands of these receptors (angiotensin II and endothelin-1) have been shown to upregulate PTHrP expression. Angiotensin II increased PTHrP production in vascular smooth muscle cells and kidney cells [114,115]. The effect of angiotensin II on PTHrP in aortic smooth muscle cells could be further enhanced by applying mechanical force [116]. The synergistic activity of stretching and angiotensin II could be inhibited by staurosporine suggesting an involvement of PKC. PKC may either act through ADAMs [113] or take a shorter way through Raf to activate ERK1/2 and, consequently, upregulate PTHrP expression (Figure 2). Endothelin-1 has been shown to raise PTHrP levels in endometrial stromal cells [76].

Four other GPCR ligands, calcitonin, gastrin, parathyroid hormone (PTH) and prostaglandin E1 (PGE_1), were shown to induce PTHrP upregulation in BEN lung carinoma cells, parietal stomach cells, SaOS-2 osteosarcoma cells and MT-2 T-leukemia cells, respectively [36,117-122]. In BEN lung carcinoma cells, the calcitonin effect on PTHrP could be mimicked by adenylate cyclase stimulator forskolin suggesting the involvement of cAMP [120]. The P1 and P3 promoters were shown to be the major targets of calcitonin. Of these, the P1 promoter which was demonstrated to harbor a cAMP regulatory element. PTH and PGE are also known to induce a rise in the intracellular cAMP level [123,124].

Another GPCR that has an impact on PTHrP expression is Smo (Smoothened). Smo is activated following ligand-dependent inactivation of its inhibitor, the plasma membrane receptor Patched (Ptc). Mutations of the Patched gene have been associated with the development of cancers, such as cutaneous basal cell carcinoma and medullablastoma [125]. Patched ligands are hedgehog proteins, such as Indian hegdehog (Ihh) and Sonic hedgehog (Shh). Ihh is important for the regulation of PTHrP activity in fetal growth plate during endochondral bone development. PTHrP, which is expressed by perichondral cells and proliferating chondrocytes in the periarticular region, interacts with the PTH/PTHrP receptor of prehypertrophic chondrocytes and columnar proliferating chondrocytes to delay mineralization of the cartilage matrix [126,127]. Ihh, which is expressed in the transition zone between proliferating and hypertrophic cells and in the upper hypertrophic chondrocytes, upregulates PTHrP expression. The signaling pathway that mediates the effect of Ihh on PTHrP is not fully understood. There is evidence that TGFβ2 may be involved in the Ihh-induced upregulation of PTHrP in the perichondrium [80]. Also, Ihh-target WSB-1 has been proposed to contribute to PTHrP upregulation [128]. WSB-1 is a component of an E3 ubiquitin ligase complex that specifically recognizes iodothyronine deiodinase (D2) and triggers its degradation in proteasomes. D2 converts the pro-hormone thyroid hormone T4 to the thyroid hormone T3. Hence, an increase in WSB-1 expression results in a decrease in T3 activity which is associated with an upregulation of PTHrP expression. In osteoblasts, the transcription factor Gli-1 seems to be important for Ihh-induced PTHrP expression [129]. Its relative Gli-2, also a hegdehog downstream target and an even more powerful gene activator, has been shown to be an important regulator for PTHrP expression in breast cancer cells [130]. Interestingly, Gli-2 expression correlates with the capacity of breast cancer cells to secrete PTHrP and to induce osteolytic lesions. As a PTHrP promoter fragment could be activated by Gli-2, it is likely that Gli-2 increases PTHrP expression by directly acting on PTHrP transcription.

It seems that GPCR ligands upregulate PTHrP in different ways. One major pathway involves ERK1/2, another cAMP. The downstream target that hedgehog proteins utilizes to regulate PTHrP seems to vary and to be dependent on the cell type.

Nuclear Receptor Ligands

A class of receptor agonists that also interfere with PTHrP expression are ligands of nuclear receptors. Nuclear receptors are ligand-regulated transcription factors that usually dimerizes to modulate transcription [131]. Classically, they bind to nuclear receptor response elements (also known as hormone response elements, HRE) consisting of two repeats (half-sites) of a RGGTCA recognition sequence. The way these half-sites are positioned to each other and how far they are separated from each other determines which type of nuclear receptor will preferentially bind to a HRE. For their transcriptional activity, nuclear receptors either bind to co-activators or co-repressors. The type of ligand and the cooperating transcription factors determines whether a nuclear receptor actually activates or represses transcription. Heterodimerization, e.g. with retinoid X receptor (RxR), and modifications, such as phosphorylation, further influence the transcriptional activities of many nuclear receptors. Nuclear receptor ligands, such as estrogen, glucocorticoids, vitamin D, progesterone and retinoic acid, have been shown to affect PTHrP expression.

Vitamin D

The effect of vitamin D and vitamin D analogs on PTHrP have received much attention because of their repressive effect on osteolysis and carcinogenesis [132]. Many cancer cells produce the vitamin D receptor (VDR) and 1α-hydroxylase, the enzyme that converts 25-hydroxy-vitamin D_3 to the more potent 1,25-dihydroxy-vitamin D_3 (calcitriol), making these cancer cells susceptible to vitamin D treatment. The large literature about the vitamin D effect on PTHrP expression shows that, with one exception, 1,25-dihydroxy-vitamin D_3 and its non-calcemic analogs EB1089 and 22-oxa-1,25-dihydroxy-vitamin D_3 (22-oxacalcitriol) downregulates PTHrP synthesis in many normal and cancerous cells (Table 1). The mechanism underlying vitamin D transrepression in human cells has been studied by using MT-2 HTLV-I transformed T-leukemia cells and LNCaP prostate cancer cells [133-135]. In MT-2 cells, vitamin D is able to repress all three PTHrP promoters [136]. In the P1 promoter, an atypical vitamin D-responsive element ($VDRE_{PTHrP}$), consisting of only one half-site of a HRE-related sequence, was identified at -535 base pairs upstream of its transcriptional start site [133]. In MT-2 cells, this sequence can be recognized by VDR, but not by RxR [133]. Unusually, binding of VDR to $VDRE_{PTHrP}$ is reduced when vitamin D is added. This suggests that vitamin D represses P1-dependent PTHrP transcription by preventing VDR from interacting with the P1 promoter. The binding activity of VDR to $VDRE_{PTHrP}$ seems to be controlled by phosphorylation [134]. The kinase that has been proposed to be responsible for this phosphorylation is the DNA dependent protein kinase (DNA-PK) [134]. A component of the DNA-PK holoenzyme, the Ku-antigen [137], was found to be attached to VDR-$VDRE_{PTHrP}$ complex [133]. In LNCaP prostate cancer cells, the same DNA element was shown to be required for the vitamin D response of the P1 promoter [135]. However, in this case, the complex formed on $VDRE_{PTHrP}$ contains RxR, but lacks the Ku-antigen. It may be that different cell types use different strategies to control P1-dependent PTHrP transcription via vitamin D.

Vitamin D also suppresses PTHrP expression in rat cells [86,138-140]. By using rat ROS 17/2.8 osteosarcoma cells and a 1.2 kbp fragment of the 5' flanking region of the rat PTHrP gene, Falzon identified a vitamin D-responsive area in the PTHrP gene between -833 and -648 upstream of the transcriptional start site [141]. This sequence harbors two VDR binding elements, one at -799 containing two HRE half sites, the other at -713 consisting of only one HRE half site. By analyzing a rat PTHrP promoter fragment of similar length in human keratinocytes, Kremer et al. found a sequence between -1121 and -1075 upstream of the transcriptional start site to be responsible for vitamin D-dependent promoter activation [93]. This rat $VDRE_{PTHrP}$ contains two complete HRE half-sites which are separated by three base pairs and binds VDR as well as RxR. How VDR regulates PTHrP transcription through these three sites is not known.

Retinoic Acid

Like vitamin D, retinoic acid, a derivative of vitamin A, shows anti-cancer activities [142] and is able to suppress PTHrP expression in human cancer cells [135,143]. In human LNCaP prostate cancer cells, the $VDRE_{PTHrP}$ not only confers responsiveness of the P1 promoter to vitamin D but also to 9-cis-retinoic acid, probably by binding to the RxR half of the VDR/RxR heterodimer [135]. The classical way by which retinoic acid affects gene transcription is by acting on a heterodimer of the retinoid acid receptor (RAR) and RxR. This RAR/RxR dimer regulates transcription through retinoic acid response elements (RAREs) [144]. However, retinoic acid response elements have not been identified in the PTHrP gene so far. Besides the negative effect, also a positive effect of retinoic acid on PTHrP expression has been found in studies that used murine P19 embryonal carcinoma cells and chicken epiphyseal chondrocytes [77,145]. In P19 cells, retinoic acid, that also forces these cells to differentiate, upregulates the level of PTHrP mRNA by stimulating transcription from the P2 promoter, the murine equivalent of the human P3 promoter [145]. For this effect, the Ets and the Sp1 binding sites were found to be essential. In the presence of retinoic acid, both Ets1 and Ets2 were able to transactivate the murine P2 promoter. As Ets1 expression can be upregulated by retinoic acid [146], the retinoic acid effect on PTHrP transcription may partially be a result of increased recruitment of Ets1 to the promoter.

Whether retinoic acid decreases or increases PTHrP expression may depend upon the cellular environment that either forces retinoic acid to target $VDRE_{PTHrP}$ or a yet to be defined $RARE_{PTHrP}$ or to upregulate PTHrP transcription via the P3 promoter.

Table 1. Factors that regulate PTHrP expression

Factor	Cooperating Partner	Promoter Involved	Effect	Cell Type	Organism	References
VIRAL PROTEINS						
HTLV-I Tax	Ets1	P3	up	Jurkat T-leukemia	human	[15, 23]
	Ets1, Sp1	P3	up	OsA-CL osteosarcoma	human	[25]
HTLV-I/II Tax		P3	up	MLA 144 T	gibbon	[181]
adenovir. E1A	Ets	P3	down	Pam212K keratinocytes	mouse	[182]
TRANSCRIPTION FACTORS (except nuclear receptors)						
Ets1/2	Sp1/MEK-1	P3	up	Jurkat T-leukemia	human	[32, 57]
	PKCε	P3	up	MCF-7 breast cancer	human	[39]
	Ras, MAPK	P3	up	primary keratinocytes	human	[60]
		P3	up	OsA-CL osteosarcoma	human	[25]
		P3	up	$NS_2T_2A_1$ breast cancer	human	[40]
		P2(mur)	up	P19 embryonal carcinoma	mouse	[145]
Sp1		P3	up	Jurkat T-leukemia	human	[32]
		P2(mur)	up	P19 embryonal carcinoma	mouse	[145]
Smad3/4	Ets1	P3	up	MDA-MB-231 breast canc	human	[38]
Gli-2			up	MDA-MB-231 breast canc	human	[130]
c-Jun			up	MLA 144 T-cells	gibbon	[181]
p53			down	squamous carcinoma cell	human	[183]
mutant p53		P1, P3	up	squamous carcinoma	human	[183, 184]
	Ras		up	embryo fibroblasts	rat	[52]
MEMBRANE RECEPTORS AND THEIR LIGANDS						
receptor tyrosine kinases and their ligands						
EGF		P1	up	NCI H520 lung cancer	human	[84]
			up	Saos-2/B-10 osteosarcoma	human	[85]
			up	PC-3 prostate cancer	human	[91]
			up	prostatic epithelial	human	[92]
			up	Leydig H-500 tumor	rat	[86]
			up	mammary epithelial	human,rat	[56, 87]
		rat	up	keratinocytes	human	[93]
		P2, P3	up	HaCaT keratinocytes	human	[88]
EGF-like ligands	Ets1/2, Ras,	P3	up	primary keratinocytes	human	[60]
			up	BEN-57 lung carcinoma	human	[89]
bFGF			down	MCT chondrocytes	mouse	[82]
mut. FGFR3			down	ATDC5 chondrogenic	mouse	[185]
IGF-I/II			up	BEN lung carcinoma cells	human	[94]
			up	mammary epithelial cells	human	[87]
insulin	MKP-1, JNK		up	MIN6 beta-cell line	mouse	[90]
			up	mammary epithelial cells	human	[87]

Table 1. Continued

Factor	Cooperating Partner	Promoter Involved	Effect	Cell Type	Organism	References
Tpr-Met	Ras		up	Fischer 3T3 cells	rat	[49]
members of the TGFβ family						
TGFβ1	Smads, Ets1	P3	up	MDA-MB-231 breast canc	human	[38]
	Smads, ERK	P3	up	MDA-MB-231 breast canc	human	[53]
			up	HOC21 ovarian cancer	human	[69]
			up	COLO16 carcinoma	human	[68]
			up	prostate epith.and carcino.	dog	[71]
			up	SCC2/88 carcinoma	dog	[65-67, 81]
			up	Walker 256 sarcoma cells	rat	[70]
			up	foreskin keratinocytes	human	[74]
			up	granulosa cells	pig	[73]
		P2	up	chondrocytes	human	[79]
			down	MCT chondrocytes	mouse	[82]
			up	epiphyseal chondrocytes	chicken	[77]
			up	embryonic metatarsal bone	mouse	[78]
			down	prostate stromal cells	dog	[71]
			up	endometrial stromal cells	human	[76]
			up	OK kidney cells	opossum	[75]
			up	primary mammary cells	rat	[72]
TGFβ-I-Rec			up	MDA-MB-231 breast canc	human	[61]
BMP-2, -4, -7			up	epiphyseal chondrocytes	chicken	[77]
			down	MCT chondrocytes	mouse	[82]
GPCRs and their ligands						
adrenoceptor			up	coronary endothelial	rat	[186]
angiotensin II			up	vascular smooth muscle	rat	[114]
			up	kidney	rat, mouse	[115]
			up	aortic smooth muscle	rat	[116]
Ca^{2+}_o (CaR)			down	8701-BC breast cancer	human	[112]
			up	MCF-7, MDA-MB-231	human	[103]
	EGFR, ERK		up	PC-3 prostate carcinoma	human	[105, 106]
	ERK1/2, p38, JNK, PKC		up	H-500 Leydig cells	rat	[104, 107, 110]
	EGFR, ERK		up	HEK293-CaR kidney	human	[102]
calcimimetic agents (CaR)			up	H-500 Leydig cells	rat	[104, 110]
			up	brain tumor	human	[108]
			up	chondrocytes	hum.,bov.	[109]
			up	MCF-7, MDA-MB-231	human	[103]
	EGFR, ERK		up	PC-3 prostate carcinoma	human	[105]
calcitonin			down	MCF-7 breast cancer	human	[187]
	cAMP	P1, P3	up	BEN lung carcinoma	human	[117-120]
endothelin-1			up	endometrial stromal	human	[76]
gastrin			up	stomach	mouse	[122]
PGE_1	cAMP		up	MT-2 T-leukemia cells	human	[36]
parathyroid hormone			up	SaOS-2 osteosarcoma cells, primary osteoblasts	human	[121]

Table 1. Continued

Factor	Cooperating Partner	Promoter Involved	Effect	Cell Type	Organism	References
cytokines						
IL-1β			up	primary osteoblasts	human	[167]
			up	synoviocytes	human	[150]
			up	umbilical vein endothelial	human	[58,168]
			up	endometrial stromal	human	[76]
			up	spleen	mouse	[169]
IL-2			up	MT-2 T-leukemia	human	[35]
IL-4			up	umbilical vein endothelial	human	[58]
			up	spleen	mouse	[170]
IL-6			up	BEN lung carcinoma	human	[94]
	Ras, ERK1/2		up	osteosarcoma, osteoblasts	human	[54]
IFNγ			down	synoviocytes	human	[150]
TNFα			up	BEN lung carcinoma	human	[94]
			up	endothelial	human	[168]
			up	synoviocytes	human	[150]
			up	endometrial stromal	human	[76]
patched ligands						
Ihh/Shh	WSB-1		up	tibial growth plate	chicken	[128]
	TGFβ2		up	embryonic bones	mouse	[80]
	Gli-1		up	osteoblasts	human	[129]
RAS PATHWAY						
Raf	JNK		up	Leydig H-500 tumor	rat	[48]
Ras	ERK1/2		up	Leydig H-500 tumor	rat	[48]
			up	Fisher 3T3 fibroblasts	rat	[47]
			up	prostate cell lines	human	[50]
	v-src		up	kidney fibroblasts	rat	[51]
	mutant p53		up	embryo fibroblasts	rat	[52]
PKC PATHWAY						
active PKCα	Ets1	P3	up	MCF-7 breast cancer	human	[44]
phorbol ester	Ets2, PKCε	P3	up	MCF-7 breast cancer	human	[39]
			up	NCI-H727 lung carcinoid	human	[55]
			up	Saos-2/B-10 osteosarcoma	human	[85]
			up	BEN lung carcinoma	human	[118]
	ionomyc, Ets1	P3	up	T-leukemia cells	human	[57]
			up	umbilical vein endothelial	human	[58 , 59]
			up	mammary epithelial cells	rat	[56]
cAMP PATHWAY						
cAMP		P1, P3	up	BEN lung carcinoma	human	[119, 120, 188]
			up	MT-2 T-leukemia	human	[36]
forskolin		P1, P3	up	BEN lung carcinoma	human	[120]

Table 1. Continued

Factor	Cooperating Partner	Promoter Involved	Effect	Cell Type	Organism	References
LIGANDS OF NUCLEAR RECEPTORS						
Estrogen receptor ligands						
estradiol			up	endometrial stromal	human	[76]
			up	kidney	rat	[155]
			up	uterus	rat	[156, 157]
			up	MCF-7 breast cancer	human	[160]
			down	MDA-MB-231/ERα$^+$	human	[158]
			down	KPL-3C breast cancer	human	[159]
Faslodex			up	KPL-3C breast cancer cells	human	[159]
tamoxifen			up	MDA-MB-231/ERα$^+$	human	[158]
			up	KPL-3C breast cancer	human	[159]
			up	MCF-7 breast cancer	human	[160]
Androgen receptor ligands						
testosterone			up	LnCaP prostate cancer	human	[163]
			down	PC-3T prostate cancer	human	[162]
			down	Leydig H-500 tumor	rat	[86]
Glucocorticoid receptor ligands						
dexamethasone			down	medullary thyroid carcino	human	[147]
			down	COLO 16 carcinoma	human	[148]
			down	Leydig H-500 tumor	rat	[86]
			down	Walker 256 sarcoma	rat	[140, 149]
			down	synoviocytes	human	[150]
			down	lactating mammary gland	rat	[151]
hydrocortisone			down	mammary epithelial cells	human	[87]
			up	8701-BC breast carcinoma	human	[112]
triamcinolone			down	NCI-H727 lung carcinoid	human	[152]
Progesterone receptor ligands						
progesterone			down	breast cancer tissue	human	[161]
			down	8701-BC breast carcinoma	human	[112]
			down	lactating mammary gland	rat	[151]
Vitamin D receptor ligands						
1,25-$(OH)_2$-vitamin D_3	Ku/VDR	P1	down	MT2 T-leukemia	human	[133]
	VDR/RxR	P1	down	LNCaP and PC-3 prostate cancer	human	[91, 135, 189]
		P1	down	NCI H520 lung cancer	human	[84]
			down	medullary thyroid carcino	human	[147]
			down	HSC-3 oral carcinoma	human	[143]
			down	Walker 256 cells	rat	[140]
	VDR	rat	down	ROS 17/2.8 osteosarcoma	rat	[138]
			down	Leydig H-500 tumor	rat	[86]
			down	mammary epithelial	human	[87]
			down	keratinocytes	human	[190]
			down	fetal long bones	rat	[139]
			down	vascular smooth muscle	cow	[191]
			down	mammary epithelial	human	[87]
			up	SCC2/88 carcinoma	dog	[66]

Table 1. Continued

Factor	Cooperating Partner	Promoter Involved	Effect	Cell Type	Organism	References
22-oxa-1,25-$(OH)_2$-vitamin D_3			down	MT2 T-leukemia	human	[192]
		P1	down	NCI H520 lung cancer	human	[84]
			down	FA-6 pancreatic carcinoma	human	[136]
EB1089	VDR/RxR	P1	down	LNCaP and PC-3 prostate	human	[135, 189]
		P1	down	NCI H520 lung cancer	human	[84]
EB1089			down	HPK1A carcinoma	human	[193]
			down	Leydig H-500 tumor	rat	[194]
Vitamin D deficiency			up/ down	keratinocytes, fibroblasts	rat	[195]
25-OH vitamin D-1α-OH-ase			up kidney	rats inoculated with human infantile fibrosarcoma	rat	[196]
Retinoic acid						
retinoic acid		P1	down	LNCaP prostate cancer	human	[135]
			down	HSC-3 oral carcinoma	human	[143]
	Ets1, Ets2	P2(mur)	up	P19 embryonal carcinoma	mouse	[145]
			up	epiphyseal chondrocytes	chicken	[77]
ECM PROTEINS						
collagen			up	8701-BC breast carcinoma	human	[178]
collagen I	$\alpha_2\beta_1$-integrin		down	pancreatic carcinoma	human	[175, 176]
collagen IV			down	FG pancreatic carcinoma	human	[175]
fibronectin	$\alpha_5\beta_1$-integrin		up	FG pancreatic carcinoma	human	[175, 177]
laminin			down	FG pancreatic carcinoma	human	[175]
vitronectin			up	FG pancreatic carcinoma	human	[175]
MECHANICAL FORCE						
low-frequency			up	blood vessel of muscle	rat	[197]
stretching	TREK-2		up	osteoblast-like cells	rat	[198]
	calcium		up	chondrocytes	rat	[199]
			up	vascular smooth muscle	rat	[200]
			up	aortic smooth muscle	rat	[201]
			up	preterm myometrium	rat	[202]
			up	smooth muscle	rat	[203]
	Ang II, PKC		up	aortic smooth muscle	rat	[116]
MISCELLANEOUS						
IFNγ			up	spleen	mouse	[170]
KCl			up	cerebellar granule neurons	rat	[204]
LPS	TNFα		up	spleen	mouse	[169]
NMDA			up	cerebellar granule neurons	rat	[204]
pVHL			down	Clear cell renal carcinoma	human	[205]
calcium	Ca^{2+} channels		up	cerebellar granule neurons	rat	[206]
ionomycin	PMA, Ets1	P3	up	T-leukemia cells	human	[57]
			up	NCI-H727 lung carcinoid	human	[55]

Glucocorticoids

Glucocorticoids, such as dexamethasone, have also been reported to downregulate PTHrP expression in cancerous and non-cancerous cells alike [86,87,140,147-152]. In one study using 8701 breast carcinoma cells, the glucocorticoid hydrocortisone was found to upregulate PTHrP production [112]. Little is known about the mechanism by which glucocorticoids regulate PTHrP expression. In MDA-MB-231 cells, a P2- and P3-containing 1.1 kbp promoter fragment strongly responded to dexamethasone [153]. In COLO 16 carcinoma cells, dexamethasone downregulated the levels of all PTHrP transcripts without changing the stability of these RNAs [148]. This suggests that dexamethasone affects PTHrP expression on the transcriptional level by modulating the activities of all three promoters. However, an attempt to identify a glucocorticoid hormone responsive element (GRE) within a 3.5 kbp 5' flanking region of the human PTHrP gene, encompassing the P2, P3 and the proximal part of the P1 promoter, has failed [148].

Gonadal Steroids

Of the gonadal steroids, estradiol-17β (E2), progesterone, testosterone and dihydro-testosterone have been shown to modulate PTHrP synthesis and/or secretion. E2 typically acts through estrogen receptor α (ERα) which normally activates genes via estrogen responsive elements (EREs) [131]. ERα is expressed in many cells, including mammary epithelial, endometrial and breast cancer cells. ERα-positive breast cancer cells usually depend on estrogen for proliferation. Based on this finding, anti-estrogens, such as tamoxifen, are routinely used to treat patients with ERα-positive breast cancer. In some cells, such as endometrial cells, tamoxifen can also act as an ERα agonist, probably as a result of a higher level of ERα co-activators in these cells [131]. The complexity of estrogen action is further increased by the existence of a second estrogen receptor, ERβ, which often antagonizes the action of ERα and which can use tamoxifen as an agonist. Furthermore, the transcriptional effect of ERα does not rely on the presence of an ERE within the regulatory sequence of a gene, but can also be mediated by other transcription factors, such as AP1 or Sp1, to which ERα is able to bind [154]. Finally, ERα can act in a non-genomically way by activating signaling cascades, such as the Ras/Raf/MEK-1/ERK1/2. In the light of this complexity, it is not surprising that both down- and upregulating effects of estrogen on PTHrP expression have been reported [76,155-160]. In ERα-positive MCF-7 breast cancer cells, E2 as well as tamoxifen was found to increase PTHrP expression [160]. In contrast in MDA-MB-231/ERα$^+$ breast cancer cells, a ERα-expressing derivative of the ERα-negative parental cell line, only tamoxifen upregulated the PTHrP level, whereas E2 had a suppressive effect [158]. A similar inverse effect of E2 and tamoxifen on PTHrP expression was found with ERα-positive KPL-3C breast cancer cells [159]. In human endometrial stromal cells, in rat kidney and uterus, estrogen increased PTHrP expression [76,155-157]. Interestingly, the upregulating effect of estrogen on the rat uterus could be inhibited by dexamethasone [156] indicating counteracting activities of steroids on PTHrP expression.

Progesterone and testosterone showed mostly negative effects on PTHrP expression. Progesterone downregulated PTHrP levels in breast cancer cells/tissues and in lactating mammary gland [112,151,161] while testosterone attenuated PTHrP production in PC-3T prostate cancer and Leydig H-500 cancer cells [86,162]. However, in the androgen-dependent LnCaP prostate cancer cells, dihydro-testosterone increased the PTHrP mRNA level which coincided with an increase in PTHrP-dependent expression of ornithine decarboxylase, an enzyme that is involved in the regulation of cell growth [163].

It can be concluded that, in the vast majority of cases, steroids have a suppressive effect on PTHrP synthesis. Hence, steroids may be suitable to treat PTHrP-related diseases, such as hypercalcaemia of malignancy. Two studies addressed this issue by treating tumor-bearing rats with dexamethasone [140,149]. At least one of the study revealed a reducing effect of the glucocorticoid on tumor burden and PTHrP blood levels [140]. However, dexamethasone did not change the PTHrP level per tumor cell suggesting that the effect of dexamethasone on PTHrP blood levels was not due to downregulating cellular PTHrP expression but rather as a result of a diminished tumor mass.

Because of the immunosuppressive effect of glucocorticoids, vitamin D may be a better choice for treating PTHrP-related diseases. The hypercalcaemic activity of vitamin D can be avoided by using non-calcemic analogs, such as 22-oxa-1,25-dihydroxy-vitamin D_3 (OCT). This compound was shown to be able to target FA-6 cancer cells that were inoculated into nude mice [164]. OCT was also demonstrated to repress PTHrP expression in Lewis lung carcinoma cells implanted into C57BL/6 mice and to reduce the ability of these tumor cells to metastasize and induce neo-angiogenesis [165]. Another non-calcemic vitamin D derivative analog V was able to reduce tumor growth in nude mice bearing canine adenocarcinoma CAC-8 cells and to help these mice to maintain their body weight [166].

Cytokines

Various cytokines, including IL-1β (interleukin-1β), IL-2, IL-4, IL-6 and TNFα (tumor necrosis factor α) have been found to increase PTHrP expression [35,54,58,76,94,150,167-170]. IL-1β induces PTHrP expression in osteoblasts, synoviocytes, endothelial and endometrial stromal cells [58,150,167,168]. Similarly, IL-4 and IL-6 affects PTHrP levels in endothelial and osteoblastic cells [54,58]. In addition, IL-6 also upregulates PTHrP expression in carcinogenic BEN lung carcinoma and MG-63 osteosarcoma cells [54,94]. Inhibition of MEK-1 or Ras abrogated the effect of IL-6 on PTHrP mRNA levels in osteosarcoma cells suggesting that the Ras/Raf/MEK-1/ERK1/2 pathway is important for IL-6 to upregulate PTHrP (Figure 2). IL-6 can act on cells by interacting with the membrane-bound form of IL-6 receptor (IL-6R) and its co-receptor gp130 [171]. However, cells are more sensitive to IL-6, when, prior to the interaction with gp130, IL-6 formed a complex with a version of the IL-6R protein that was solubilized by ADAM17-induced limited proteolysis. Through this mechanism, termed trans-signaling, IL-6 has been shown to stimulate tumor growth. As IL-6 is an inflammatory cytokine, IL-6 may play a role in upregulating PTHrP expression particularly in inflammatory cancers.

Extracellular Matrix

The extracellular matrix (ECM) plays an important role in carcinogenesis. Increased ECM stiffness has been associated with the augmented responsiveness of cells to growth factors, activation of ERK1/2 and tumor progression [172,173]. In addition, ECM composition is different in cancer tissue versus normal tissue. In invasive breast cancer, stromal cells overexpress fibronectin and collagen I [174]. Fibronectin and collagen I have been found to modulate PTHrP expression when interacting with pancreatic carcinoma cells via $\alpha_5\beta_1$ and $\alpha_2\beta_1$ integrins, respectively [175-177]. Fibronectin increased PTHrP production. A similar effect was also found with vitronectin. In contrast, collagen I, and also collagen IV and laminin, downregulated PTHrP expression. However, collagen had a positive effect on PTHrP production when 8701 breast carcinoma cells were attached to this ECM protein [178]. It seems that, depending on the cell type, the composition of the ECM influences PTHrP expression differently. As a stiffer extracellular matrix with an increased protein density causes activation of ERK1/2 in the ECM-attached cell, it is possible that upregulation of PTHrP expression by ECM proteins is mediated by the Ras/Raf/MEK-1/ERK1/2 pathway.

Conclusion

A plethora of factors are able to regulate PTHrP expression. Almost all of them do so by interfering with the transcription of the PTHrP gene. Many PTHrP activators have in common to stimulate PTHrP transcription through the Ras/Raf/MEK-1/ERK1/2 pathway which is able to target the major P3-activators Ets1 or Ets2. Hence, the proximal TATA-box containing P3 promoter may be responsible for mediating most of the activator-induced upregulations of PTHrP expression. In contrast, though able to response to activating factors, the second TATA-box containing P1 promoter seems to be primarily engaged in steroid-dependent repression of PTHrP transcription. And last, but not least, the P2 promoter may be considered as a “house-keeping” promoter that maintains low level of PTHrP expression [22]. Whether and how these different promoters communicate with one another is not known. Theoretically, no crosstalk is required in the case of an activation event. Each promoter could be activated independently and contribute to the increase in PTHrP expression. However, the effect of an inhibitor leading to a shut-down of PTHrP transcription in general cannot be achieved without an interplay between the promoters unless all of the promoters are similarly affected by the inhibitor. In the case of vitamin D, it seems that the inhibitor targets primarily the P1 promoter to suppress PTHrP expression. It is possible that P1 acts as a master promoter that influences the activities of the others. It has been shown that binding of liganded VDR to a distant site is able to modulate chromatin remodeling at a proximal promoter [179]. Such chromatin remodeling activities might be used by the PTHrP promoters to interact with each other.

Unterstanding the mechanismen underlying the transcriptional regulation of the PTHrP gene may help to find new therapeutics for treatment of diseases, such as hypercalcemia of malignancy, that are caused by aberrant expression of PTHrP. A non-calcemic vitamin D analog may be one agent to suppress PTHrP transcription. Another may be 6-thioguanosine (S6G). This anti-leukemic nucleoside analog was shown to reduce PTHrP mRNA levels in breast cancer cells [153]. Converted into deoxy-thioguanosine, S6G is incorporated into DNA where it causes localized distortion of the DNA duplex due to instabile base pairing with either cytosine or thymine [180]. This may affect binding of transcription factors to its DNA-recognition sequence, especially if this DNA element contains a high percentage of guanines, such as the Ets or Sp1 binding site. S6G-modified DNA in promoter regions of the PTHrP gene may, therefore, interfere with the DNA-binding of transcriptional activators, such as Ets1 or Ets2, that are important for PTHrP transcription.

REFERENCES

[1] dePapp, A. E. & Stewart, A. F. (1993). Parathyroid hormone-related protein: a peptide of diverse physiologic functions. *Trends Endocrinol Metab, 4*, 181-183.

[2] Moseley, J. M. & Gillespie, M. T. (1995). Parathyroid hormone-related protein. *Crit Rev Clin Lab Sci, 32*, 299-343.

[3] Philbrick, W. M., Wysolmerski, J. J., Galbraith, S., Holt, E., Orloff, J. J., Yang, K. H., Vasavada, R. C., Weir, E. C., Broadus, A. E. & Stewart, A. F. (1996). Defining the roles of parathyroid hormone-related protein in normal physiology. *Physiol Rev, 76*, 127-173.

[4] Strewler, G. J. (2000). The physiology of parathyroid hormone-related protein. *N Engl J Med, 342*, 177-185.

[5] Dittmer, J. (2004). Importance of PTHrP for cancer development. *Gene Ther Mol Biol, 8*, 451-464.

[6] Tsigelny, I., Burton, D. W., Sharikov, Y., Hastings, R. H. & Deftos, L. J. (2005). Coherent expression chromosome cluster analysis reveals differential regulatory functions of amino-terminal and distal parathyroid hormone-related protein domains in prostate carcinoma. *J Biomed Biotechnol.*, 2005, 353-363.

[7] Dittmer, A., Vetter, M., Schunke, D., Span, P. N., Sweep, F., Thomssen, C. & Dittmer, J. (2006). Parathyroid hormone-related protein regulates tumor-relevant genes in breast cancer cells. *J Biol Chem., 281*, 14563-14572.

[8] Guise, T. A., Yin, J. J., Taylor, S. D., Kumagai, Y., Dallas, M., Boyce, B. F., Yoneda, T. & Mundy, G. R. (1996). Evidence for a causal role of parathyroid hormone-related protein in the pathogenesis of human breast cancer-mediated osteolysis. *J Clin Invest, 98*, 1544-1549.

[9] Vasuda, T., Banville, D., Hendy, G. N. & Goltzman, D. (1989). Characterization of the human parathyroid hormone-like peptide gene. *J Biol Chem, 264*, 7720-7725.

[10] Vasavada, R. C., Wysolmerski, J. J., Broadus, A. E. & Philbrick, W. M. (1993). Identification and characterization of a GC-rich promoter of the human parathyroid hormone-related peptide gene. *Mol Endocrinol, 7*, 273-282.

[11] Mangin, M., Ikeda, K., Dreyer, B. E. & Broadus, A. E. (1990). Identification of an up-stream promoter of the human parathyroid hormone-related peptide gene. *Mol Endocrinol, 4*, 851-858.

[12] Suva, L. J., Mather, K. A., Gillespie, M. T., Webb, G. C., Ng, K. W., Winslow, G. A., Wood, W. I., Martin, T. J. & Hudson, P. J. (1989). Structure of the 5' flanking region of the gene encoding human parathyroid-hormone-related protein (PTHrP). *Gene, 77*, 95-105.

[13] Mangin, M., Ikeda, K., Dreyer, B. E. & Broadus, A. E. (1989). Isolation and characterization of the human parathyroid hormone-like peptide gene. *Proc Natl Acad Sci U S A., 86*, 2408-2412.

[14] Nakamura, M., Hashimoto, T., Furuyama, J. & Kakudo, K. (1995). Multiple alternative splice isoforms of parathyroid hormone-related peptide mRNA in human cell lines. *J Mol Endocrinol., 15*, 245-249.

[15] Dittmer, J., Gitlin, S. D., Reid, R. L. & Brady, J. N. (1993). Transactivation of the P2 promoter of parathyroid hormone-related protein by human T-cell lymphotropic virus type I Tax1: evidence for the involvement of transcription factor Ets1. *J Virol, 67*, 6087-6095.

[16] Ganderton, R. H. & Briggs, R. S. (2000). Increased upstream methylation has no influence on the overexpression of the parathyroid hormone-related protein gene in squamous cell carcinoma of the lung. *Eur J Cancer, 36*, 2128-2136.

[17] Southby, J., O'Keeffe, L. M., Martin, T. J. & Gillespie, M. T. (1995). Alternative promoter usage and mRNA splicing pathways for parathyroid hormone-related protein in normal tissues and tumours. *Br J Cancer, 72*, 702-707.

[18] Wade, P. A. (2001). Methyl CpG-binding proteins and transcriptional repression. *Bioessays., 23*, 1131-1137.

[19] Jones, P. A. & Laird, P. W. (1999). Cancer epigenetics comes of age. *Nat Genet, 21*, 163-167.

[20] Feinberg, A. P. & Tycko, B. (2004). The history of cancer epigenetics. *Nat Rev Cancer., 4*, 143-153.

[21] Holt, E. H., Vasavada, R. C., Bander, N. H., Broadus, A. E. & Philbrick, W. M. (1993). Region-specific methylation of the parathyroid hormone-related peptide gene determines its expression in human renal carcinoma cell lines. *J Biol Chem, 268*, 20639-45.

[22] Ganderton, R. H., Day, I. N. & Briggs, R. S. (1995). Patterns of DNA methylation of the parathyroid hormone-related protein gene in human lung carcinoma. *Eur J Cancer, 31A*, 1697-1700.

[23] Watanabe, T., Yamaguchi, K., Takatsuki, K., Osame, M. & Yoshida, M. (1990). Constitutive expression of parathyroid hormone-related protein gene in human T cell leukemia virus type 1 (HTLV-1) carriers and adult T cell leukemia patients that can be trans-activated by HTLV-1 tax gene. *J Exp Med, 172*, 759-765.

[24] Yamaguchi, K., Kiyokawa, T., Watanabe, T., Ideta, T., Asayama, K., Mochizuki, M., Blank, A. & Takatsuki, K. (1994). Increased serum levels of C-terminal parathyroid hormone-related protein in different diseases associated with HTLV-1 infection. *Leukemia, 8*, 1708-1711.

[25] Dittmer, J., Pise-Masison, C. A., Clemens, K. E., Choi, K. S. & Brady, J. N. (1997). Interaction of human T-cell lymphotropic virus type I Tax, Ets1, and Sp1 in transactivation of the PTHrP P2 promoter. *J Biol Chem, 272*, 4953-4958.

[26] Muthusamy, N., Barton, K. & Leiden, J. M. (1995). Defective activation and survival of T cells lacking the Ets-1 transcription factor. *Nature, 377*, 639-642.

[27] Barton, K., Muthusamy, N., Fischer, C., Ting, C. N., Walunas, T. L., Lanier, L. L. & Leiden, J. M. (1998). The Ets-1 transcription factor is required for the development of natural killer cells in mice. *Immunity, 9*, 555-563.

[28] Wang, D., John, S. A., Clements, J. L., Percy, D. H., Barton, K. P. & Garrett-Sinha, L. A. (2005). Ets-1 deficiency leads to altered B cell differentiation, hyperresponsiveness to TLR9 and autoimmune disease. *Int Immunol., 17*, 1179-1191.

[29] Dittmer, J. (2003). The Biology of the Ets1 Proto-Oncogene. *Mol Cancer, 2*, 29.

[30] Span, P. N., Manders, P., Heuvel, J. J., Thomas, C. M., Bosch, R. R., Beex, L. V. & Sweep, C. G. (2002). Expression of the transcription factor Ets-1 is an independent prognostic marker for relapse-free survival in breast cancer. *Oncogene, 21*, 8506-8509.

[31] Dittmer, J. & Nordheim, A. (1998). Ets transcription factors and human disease. *Biochim Biophys Acta, 1377*, F1-11.

[32] Dittmer, J., Gegonne, A., Gitlin, S. D., Ghysdael, J. & Brady, J. N. (1994). Regulation of parathyroid hormone-related protein (PTHrP) gene expression. Sp1 binds through an inverted CACCC motif and regulates promoter activity in cooperation with Ets1. *J Biol Chem, 269*, 21428-21434.

[33] Gitlin, S. D., Dittmer, J., Shin, R. C. & Brady, J. N. (1993). Transcriptional activation of the human T-lymphotropic virus type I long terminal repeat by functional interaction of Tax1 and Ets1. *J Virol, 67*, 7307-7316.

[34] Gegonne, A., Bosselut, R., Bailly, R. A. & Ghysdael, J. (1993). Synergistic activation of the HTLV1 LTR Ets-responsive region by transcription factors Ets1 and Sp1. *Embo J, 12*, 1169-1178.

[35] Ikeda, K., Okazaki, R., Inoue, D., Ohno, H., Ogata, E. & Matsumoto, T. (1993). Interleukin-2 increases production and secretion of parathyroid hormone-related peptide by human T cell leukemia virus type I-infected T cells: possible role in hypercalcemia associated with adult T cell leukemia. *Endocrinology., 132*, 2551-2556.

[36] Ikeda, K., Okazaki, R., Inoue, D., Ogata, E. & Matsumoto, T. (1993). Transcription of the gene for parathyroid hormone-related peptide from the human is activated through a cAMP-dependent pathway by prostaglandin E1 in HTLV-I-infected T cells. *J Biol Chem, 268*, 1174-1179.

[37] Kozlow, W. & Guise, T. A. (2005). Breast cancer metastasis to bone: mechanisms of osteolysis and implications for therapy. *J Mammary Gland Biol Neoplasia., 10*, 169-180.

[38] Lindemann, R. K., Ballschmieter, P., Nordheim, A. & Dittmer, J. (2001). Transforming growth factor beta regulates parathyroid hormone-related protein expression in MDA-MB-231 breast cancer cells through a novel Smad/Ets synergism. *J Biol Chem, 276*, 46661-46670.

[39] Lindemann, R. K., Braig, M., Hauser, C. A., Nordheim, A. & Dittmer, J. (2003). Ets2 and PKCepsilon are important regulators of parathyroid hormone-related protein expression in MCF-7 breast cancer cells. *Biochem J, 372*, 787-797.

[40] Cataisson, C., Gordon, J., Roussiere, M., Abdalkhani, A., Lindemann, R., Dittmer, J., Foley, J. & Bouizar, Z. (2003). Ets-1 activates parathyroid hormone-related protein gene expression in tumorigenic breast epithelial cells. *Mol Cell Endocrinol., 204*, 155-68.

[41] Mellor, H. & Parker, P. J. (1998). The extended protein kinase C superfamily. *Biochem J, 332 (Pt 2)*, 281-292.

[42] Ways, D. K., Kukoly, C. A., deVente, J., Hooker, J. L., Bryant, W. O., Posekany, K. J., Fletcher, D. J., Cook, P. P. & Parker, P. J. (1995). MCF-7 breast cancer cells transfected with protein kinase C-alpha exhibit altered expression of other protein kinase C isoforms and display a more aggressive neoplastic phenotype. *J Clin Invest, 95*, 1906-1915.

[43] Vetter, M., Blumenthal, S. G., Lindemann, R. K., Manns, J., Wesselborg, S., Thomssen, C. & Dittmer, J. (2005). Ets1 is an effector of protein kinase Calpha in cancer cells. *Oncogene, 24*, 650-661.

[44] Lindemann, R. K., Braig, M., Ballschmieter, P., Guise, T. A., Nordheim, A. & Dittmer, J. (2003). Protein kinase Calpha regulates Ets1 transcriptional activity in invasive breast cancer cells. *Int J Oncol, 22*, 799-805.

[45] Yang, B. S., Hauser, C. A., Henkel, G., Colman, M. S., Van Beveren, C., Stacey, K. J., Hume, D. A., Maki, R. A. & Ostrowski, M. C. (1996). Ras-mediated phosphorylation of a conserved threonine residue enhances the transactivation activities of c-Ets1 and c-Ets2. *Mol Cell Biol, 16*, 538-547.

[46] Soh, J. W., Lee, E. H., Prywes, R. & Weinstein, I. B. (1999). Novel roles of specific isoforms of protein kinase C in activation of the c-fos serum response element. *Mol Cell Biol, 19*, 1313-1324.

[47] Aklilu, F., Park, M., Goltzman, D. & Rabbani, S. A. (1997). Induction of parathyroid hormone-related peptide by the Ras oncogene: role of Ras farnesylation inhibitors as potential therapeutic agents for hypercalcemia of malignancy. *Cancer Res, 57*, 4517-4522.

[48] Aklilu, F., Gladu, J., Goltzman, D. & Rabbani, S. A. (2000). Role of mitogen-activated protein kinases in the induction of parathyroid hormone-related peptide. *Cancer Res, 60*, 1753-1760.

[49] Aklilu, F., Park, M., Goltzman, D. & Rabbani, S. A. (1996). Increased PTHRP production by a tyrosine kinase oncogene, Tpr-Met: role of the Ras signaling pathway. *Am J Physiol., 271*, E277-E283.

[50] Kremer, R., Goltzman, D., Amizuka, N., Webber, M. M. & Rhim, J. S. (1997). ras Activation of human prostate epithelial cells induces overexpression of parathyroid hormone-related peptide. *Clin Cancer Res., 3*, 855-859.

[51] Li, X. & Drucker, D. J. (1994). Parathyroid hormone-related peptide is a downstream target for ras and src activation. *J Biol Chem, 269*, 6263-6266.

[52] Motokura, T., Endo, K., Kumaki, K., Ogata, E. & Ikeda, K. (1995). Neoplastic transformation of normal rat embryo fibroblasts by a mutated p53 and an activated ras oncogene induces parathyroid hormone-related peptide gene expression and causes hypercalcemia in nude mice. *J Biol Chem, 270*, 30857-30861.

[53] Kakonen, S. M., Selander, K. S., Chirgwin, J. M., Yin, J. J., Burns, S., Rankin, W. A., Grubbs, B. G., Dallas, M., Cui, Y. & Guise, T. A. (2002). Transforming growth factor-beta stimulates parathyroid hormone-related protein and osteolytic metastases via Smad and mitogen-activated protein kinase signaling pathways. *J Biol Chem, 277*, 24571-24578.

[54] Guillen, C., de Gortazar, A. R. & Esbrit, P. (2004). The interleukin-6/soluble interleukin-6 receptor system induces parathyroid hormone-related protein in human osteoblastic cells. *Calcif Tissue Int., 75*, 153-159.

[55] Brandt, D. W., Pandol, S. J. & Deftos, L. J. (1991). Calcium-stimulated parathyroid hormone-like protein secretion: potentiation through a protein kinase-C pathway. *Endocrinology., 128*, 2999-3004.

[56] Ferrari, S. L., Rizzoli, R. & Bonjour, J. P. (1994). Effects of epidermal growth factor on parathyroid hormone-related protein production by mammary epithelial cells. *J Bone Miner Res, 9*, 639-644.

[57] Richard, V., Nadella, M. V., Green, P. L., Lairmore, M. D., Feuer, G., Foley, J. G. & Rosol, T. J. (2005). Transcriptional regulation of parathyroid hormone-related protein promoter P3 by ETS-1 in adult T-cell leukemia/lymphoma. *Leukemia., 19*, 1175-1183.

[58] Ferguson, J. E., 2nd, Seaner, R. M., Bruns, D. E. & Bruns, M. E. (1995). Interleukin-1 beta and interleukin-4 increase parathyroid hormone-related protein secretion by human umbilical vein endothelial cells in culture. *Am J Obstet Gynecol., 173*, 448-455.

[59] Rian, E., Jemtland, R., Olstad, O. K., Endresen, M. J., Grasser, W. A., Thiede, M. A., Henriksen, T., Bucht, E. & Gautvik, K. M. (1994). Parathyroid hormone-related protein is produced by cultured endothelial cells: a possible role in angiogenesis. *Biochem Biophys Res Commun., 198*, 740-747.

[60] Cho, Y. M., Lewis, D. A., Koltz, P. F., Richard, V., Gocken, T. A., Rosol, T. J., Konger, R. L., Spandau, D. F. & Foley, J. (2004). Regulation of parathyroid hormone-related protein gene expression by epidermal growth factor-family ligands in primary human keratinocytes. *J Endocrinol, 181*, 179-190.

[61] Yin, J. J., Selander, K., Chirgwin, J. M., Dallas, M., Grubbs, B. G., Wieser, R., Massague, J., Mundy, G. R. & Guise, T. A. (1999). TGF-beta signaling blockade inhibits PTHrP secretion by breast cancer cells and bone metastases development. *J Clin Invest, 103*, 197-206.

[62] Jinnin, M., Ihn, H., Asano, Y., Yamane, K., Trojanowska, M. & Tamaki, K. (2004). Tenascin-C upregulation by transforming growth factor-beta in human dermal fibroblasts involves Smad3, Sp1, and Ets1. *Oncogene, 23*, 1656-1667.

[63] Van Beek, J. P., Kennedy, L., Rockel, J. S., Bernier, S. M. & Leask, A. (2006). The induction of CCN2 by TGFbeta1 involves Ets-1. *Arthritis Res Ther., 8*, R36.

[64] Lindemann, R. K., Nordheim, A. & Dittmer, J. (2003). Interfering with TGFbeta-induced Smad3 nuclear accumulation differentially affects TGFbeta-dependent gene expression. *Mol Cancer, 2*, 20.

[65] Merryman, J. I., DeWille, J. W., Werkmeister, J. R., Capen, C. C. & Rosol, T. J. (1994). Effects of transforming growth factor-beta on parathyroid hormone-related protein production and ribonucleic acid expression by a squamous carcinoma cell line in vitro. *Endocrinology., 134*, 2424-2430.

[66] Kunakornsawat, S., Rosol, T. J., Capen, C. C., Middleton, R. P., Hannah, S. S. & Inpanbutr, N. (2001). Effects of 1,25(OH)2D3, EB1089, and analog V on PTHrP production, PTHrP mRNA expression and cell growth in SCC 2/88. *Anticancer Res., 21*, 3355-3363.

[67] Sellers, R. S., Capen, C. C. & Rosol, T. J. (2002). Messenger RNA stability of parathyroid hormone-related protein regulated by transforming growth factor-beta1. *Mol Cell Endocrinol, 188*, 37-46.

[68] Kiriyama, T., Gillespie, M. T., Glatz, J. A., Fukumoto, S., Moseley, J. M. & Martin, T. J. (1993). Transforming growth factor beta stimulation of parathyroid hormone-related protein (PTHrP): a paracrine regulator? *Mol Cell Endocrinol., 92*, 55-62.

[69] Yasui, T., Uemura, H., Irahara, M. & Aono, T. (1997). Effects of transforming growth factor-beta on the production of parathyroid hormone-related peptide in a human ovarian cancer cell line in vitro. *J Obstet Gynaecol Res., 23*, 231-238.

[70] Benitez-Verguizas, J., Loarte, D., de Miguel, F. & Esbrit, P. (1999). Effects of transforming growth factor beta1 on cell growth and parathyroid hormone-related protein in Walker 256 tumor cells. *Life Sci., 65*, 1807-1816.

[71] Sellers, R. S., LeRoy, B. E., Blomme, E. A., Tannehill-Gregg, S., Corn, S. & Rosol, T. J. (2004). Effects of transforming growth factor-beta1 on parathyroid hormone-related protein mRNA expression and protein secretion in canine prostate epithelial, stromal, and carcinoma cells. *Prostate., 58*, 366-373.

[72] Ferrari, S. L., Rizzoli, R. & Bonjour, J. P. (1992). Parathyroid hormone-related protein production by primary cultures of mammary epithelial cells. *J Cell Physiol., 150*, 304-311.

[73] Garmey, J. C., Schnorr, J. A., Bruns, M. E., Bruns, D. E., Seaner, R. M., Ferguson, I. J., Luking Jayes, F. C., Aguirre, C. & Veldhuis, J. D. (2000). Expression of parathyroid hormone-related peptide (PTH-rp) and its receptorin the porcine ovary: regulation by transforming growth factor-beta and possible paracrine effects of granulosa cell PTH-rp secretion on theca cells. *Biol Reprod., 62*, 334-339.

[74] Werkmeister, J. R., Blomme, E. A., Weckmann, M. T., Grone, A., McCauley, L. K., Wade, A. B., O'Rourke, J., Capen, C. C. & Rosol, T. J. (1998). Effect of transforming growth factor-beta1 on parathyroid hormone-related protein secretion and mRNA expression by normal human keratinocytes in vitro. *Endocrine., 8*, 291-299.

[75] Law, F., Rizzoli, R. & Bonjour, J. P. (1993). Transforming growth factor-beta modulates the parathyroid hormone-related protein-induced responses in renal epithelial cells. *Endocrinology., 133*, 145-151.

[76] Casey, M. L., Mibe, M. & MacDonald, P. C. (1993). Regulation of parathyroid hormone-related protein gene expression in human endometrial stromal cells in culture. *J Clin Endocrinol Metab., 77*, 188-194.

[77] Pateder, D. B., Rosier, R. N., Schwarz, E. M., Reynolds, P. R., Puzas, J. E., D'Souza, M. & O'Keefe, R. J. (2000). PTHrP expression in chondrocytes, regulation by TGF-beta, and interactions between epiphyseal and growth plate chondrocytes. *Exp Cell Res., 256*, 555-562.

[78] Serra, R., Karaplis, A. & Sohn, P. (1999). Parathyroid hormone-related peptide (PTHrP)-dependent and -independent effects of transforming growth factor beta (TGF-beta) on endochondral bone formation. *J Cell Biol., 145*, 783-794.

[79] Terkeltaub, R., Lotz, M., Johnson, K., Deng, D., Hashimoto, S., Goldring, M. B., Burton, D. & Deftos, L. J. (1998). Parathyroid hormone-related proteins is abundant in osteoarthritic cartilage, and the parathyroid hormone-related protein 1-173 isoform is

selectively induced by transforming growth factor beta in articular chondrocytes and suppresses generation of extracellular inorganic pyrophosphate. *Arthritis Rheum., 41*, 2152-2164.

[80] Alvarez, J., Sohn, P., Zeng, X., Doetschman, T., Robbins, D. J. & Serra, R. (2002). TGFbeta2 mediates the effects of hedgehog on hypertrophic differentiation and PTHrP expression. *Development, 129*, 1913-1924.

[81] Sellers, R. S., Luchin, A. I., Richard, V., Brena, R. M., Lima, D. & Rosol, T. J. (2004). Alternative splicing of parathyroid hormone-related protein mRNA: expression and stability. *J Mol Endocrinol., 33*, 227-241.

[82] Terkeltaub, R. A., Johnson, K., Rohnow, D., Goomer, R., Burton, D. & Deftos, L. J. (1998). Bone morphogenetic proteins and bFGF exert opposing regulatory effects on PTHrP expression and inorganic pyrophosphate elaboration in immortalized murine endochondral hypertrophic chondrocytes (MCT cells). *J Bone Miner Res., 13*, 931-41.

[83] Kolibaba, K. S. & Druker, B. J. (1997). Protein tyrosine kinases and cancer. *Biochim Biophys Acta, 1333*, F217-F248.

[84] Falzon, M. & Zong, J. (1998). The noncalcemic vitamin D analogs EB1089 and 22-oxacalcitriol suppress serum-induced parathyroid hormone-related peptide gene expression in a lung cancer cell line. *Endocrinology., 139*, 1046-1053.

[85] Rodan, S. B., Wesolowski, G., Ianacone, J., Thiede, M. A. & Rodan, G. A. (1989). Production of parathyroid hormone-like peptide in a human osteosarcoma cell line: stimulation by phorbol esters and epidermal growth factor. *J Endocrinol., 122*, 219-227.

[86] Liu, B., Goltzman, D. & Rabbani, S. A. (1993). Regulation of parathyroid hormone-related peptide production in vitro by the rat hypercalcemic Leydig cell tumor H-500. *Endocrinology., 132*, 1658-1664.

[87] Sebag, M., Henderson, J., Goltzman, D. & Kremer, R. (1994). Regulation of parathyroid hormone-related peptide production in normal human mammary epithelial cells in vitro. *Am J Physiol., 267*, C723-C730.

[88] Heath, J. K., Southby, J., Fukumoto, S., O'Keeffe, L. M., Martin, T. J. & Gillespie, M. T. (1995). Epidermal growth factor-stimulated parathyroid hormone-related protein expression involves increased gene transcription and mRNA stability. *Biochem J, 307 (Pt 1)*, 159-167.

[89] Burton, P. B. & Knight, D. E. (1992). Parathyroid hormone-related peptide can regulate the growth of human lung cancer cells, and may form part of an autocrine TGF-alpha loop. *FEBS Lett, 305*, 228-232.

[90] Zhang, B., Hosaka, M., Sawada, Y., Torii, S., Mizutani, S., Ogata, M., Izumi, T. & Takeuchi, T. (2003). Parathyroid hormone-related protein induces insulin expression through activation of MAP kinase-specific phosphatase-1 that dephosphorylates c-Jun NH2-terminal kinase in pancreatic beta-cells. *Diabetes., 52*, 2720-2730.

[91] Tovar Sepulveda, V. A. & Falzon, M. (2002). Regulation of PTH-related protein gene expression by vitamin D in PC-3 prostate cancer cells. *Mol Cell Endocrinol, 190*, 115-124.

[92] Cramer, S. D., Peehl, D. M., Edgar, M. G., Wong, S. T., Deftos, L. J. & Feldman, D. (1996). Parathyroid hormone--related protein (PTHrP) is an epidermal growth factor-regulated secretory product of human prostatic epithelial cells. *Prostate, 29*, 20-29.

[93] Kremer, R., Sebag, M., Champigny, C., Meerovitch, K., Hendy, G. N., White, J. & Goltzman, D. (1996). Identification and characterization of 1,25-dihydroxyvitamin D3-responsive repressor sequences in the rat parathyroid hormone-related peptide gene. *J Biol Chem., 271*, 16310-16316.

[94] Rizzoli, R., Feyen, J. H., Grau, G., Wohlwend, A., Sappino, A. P. & Bonjour, J. P. (1994). Regulation of parathyroid hormone-related protein production in a human lung squamous cell carcinoma line. *J Endocrinol, 143*, 333-241.

[95] Tamagnone, L. & Comoglio, P. M. (1997). Control of invasive growth by hepatocyte growth factor (HGF) and related scatter factors. *Cytokine Growth Factor Rev, 8*, 129-142.

[96] Bardelli, A., Longati, P., Gramaglia, D., Basilico, C., Tamagnone, L., Giordano, S., Ballinari, D., Michieli, P. & Comoglio, P. M. (1998). Uncoupling signal transducers from oncogenic MET mutants abrogates cell transformation and inhibits invasive growth. *Proc Natl Acad Sci U S A., 95*, 14379-14383.

[97] Paumelle, R., Tulasne, D., Kherrouche, Z., Plaza, S., Leroy, C., Reveneau, S., Vandenbunder, B., Fafeur, V. & Tulashe, D. (2002). Hepatocyte growth factor/scatter factor activates the ETS1 transcription factor by a RAS-RAF-MEK-ERK signaling pathway. *Oncogene, 21*, 2309-2319.

[98] Normanno, N., De Luca, A., Bianco, C., Strizzi, L., Mancino, M., Maiello, M. R., Carotenuto, A., De Feo, G., Caponigro, F. & Salomon, D. S. (2006). Epidermal growth factor receptor (EGFR) signaling in cancer. *Gene., 366*, 2-16. Epub 2005 Dec 27.

[99] Fischer, O. M., Hart, S., Gschwind, A. & Ullrich, A. (2003). EGFR signal transactivation in cancer cells. *Biochem Soc Trans., 31*, 1203-1208.

[100] Singh, A. B. & Harris, R. C. (2005). Autocrine, paracrine and juxtacrine signaling by EGFR ligands. *Cell Signal., 17*, 1183-1193.

[101] Kremer, R., Shustik, C., Tabak, T., Papavasiliou, V. & Goltzman, D. (1996). Parathyroid-hormone-related peptide in hematologic malignancies. *Am J Med, 100*, 406-411.

[102] MacLeod, R. J., Yano, S., Chattopadhyay, N. & Brown, E. M. (2004). Extracellular calcium-sensing receptor transactivates the epidermal growth factor receptor by a triple-membrane-spanning signaling mechanism. *Biochem Biophys Res Commun., 320*, 455-460.

[103] Sanders, J. L., Chattopadhyay, N., Kifor, O., Yamaguchi, T., Butters, R. R. & Brown, E. M. (2000). Extracellular calcium-sensing receptor expression and its potential role in regulating parathyroid hormone-related peptide secretion in human breast cancer cell lines. *Endocrinology, 141*, 4357-4364.

[104] Sanders, J. L., Chattopadhyay, N., Kifor, O., Yamaguchi, T. & Brown, E. M. (2000). Extracellular calcium-sensing receptor (CaR) expression and its potential role in parathyroid hormone-related peptide (PTHrP) secretion in the H-500 rat Leydig cell model of humoral hypercalcemia of malignancy. *Biochem Biophys Res Commun., 269*, 427-432.

[105] Sanders, J. L., Chattopadhyay, N., Kifor, O., Yamaguchi, T. & Brown, E. M. (2001). Ca(2+)-sensing receptor expression and PTHrP secretion in PC-3 human prostate cancer cells. *Am J Physiol Endocrinol Metab., 281*, E1267-E1274.

[106] Yano, S., Macleod, R. J., Chattopadhyay, N., Tfelt-Hansen, J., Kifor, O., Butters, R. R. & Brown, E. M. (2004). Calcium-sensing receptor activation stimulates parathyroid hormone-related protein secretion in prostate cancer cells: role of epidermal growth factor receptor transactivation. *Bone., 35*, 664-672.

[107] Tfelt-Hansen, J., MacLeod, R. J., Chattopadhyay, N., Yano, S., Quinn, S., Ren, X., Terwilliger, E. F., Schwarz, P. & Brown, E. M. (2003). Calcium-sensing receptor stimulates PTHrP release by pathways dependent on PKC, p38 MAPK, JNK, and ERK1/2 in H-500 cells. *Am J Physiol Endocrinol Metab, 285*, E329-E337.

[108] Chattopadhyay, N., Evliyaoglu, C., Heese, O., Carroll, R., Sanders, J., Black, P. & Brown, E. M. (2000). Regulation of secretion of PTHrP by Ca(2+)-sensing receptor in human astrocytes, astrocytomas, and meningiomas. *Am J Physiol Cell Physiol, 279*, C691-C699.

[109] Burton, D. W., Foster, M., Johnson, K. A., Hiramoto, M., Deftos, L. J. & Terkeltaub, R. (2005). Chondrocyte calcium-sensing receptor expression is up-regulated in early guinea pig knee osteoarthritis and modulates PTHrP, MMP-13, and TIMP-3 expression. *Osteoarthritis Cartilage., 13*, 395-404.

[110] Buchs, N., Manen, D., Bonjour, J. P. & Rizzoli, R. (2000). Calcium stimulates parathyroid hormone-related protein production in Leydig tumor cells through a putative cation-sensing mechanism. *Eur J Endocrinol, 142*, 500-505.

[111] Chattopadhyay, N. (2006). Effects of calcium-sensing receptor on the secretion of parathyroid hormone-related peptide and its impact on humoral hypercalcemia of malignancy. *Am J Physiol Endocrinol Metab., 290*, E761-E770.

[112] Luparello, C., Santamaria, F. & Schilling, T. (2000). Regulation of PTHrP and PTH/PTHrP receptor by extracellular Ca2+ concentration and hormones in the breast cancer cell line 8701-BC. *Biol Chem., 381*, 303-308.

[113] Ohtsu, H., Dempsey, P. J. & Eguchi, S. (2006). ADAMs as mediators of EGF receptor transactivation by G protein-coupled receptors. *Am J Physiol Cell Physiol., 291*, C1-10.

[114] Pirola, C. J., Wang, H. M., Kamyar, A., Wu, S., Enomoto, H., Sharifi, B., Forrester, J. S., Clemens, T. L. & Fagin, J. A. (1993). Angiotensin II regulates parathyroid hormone-related protein expression in cultured rat aortic smooth muscle cells through transcriptional and post-transcriptional mechanisms. *J Biol Chem., 268*, 1987-1994.

[115] Lorenzo, O., Ruiz-Ortega, M., Esbrit, P., Ruperez, M., Ortega, A., Santos, S., Blanco, J., Ortega, L. & Egido, J. (2002). Angiotensin II increases parathyroid hormone-related protein (PTHrP) and the type 1 PTH/PTHrP receptor in the kidney. *J Am Soc Nephrol., 13*, 1595-1607.

[116] Noda, M., Katoh, T., Takuwa, N., Kumada, M., Kurokawa, K. & Takuwa, Y. (1994). Synergistic stimulation of parathyroid hormone-related peptide gene expression by mechanical stretch and angiotensin II in rat aortic smooth muscle cells. *J Biol Chem, 269*, 17911-17917.

[117] Deftos, L. J., Hogue-Angeletti, R., Chalberg, C. & Tu, S. (1989). PTHrP secretion is stimulated by CT and inhibited by CgA peptides. *Endocrinology., 125*, 563-565.

[118] Emly, J. F., Hughes, S., Green, E. & Ratcliffe, W. A. (1994). Expression and secretion of parathyroid hormone-related protein by a human cancer cell line. *Biochim Biophys Acta., 1220*, 193-198.

[119] Chilco, P. J., Gerardi, J. M., Kaczmarczyk, S. J., Chu, S., Leopold, V. & Zajac, J. D. (1993). Calcitonin increases transcription of parathyroid hormone-related protein via cAMP. *Mol Cell Endocrinol., 94*, 1-7.

[120] Chilco, P. J., Leopold, V. & Zajac, J. D. (1998). Differential regulation of the parathyroid hormone-related protein gene P1 and P3 promoters by cAMP. *Mol Cell Endocrinol, 138*, 173-184.

[121] Walsh, C. A., Bowler, W. B., Bilbe, G., Fraser, W. D. & Gallagher, J. A. (1997). Effects of PTH on PTHrP gene expression in human osteoblasts: up-regulation with the kinetics of an immediate early gene. *Biochem Biophys Res Commun., 239*, 155-159.

[122] Jain, R. N. & Samuelson, L. C. (2006). Transcriptional Profiling of Gastrin-Regulated Genes in Mouse Stomach. *Physiol Genomics, 14*, 14.

[123] Juppner, H., Abou-Samra, A. B., Freeman, M., Kong, X. F., Schipani, E., Richards, J., Kolakowski, L. F., Jr., Hock, J., Potts, J. T., Jr., Kronenberg, H. M. & et al. (1991). A G protein-linked receptor for parathyroid hormone and parathyroid hormone-related peptide. *Science, 254*, 1024-1026.

[124] Jabbour, H. N. & Sales, K. J. (2004). Prostaglandin receptor signalling and function in human endometrial pathology. *Trends Endocrinol Metab., 15*, 398-404.

[125] High, A. & Zedan, W. (2005). Basal cell nevus syndrome. Curr Opin Oncol., 17, 160-6.

[126] Vortkamp, A., Lee, K., Lanske, B., Segre, G. V., Kronenberg, H. M. & Tabin, C. J. (1996). Regulation of rate of cartilage differentiation by Indian hedgehog and PTH-related protein. *Science, 273*, 613-622.

[127] Lanske, B., Karaplis, A. C., Lee, K., Luz, A., Vortkamp, A., Pirro, A., Karperien, M., Defize, L. H., Ho, C., Mulligan, R. C., Abou-Samra, A. B., Juppner, H., Segre, G. V. & Kronenberg, H. M. (1996). PTH/PTHrP receptor in early development and Indian hedgehog-regulated bone growth. *Science., 273*, 663-666.

[128] Dentice, M., Bandyopadhyay, A., Gereben, B., Callebaut, I., Christoffolete, M. A., Kim, B. W., Nissim, S., Mornon, J. P., Zavacki, A. M., Zeold, A., Capelo, L. P., Curcio-Morelli, C., Ribeiro, R., Harney, J. W., Tabin, C. J. & Bianco, A. C. (2005). The Hedgehog-inducible ubiquitin ligase subunit WSB-1 modulates thyroid hormone activation and PTHrP secretion in the developing growth plate. *Nat Cell Biol., 7*, 698-705.

[129] Jemtland, R., Divieti, P., Lee, K. & Segre, G. V. (2003). Hedgehog promotes primary osteoblast differentiation and increases PTHrP mRNA expression and iPTHrP secretion. *Bone., 32*, 611-620.

[130] Sterling, J. A., Oyajobi, B. O., Grubbs, B., Padalecki, S. S., Munoz, S. A., Gupta, A., Story, B., Zhao, M. & Mundy, G. R. (2006). The hedgehog signaling molecule gli2 induces parathyroid hormone-related Peptide expression and osteolysis in metastatic human breast cancer cells. *Cancer Res., 66*, 7548-7553.

[131] Gronemeyer, H., Gustafsson, J. A. & Laudet, V. (2004). Principles for modulation of the nuclear receptor superfamily. *Nat Rev Drug Discov., 3*, 950-964.

[132] McCarty, M. F. & Block, K. I. (2006). Toward a core nutraceutical program for cancer management. *Integr Cancer Ther., 5*, 150-171.

[133] Nishishita, T., Okazaki, T., Ishikawa, T., Igarashi, T., Hata, K., Ogata, E. & Fujita, T. (1998). A negative vitamin D response DNA element in the human parathyroid hormone-related peptide gene binds to vitamin D receptor along with Ku antigen to mediate negative gene regulation by vitamin D. *J Biol Chem., 273*, 10901-10907.

[134] Okazaki, T., Nishimori, S., Ogata, E. & Fujita, T. (2003). Vitamin D-dependent recruitment of DNA-PK to the chromatinized negative vitamin D response element in the PTHrP gene is required for gene repression by vitamin D. *Biochem Biophys Res Commun., 304*, 632-637.

[135] Sepulveda, V. A., Weigel, N. L. & Falzon, M. (2006). Prostate cancer cell type-specific involvement of the VDR and RXR in regulation of the human PTHrP gene via a negative VDRE. *Steroids., 71*, 102-115.

[136] Endo, K., Ichikawa, F , Uchiyama, Y., Katsumata, K., Ohkawa, H., Kumaki, K., Ogata, E. & Ikeda, K. (1994). Evidence for the uptake of a vitamin D analogue (OCT) by a human carcinoma and its effect of suppressing the transcription of parathyroid hormone-related peptide gene in vivo. *J Biol Chem, 269*, 32693-32699.

[137] Gullo, C., Au, M., Feng, G. & Teoh, G. (2006). The biology of Ku and its potential oncogenic role in cancer. *Biochim Biophys Acta., 1765*, 223-34. Epub 2006 Jan 25.

[138] Falzon, M. (1996). DNA sequences in the rat parathyroid hormone-related peptide gene responsible for 1,25-dihydroxyvitamin D3-mediated transcriptional repression. *Mol Endocrinol., 10*, 672-681.

[139] Karmali, R., Nijs-De Wolf, N., Beyer, I., Hendy, G. N. & Bergmann, P. (1999). 1,25-dihydroxyvitamin D3 inhibits parathyroid hormone-related peptide mRNA expression in fetal rat long bones in culture. *In Vitro Cell Dev Biol Anim., 35*, 296-298.

[140] Cohen-Solal, M. E., Bouizar, Z., Denne, M. A., Graulet, A. M., Gueris, J., Bracq, S., Jullienne, A. & de Vernejoul, M. C. (1995). 1,25 dihydroxyvitamin D and dexamethasone decrease in vivo Walker carcinoma growth, but not parathyroid hormone related protein secretion. *Horm Metab Res, 27*, 403-407.

[141] Falzon, M. (1997). The noncalcemic vitamin D analogues EB1089 and 22-oxacalcitriol interact with the vitamin D receptor and suppress parathyroid hormone-related peptide gene expression. *Mol Cell Endocrinol, 127*, 99-108.

[142] Freemantle, S. J., Spinella, M. J. & Dmitrovsky, E. (2003). Retinoids in cancer therapy and chemoprevention: promise meets resistance. *Oncogene., 22*, 7305-7315.

[143] Abe, M., Akeno, N., Ohida, S. & Horiuchi, N. (1998). Inhibitory effects of 1,25-dihydroxyvitamin D3 and 9-cis-retinoic acid on parathyroid hormone-related protein expression by oral cancer cells (HSC-3). *J Endocrinol., 156*, 349-357.

[144] Balmer, J. E. & Blomhoff, R. (2002). Gene expression regulation by retinoic acid. *J Lipid Res., 43*, 1773-1808.

[145] Karperien, M., Farih-Sips, H., Lowik, C. W., de Laat, S. W., Boonstra, J. & Defize, L. H. (1997). Expression of the parathyroid hormone-related peptide gene in retinoic acid-induced differentiation: involvement of ETS and Sp1. *Mol Endocrinol, 11*, 1435-1448.

[146] Raouf, A. & Seth, A. (2000). Ets transcription factors and targets in osteogenesis. *Oncogene, 19*, 6455-5463.

[147] Ikeda, K., Lu, C., Weir, E. C., Mangin, M. & Broadus, A. E. (1989). Transcriptional regulation of the parathyroid hormone-related peptide gene by glucocorticoids and vitamin D in a human C-cell line. *J Biol Chem., 264*, 15743-15746.

[148] Glatz, J. A., Heath, J. K., Southby, J., O'Keeffe, L. M., Kiriyama, T., Moseley, J. M., Martin, T. J. & Gillespie, M. T. (1994). Dexamethasone regulation of parathyroid hormone-related protein (PTHrP) expression in a squamous cancer cell line. *Mol Cell Endocrinol, 101*, 295-306.

[149] Schilling, T., Pecherstorfer, M., Blind, E., Kohl, B., Wagner, H., Ziegler, R. & Raue, F. (1996). Glucocorticoids decrease the production of parathyroid hormone-related protein in vitro but not in vivo in the Walker carcinosarcoma 256 rat model. *Bone., 18*, 315-319.

[150] Funk, J. L., Cordaro, L. A., Wei, H., Benjamin, J. B. & Yocum, D. E. (1998). Synovium as a source of increased amino-terminal parathyroid hormone-related protein expression in rheumatoid arthritis. A possible role for locally produced parathyroid hormone-related protein in the pathogenesis of rheumatoid arthritis. *J Clin Invest., 101*, 1362-1371.

[151] Uemura, H., Yasui, T., Umino, Y., Yamada, M., Kuwahara, A., Matsuzaki, T., Maegawa, M. & Irahara, M. (2005). Regulatory factors on parathyroid hormone-related peptide production by primary culture of lactating rat mammary gland. *Horm Metab Res., 37*, 463-467.

[152] Lu, C., Ikeda, K., Deftos, L. J., Gazdar, A. F., Mangin, M. & Broadus, A. E. (1989). Glucocorticoid regulation of parathyroid hormone-related peptide gene transcription in a human neuroendocrine cell line. *Mol Endocrinol., 3*, 2034-2040.

[153] Gallwitz, W. E., Guise, T. A. & Mundy, G. R. (2002). Guanosine nucleotides inhibit different syndromes of PTHrP excess caused by human cancers in vivo. *J Clin Invest, 110*, 1559-1572.

[154] Milano, A., Lago, L. D., Sotiriou, C., Piccart, M. & Cardoso, F. (2006). What clinicians need to know about antioestrogen resistance in breast cancer therapy. *Eur J Cancer, 8*, 8.

[155] Cros, M., Silve, C., Graulet, A. M., Morieux, C., Urena, P., de Vernejoul, M. C. & Bouizar, Z. (1998). Estrogen stimulates PTHrP but not PTH/PTHrP receptor gene expression in the kidney of ovariectomized rat. *J Cell Biochem., 70*, 84-93.

[156] Paspaliaris, V., Petersen, D. N. & Thiede, M. A. (1995). Steroid regulation of parathyroid hormone-related protein expression and action in the rat uterus. *J Steroid Biochem Mol Biol., 53*, 259-265.

[157] Thiede, M. A., Harm, S. C., Hasson, D. M. & Gardner, R. M. (1991). In vivo regulation of parathyroid hormone-related peptide messenger ribonucleic acid in the rat uterus by 17 beta-estradiol. *Endocrinology., 128*, 2317-2323.

[158] Rabbani, S. A., Khalili, P., Arakelian, A., Pizzi, H., Chen, G. & Goltzman, D. (2005). Regulation of parathyroid hormone-related peptide by estradiol: effect on tumor growth and metastasis in vitro and in vivo. *Endocrinology., 146*, 2885-94. Epub 2005 Apr 14.

[159] Kurebayashi, J. & Sonoo, H. (1997). Parathyroid hormone-related protein secretion is inhibited by oestradiol and stimulated by antioestrogens in KPL-3C human breast cancer cells. *Br J Cancer, 75*, 1819-1825.

[160] Funk, J. L. & Wei, H. (1998). Regulation of parathyroid hormone-related protein expression in MCF-7 breast carcinoma cells by estrogen and antiestrogens. *Biochem Biophys Res Commun, 251*, 849-854.

[161] Sugimoto, T., Shiba, E., Watanabe, T. & Takai, S. (1999). Suppression of parathyroid hormone-related protein messenger RNA expression by medroxyprogesterone acetate in breast cancer tissues. *Breast Cancer Res Treat., 56*, 11-23.

[162] Pizzi, H., Gladu, J., Carpio, L., Miao, D., Goltzman, D. & Rabbani, S. A. (2003). Androgen regulation of parathyroid hormone-related peptide production in human prostate cancer cells. *Endocrinology, 144*, 858-867.

[163] Asadi, F., Faraj, M., Malakouti, S. & Kukreja, S. C. (2001). Effect of parathyroid hormone related protein, and dihydrotestosterone on proliferation and ornithine decarboxylase mRNA in human prostate cancer cell lines. *Int Urol Nephrol, 33*, 417-422.

[164] Koike, N., Endo, K., Kubodera, N., Kumaki, K., Ikeda, K., Ogata, E. & Stumpf, W. E. (1999). In vivo nuclear uptake of a vitamin D analog (OCT) in different tumor cell populations of FA-6 cancer xenograft in nude mice by receptor autoradiography. *Anticancer Res., 19*, 4955-4958.

[165] Nakagawa, K., Sasaki, Y., Kato, S., Kubodera, N. & Okano, T. (2005). 22-Oxa-1alpha,25-dihydroxyvitamin D3 inhibits metastasis and angiogenesis in lung cancer. *Carcinogenesis., 26*, 1044-1054.

[166] Kunakornsawat, S., Rosol, T. J., Capen, C. C., Reddy, G. S., Binderup, L. & Inpanbutr, N. (2002). Effects of 1,25-dihydroxyvitamin D3 [1,25(OH)2D3] and its analogues (EB1089 and analog V) on canine adenocarcinoma (CAC-8) in nude mice. *Biol Pharm Bull., 25*, 642-647.

[167] Tsai, J. A., Rong, H., Torring, O., Matsushita, H. & Bucht, E. (2000). Interleukin-1beta upregulates PTHrP-mRNA expression and protein production and decreases TGF-beta in normal human osteoblast-like cells. *Calcif Tissue Int., 66*, 363-369.

[168] Eto, M., Akishita, M., Ishikawa, M., Kozaki, K., Yoshizumi, M., Hashimoto, M., Ako, J., Sugimoto, N., Nagano, K., Sudoh, N., Toba, K. & Ouchi, Y. (1998). Cytokine-induced expression of parathyroid hormone-related peptide in cultured human vascular endothelial cells. *Biochem Biophys Res Commun., 249*, 339-343.

[169] Funk, J. L., Krul, E. J., Moser, A. H., Shigenaga, J. K., Strewler, G. J., Grunfeld, C. & Feingold, K. R. (1993). Endotoxin increases parathyroid hormone-related protein mRNA levels in mouse spleen. Mediation by tumor necrosis factor. *J Clin Invest., 92*, 2546-2552.

[170] Funk, J. L., Shigenaga, J. K., Moser, A. H., Krul, E. J., Strewler, G. J., Feingold, K. R. & Grunfeld, C. (1994). Cytokine regulation of parathyroid hormone-related protein messenger ribonucleic acid levels in mouse spleen: paradoxical effects of interferon-gamma and interleukin-4. *Endocrinology., 135*, 351-358.

[171] Scheller, J., Ohnesorge, N. & Rose-John, S. (2006). Interleukin-6 trans-signalling in chronic inflammation and cancer. *Scand J Immunol., 63*, 321-329

[172] Paszek, M. J. & Weaver, V. M. (2004). The tension mounts: mechanics meets morphogenesis and malignancy. *J Mammary Gland Biol Neoplasia., 9*, 325-342.

[173] Paszek, M. J., Zahir, N., Johnson, K. R., Lakins, J. N., Rozenberg, G. I., Gefen, A., Reinhart-King, C. A., Margulies, S. S., Dembo, M., Boettiger, D., Hammer, D. A. & Weaver, V. M. (2005). Tensional homeostasis and the malignant phenotype. *Cancer Cell., 8*, 241-254.

[174] Brown, L. F., Guidi, A. J., Schnitt, S. J., Van De Water, L., Iruela-Arispe, M. L., Yeo, T. K., Tognazzi, K. & Dvorak, H. F. (1999). Vascular stroma formation in carcinoma in situ, invasive carcinoma, and metastatic carcinoma of the breast. *Clin Cancer Res., 5*, 1041-1056.

[175] Grzesiak, J. J., Clopton, P., Chalberg, C., Smith, K., Burton, D. W., Silletti, S., Moossa, A. R., Deftos, L. J. & Bouvet, M. (2004). The extracellular matrix differentially regulates the expression of PTHrP and the PTH/PTHrP receptor in FG pancreatic cancer cells. *Pancreas, 29*, 85-92.

[176] Grzesiak, J. J., Smith, K. C., Chalberg, C., Burton, D. W., Deftos, L. J. & Bouvet, M. (2005). Type I collagen and divalent cation shifts disrupt cell-cell adhesion, increase migration, and decrease PTHrP, IL-6, and IL-8 expression in pancreatic cancer cells. *Int J Gastrointest Cancer., 36*, 131-146.

[177] Grzesiak, J. J., Smith, K. C., Burton, D. W., Deftos, L. J. & Bouvet, M. (2005). GSK3 and PKB/Akt are associated with integrin-mediated regulation of PTHrP, IL-6 and IL-8 expression in FG pancreatic cancer cells. *Int J Cancer., 114*, 522-530.

[178] Luparello, C., Schilling, T., Cirincione, R. & Pucci-Minafra, I. (1999). Extracellular matrix regulation of PTHrP and PTH/PTHrP receptor in a human breast cancer cell line. *FEBS Lett., 463*, 265-269.

[179] Gutierrez, S., Liu, J., Javed, A., Montecino, M., Stein, G. S., Lian, J. B. & Stein, J. L. (2004). The vitamin D response element in the distal osteocalcin promoter contributes to chromatin organization of the proximal regulatory domain. *J Biol Chem., 279*, 43581-43588.

[180] Bohon, J. & de los Santos, C. R. (2005). Effect of 6-thioguanine on the stability of duplex DNA. *Nucleic Acids Res., 33*, 2880-2886.

[181] Ejima, E., Rosenblatt, J. D., Massari, M., Quan, E., Stephens, D., Rosen, C. A. & Prager, D. (1993). Cell-type-specific transactivation of the parathyroid hormone-related protein gene promoter by the human T-cell leukemia virus type I (HTLV-I) tax and HTLV-II tax proteins. *Blood., 81*, 1017-1024.

[182] Foley, J., Wysolmerski, J. J., Missero, C., King, C. S. & Philbrick, W. M. (1999). Regulation of parathyroid hormone-related protein gene expression in murine keratinocytes by E1A isoforms: a role for basal promoter and Ets-1 site. *Mol Cell Endocrinol, 156*, 13-23.

[183] Foley, J., Wysolmerski, J. J., Broadus, A. E. & Philbrick, W. M. (1996). Parathyroid hormone-related protein gene expression in human squamous carcinoma cells is repressed by mutant isoforms of p53. *Cancer Res, 56*, 4056-4062.

[184] Foley, J., King, C. S., Jimenez, J. A., Wysolmerski, J. J. & Philbrick, W. M. (2000). Activation of PTHrP gene expression in squamous carcinoma cell lines by mutant isoforms of the tumor suppressor p53. *Oncol Res., 12*, 71-81.

[185] Yamanaka, Y., Tanaka, H., Koike, M., Nishimura, R. & Seino, Y. (2003). PTHrP rescues ATDC5 cells from apoptosis induced by FGF receptor 3 mutation. *J Bone Miner Res., 18*, 1395-1403.

[186] Schorr, K., Taimor, G., Degenhardt, H., Weber, K. & Schluter, K. D. (2003). Parathyroid hormone-related peptide is induced by stimulation of alpha 1A-adrenoceptors and improves resistance against apoptosis in coronary endothelial cells. *Mol Pharmacol., 63*, 111-118.

[187] Rong, H., Ji, H., Tsai, J. A., Pernow, Y. & Bucht, E. (1999). Calcitonin-suppressed expression of parathyroid hormone-related protein in breast cancer cells. *Biochem Biophys Res Commun., 265*, 260-264.

[188] Rizzoli, R., Aubert, M. L., Sappino, A. P. & Bonjour, J. P. (1994). Cyclic AMP increases the release of parathyroid hormone-related protein from a lung-cancer cell line. *Int J Cancer., 56*, 422-426.

[189] Tovar Sepulveda, V. A. & Falzon, M. (2003). Prostate cancer cell type-specific regulation of the human PTHrP gene via a negative VDRE. *Mol Cell Endocrinol, 204*, 51-64.

[190] Kremer, R., Karaplis, A. C., Henderson, J., Gulliver, W., Banville, D., Hendy, G. N. & Goltzman, D. (1991). Regulation of parathyroid hormone-like peptide in cultured normal human keratinocytes. Effect of growth factors and 1,25 dihydroxyvitamin D3 on gene expression and secretion. *J Clin Invest., 87*, 884-893.

[191] Jono, S., Nishizawa, Y., Shioi, A. & Morii, H. (1998). 1,25-Dihydroxyvitamin D3 increases in vitro vascular calcification by modulating secretion of endogenous parathyroid hormone-related peptide. *Circulation., 98*, 1302-1306.

[192] Inoue, D., Matsumoto, T., Ogata, E. & Ikeda, K. (1993). 22-Oxacalcitriol, a noncalcemic analogue of calcitriol, suppresses both cell proliferation and parathyroid hormone-related peptide gene expression in human T cell lymphotrophic virus, type I-infected T cells. *J Biol Chem, 268*, 16730-16736.

[193] El Abdaimi, K., Papavasiliou, V., Rabbani, S. A., Rhim, J. S., Goltzman, D. & Kremer, R. (1999). Reversal of hypercalcemia with the vitamin D analogue EB1089 in a human model of squamous cancer. *Cancer Res, 59*, 3325-3328.

[194] Haq, M., Kremer, R., Goltzman, D. & Rabbani, S. A. (1993). A vitamin D analogue (EB1089) inhibits parathyroid hormone-related peptide production and prevents the development of malignancy-associated hypercalcemia in vivo. *J Clin Invest., 91*, 2416-2422.

[195] Errazahi, A., Lieberherr, M., Bouizar, Z. & Rizk-Rabin, M. (2004). PTH-1R responses to PTHrP and regulation by vitamin D in keratinocytes and adjacent fibroblasts. *J Steroid Biochem Mol Biol., 89-90*, 381-385.

[196] Michigami, T., Yamato, H., Suzuki, H., Nagai-Itagaki, Y., Sato, K. & Ozono, K. (2001). Conflicting actions of parathyroid hormone-related protein and serum calcium as regulators of 25-hydroxyvitamin D(3)-1 alpha-hydroxylase expression in a nude rat model of humoral hypercalcemia of malignancy. *J Endocrinol., 171*, 249-257.

[197] Schneider, A. G., Leuthauser, K. & Pette, D. (1999). Parathyroid hormone-related protein is rapidly up-regulated in blood vessels of rat skeletal muscle by low-frequency stimulation. *Pflugers Arch., 439*, 167-173.

[198] Chen, X., Macica, C. M., Ng, K. W. & Broadus, A. E. (2005). Stretch-induced PTH-related protein gene expression in osteoblasts. *J Bone Miner Res., 20,* 1454-1461.

[199] Tanaka, N., Ohno, S., Honda, K., Tanimoto, K., Doi, T., Ohno-Nakahara, M., Tafolla, E., Kapila, S. & Tanne, K. (2005). Cyclic mechanical strain regulates the PTHrP expression in cultured chondrocytes via activation of the Ca2+ channel. *J Dent Res., 84,* 64-68.

[200] Schordan, E., Welsch, S., Rothhut, S., Lambert, A., Barthelmebs, M., Helwig, J. J. & Massfelder, T. (2004). Role of parathyroid hormone-related protein in the regulation of stretch-induced renal vascular smooth muscle cell proliferation. *J Am Soc Nephrol., 15,* 3016-3025.

[201] Pirola, C. J., Wang, H. M., Strgacich, M. I., Kamyar, A., Cercek, B., Forrester, J. S., Clemens, T. L. & Fagin, J. A. (1994). Mechanical stimuli induce vascular parathyroid hormone-related protein gene expression in vivo and in vitro. *Endocrinology., 134,* 2230-2236.

[202] Daifotis, A. G., Weir, E. C., Dreyer, B. E. & Broadus, A. E. (1992). Stretch-induced parathyroid hormone-related peptide gene expression in the rat uterus. *J Biol Chem., 267,* 23455-23458.

[203] Yamamoto, M., Harm, S. C., Grasser, W. A. & Thiede, M. A. (1992). Parathyroid hormone-related protein in the rat urinary bladder: a smooth muscle relaxant produced locally in response to mechanical stretch. *Proc Natl Acad Sci U S A., 89,* 5326-5330.

[204] Ono, T., Inokuchi, K., Ogura, A., Ikawa, Y., Kudo, Y. & Kawashima, S. (1997). Activity-dependent expression of parathyroid hormone-related protein (PTHrP) in rat cerebellar granule neurons. Requirement of PTHrP for the activity-dependent survival of granule neurons. *J Biol Chem., 272,* 14404-144011.

[205] Massfelder, T., Lang, H., Schordan, E., Lindner, V., Rothhut, S., Welsch, S., Simon-Assmann, P., Barthelmebs, M., Jacqmin, D. & Helwig, J. J. (2004). Parathyroid hormone-related protein is an essential growth factor for human clear cell renal carcinoma and a target for the von Hippel-Lindau tumor suppressor gene. *Cancer Res, 64,* 180-188.

[206] Holt, E. H., Broadus, A. E. & Brines, M. L. (1996). Parathyroid hormone-related peptide is produced by cultured cerebellar granule cells in response to L-type voltage-sensitive Ca2+ channel flux via a Ca2+/calmodulin-dependent kinase pathway. *J Biol Chem., 271,* 28105-28111.

In: Novel Aspects of PTHrP Physiopathology
Editor: Claudio Luparello, pp. 271-304
ISBN: 978-1-60021-857-6

Chapter XI

NOVEL MOLECULAR INTERACTIONS OF PARATHYROID HORMONE-RELATED PROTEIN IN CANCER

John J. Grzesiak[1,*], Michael Bouvet[1], Randolph H. Hastings[2], Douglas W. Burton[3], and Leonard J. Deftos[3]
Veterans Affairs San Diego Healthcare System and the Departments of [1]Surgery, [2]Anesthesiology, and [3]Medicine (Endocrinology), University of California, San Diego, California 92161, USA.

ABSTRACT

Our laboratories have studied the gene transcription, translation, secretion, and processing of parathyroid hormone-related protein (PTHrP) in a variety of human cancers, including prostate, breast, pancreas, and lung. Using immunochemical and nucleic acid probes, we have demonstrated the presence of distinct populations of PTHrP-containing cells in these cancers in vivo. We also studied PTHrP secretion in cancer cell lines in order to identify the basic pathways involved. We combined several immunochemical and biochemical approaches in concert with nucleic acid and antibody probes to assess the predominant species of PTHrP and PTHrP mRNA expression in cancer cells. Additionally, we have developed stable and transient transfection systems using expression plasmids for the three isoforms of PTHrP and mutant forms of identified and putative functional domains of the polypeptide to study the regulation of PTHrP gene expression and processing directly. Among the biological effects demonstrated for PTHrP in cancer are nuclear interactions, and interactions with cytokines, osteokines, apoptosis-regulating pathways, and the extracellular matrix

* Correspondence concerning this article should be addressed to: John J. Grzesiak, Department of Surgery, University of California, Veterans Affairs San Diego Healthcare System, Mail code: 151, 3350 La Jolla Village Drive, San Diego, California 92161. E-mail: jgrzesiak@vapop.ucsd.edu; Fax: (858)552-7436.

(ECM). In the following chapter, we will extend and discuss our studies of PTHrP and its relevance in human cancer.

INTRODUCTION

Our laboratories are interested in understanding the regulation of parathyroid hormone-related protein (PTHrP) gene expression and processing as well as its functional role in the pathobiology of several cancers, including prostate, breast, pancreas, and lung. In vitro and in vivo studies using immunochemical, biochemical, antibody, and nucleic acid probes, as well as stable and transient transfection systems indicate novel regulatory mechanisms and distinct biological functions for PTHrP and its processed peptides in cancer. These include nuclear interactions, as well as interactions with cytokines, osteokines, apoptosis-regulating pathways, and the extracellular matrix (ECM). In the following chapter, we discuss our current understanding of the regulation and functions of PTHrP in human cancers.

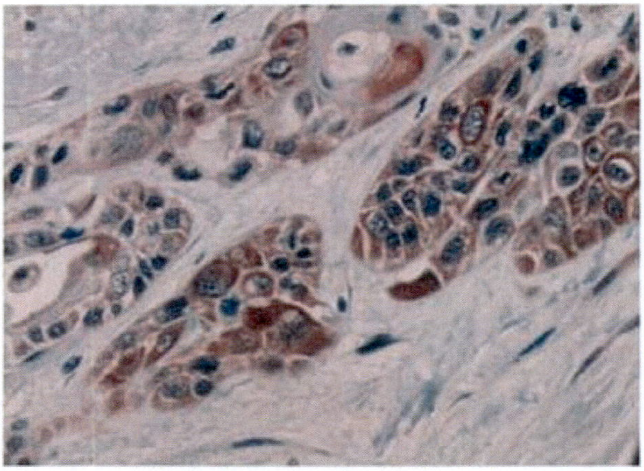

Figure 1. Pancreatic ductal adenocarcinoma: strong cytoplasmic staining of ductal cells for PTHrP. This specimen was obtained from a patient with pancreatic adenocarcinoma after surgical resection and immunostained with a monoclonal antibody against PTHrP (109-141) 400x magnification.

Regulatory Interactions between Parathyroid Hormone-Related Protein and the Extracellular Matrix in Pancreatic Cancer

Previous studies by our laboratory have demonstrated that PTHrP and its receptor (PTH/PTHrP receptor) are commonly expressed by the ductal cells in pancreatic cancer in vivo as well as in pancreatic cancer cell lines in vitro, and suggest their participation in the progression of this devastating disease (Figure 1 and Table 1) (Bouvet et al., 2001; Bouvet et al., 2002). It has also been demonstrated that one of the major hallmarks of pancreatic adenocarcinoma is a strong desmoplastic response characterized by highly up-regulated expression of the extracellular matrix (ECM) (Bardeesy and DePinho, 2002; Binkley et al., 2004; Iacobuzio-Donahue et al., 2003a; Iacobuzio-Donahue et al., 2003b; Linder et al., 2001;

Mollenhauer et al., 1987; Shimoyama et al., 1995; Stein et al., 2004), a critical regulator of diverse cellular processes such as differentiation, proliferation, and angiogenesis (Hynes, 2002; Ruoslahti, 1991; Ruoslahti et al., 1994). It has been previously shown in prostate, colon, and breast cancer that PTHrP regulates the expression of the ECM axis in vitro (Luparello et al., 1999; Shen and Falzon, 2003; Shen and Falzon, 2005; Shen et al., 2004). Using the FG pancreatic adenocarcinoma cell line, we demonstrated a significant inverse correlation between FG cell proliferation and PTHrP expression that depended on the ECM protein on which the cells were cultured (Grzesiak et al., 2004). Generally, ECM proteins that promoted the strongest proliferation, including types I and IV collagen, and laminin, resulted in decreased expression of PTHrP. Conversely, ECM proteins that promoted the weakest proliferation, including fibronectin (Fn), vitronectin, and BSA, resulted in increased PTHrP expression. A similar trend was found between FG cell proliferation and PTH/PTHrP receptor expression. Along with the results from breast, prostate, and colon cancers described above, where PTHrP regulated ECM axis expression, our observations in pancreatic cancer, where the ECM axis regulates the expression of PTHrP and the PTH/PTHrP receptor, suggest the existence of a feedback loop and a unique functional relationship between the ECM and PTHrP axes that may be important for the progression of desmoplastic cancers.

Table 1. PTHrP axis, IL-6, and IL-8 expression relative to adhesion index in pancreatic cancer cell lines[1]

Cell Line	PTHrP[2] Secreted	Intracellular	PTH/PTHrP receptor[3]	IL-6 secreted[2]	IL-8 secreted[2]	Adhesion Index[4]
AsPC-1	3.5	1.49	+	0	541	4
BxPC-3	59.6	2.8	+	0	1352	1
Capan-1	4.08	1.15	-	27	1532	5
CFPAC-1	28.8	1.72	-	62	1716	2
FG	9.3	1.4	+	NYT	NYT	6
Mia PaCa-2	1.19	0.45	+	0	1678	7
Panc-1	1.34	0.97	+	0	177	3

[1](Bouvet et al., 2001; Bouvet et al., 2002; Grzesiak and Bouvet, 2006; Grzesiak et al., 2005a; Grzesiak et al., 2005b);

[2]Data expressed as pg/94 hr/μg cellular protein;

[3]PTH/PTHrP receptor expression in various pancreatic cell lines was determined using RT-PCR;

[4]Adhesion index is derived by comparing integrin expression and strength of adhesion on types I and IV collagen, fibronectin, laminin-1, and vitronectin between the different cell lines, with 1>7 (Grzesiak et al., 2006; Grzesiak et al., 2005b);

NYT – not yet tested.

Cells attach to the ECM through integrins, the family of heterodimeric transmembrane receptor proteins that are also involved in the transmission of intracellular signals inside the cell (Hynes, 2002; Julianc, 2002; Ruoslahti, 1991; Ruoslahti, 1996; Ruoslahti et al., 1994). Examination of the potential signaling interactions between the ECM and PTHrP pathways in pancreatic cancer revealed that, under serum-free conditions, $\alpha_5\beta_1$ integrin-mediated adhesion to Fn resulted in a phenotype that included a reduction in cell proliferation, increased E-cadherin-mediated cell-cell adhesion, increased β-catenin localization throughout the cell, inhibition of cell migration, and increased expression of PTHrP, as well as interleukin-6 (IL-6), and interleukin-8 (IL-8) relative to $\alpha_2\beta_1$ integrin-mediated adhesion on type I collagen (Figure 2) (Grzesiak et al., 2005a). A phosphoprotein immunoblotting screen of FG pancreatic cancer cells grown on either Fn or type I collagen indicated that GSK3 and PKB/Akt, among others, were differentially phosphorylated on these two substrates, implicating cell-cell adhesion architecture, including E-cadherin, β-catenin, as well as downstream signaling effectors, GSK3 and PKB/Akt, in the integrin-mediated regulation of PTHrP, IL-6 and IL-8 in pancreatic cancer.

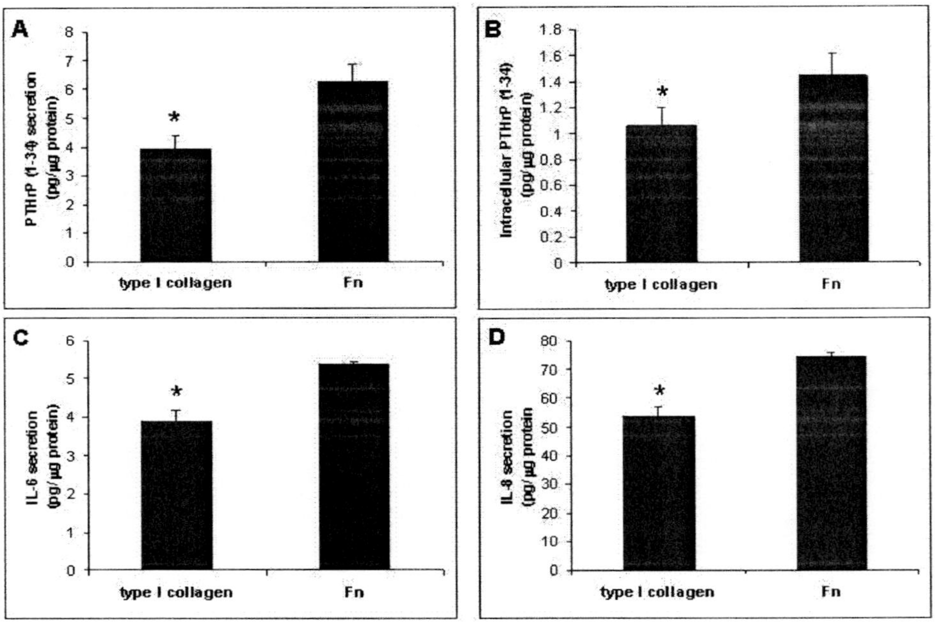

Figure 2. PTHrP, IL-8 and IL-6 are increased on Fn and decreased on type I collagen in FG pancreatic adenocarcinoma cells. Cell lysates were prepared and conditioned media from FG cells grown on Fn or type I collagen in triplicate wells were harvested after 96h. Secreted (A) and intracellular (B) PTHrP levels were measured utilizing an in-house radioimmunoassay developed using antibodies to the amino-terminus (amino acids 1-34) of PTHrP. Conditioned media were also tested for IL-6 (C) and IL-8 (D) secretion by ELISA. Results represent the mean ± SEM of triplicate wells from five experiments. * = $p < 0.05$ (Grzesiak et al., 2005a).

Extending our observations in FG cells to other pancreatic cancer cell lines we found that ECM-dependent differences in E-cadherin and β-catenin localization along with GSK3 and PKB/Akt phosphorylation occur in multiple pancreatic cancer cell lines, resulting in differences in ECM-mediated migration and IL-6, IL-8, and PTHrP expression that are generally consistent with previous observations in FG cells (Grzesiak et al., 2005b). Our functional studies with chemical inhibitors suggest further that GSK3 and PKB/Akt are involved in the integrin-mediated regulation of PTHrP, IL-6, and IL-8 expression in pancreatic cancer.

Collectively, these data indicate that $\alpha_2\beta_1$ integrin-mediated type I collagen adhesion disrupts cell-cell adhesion architecture resulting in increased migration and decreased PTHrP, IL-6, and IL-8 expression in pancreatic cancer cells. This highly proliferative and migratory phenotype on type I collagen is further characterized by increased phosphorylation of GSK3 and PKB/Akt. By contrast, $\alpha_5\beta_1$ integrin-mediated Fn adhesion increases cell-cell adhesion architecture resulting in decreased migration, increased PTHrP, IL-6, and IL-8 expression, and decreased phosphorylation of GSK3 and PKB/Akt in pancreatic cells.

Besides its function in the stabilization of E-cadherin-mediated cell-cell adherens junctions on the cytoplasmic side of the plasma membrane (Takeichi, 1991), β-catenin has also been shown to play a critical role in intracellular signaling (Wong and Pignatelli, 2002), where GSK3 is a key component in the β-catenin signaling pathway (Doble and Woodgett, 2003). Phosphorylation of β-catenin by GSK3 leads to its dissociation from the adherens complex and transfer of the protein to the cytosol, where it exists in a soluble, monomeric state (Wong and Pignatelli, 2002). Cytosolic β-catenin may subsequently be degraded or translocate to the nucleus, where it binds with a member of the lymphoid enhancer factor/T-cell factor (Lef/Tcf) family of transcription factors to form a complex that activates target genes by binding to their promoter regions (Brantjes et al., 2002; Wong and Pignatelli, 2002). The E-cadherin, Fn, and IL-8 genes all contain consensus Lef/Tcf binding domains in their promoter regions, and have been previously shown to be direct targets of β-catenin/Lef/Tcf transcriptional activator complexes (Gradl et al., 1999; Huber et al., 1996; Levy et al., 2002).

The consensus Lef/Tcf DNA binding sequence is (A/T)(A/T)CAAAGG (Huber et al., 1996; Levý et al., 2002; Mangin et al., 1990). Interestingly, the PTHrP gene also contains a potential Lef/Tcf DNA binding sequence between exons 1A and 1B (Mangin et al., 1990). In support of the involvement of Lef/Tcf and β-catenin in the mechanism of PTHrP expression, PTHrP signaling has been shown to regulate the epidermal and mesenchymal expression of Lef-1 and β-catenin during embryonic breast development (Foley et al., 2001). This indicates that such changes in cell fate involve an interaction between the PTHrP and β-catenin signaling pathways.

In light of our results, it appears that Fn, a known survival factor (Jan et al., 2004; Lee and Ruoslahti, 2005), could be promoting a slower-growing, non-migratory phenotype, at least in part, by activation of Lef/Tcf target genes, including potentially PTHrP, that appear to be upregulated in pancreatic cancer cells grown on Fn. Type I collagen, by contrast, may promote a faster-growing, migratory phenotype in pancreatic cancer cells, at least in part, by downregulation of cell-cell adhesion architecture, leading to the downregulation of Lef/Tcf target genes.

Parathyroid Hormone-Related Protein and Heat Shock Protein 70 in Cancer Cells

Recent studies indicate that the oncogenic functions of PTHrP and its derived peptides cannot be attributed solely to the G protein-coupled PTH/PTHrP receptor binding via its N-terminus. There is accumulating and compelling evidence that mid-region and C-terminal forms of PTHrP also generated through processing of native isoforms, can mediate growth-regulating effects absent binding to the classical PTH/PTHrP receptor that PTHrP shares with PTH (Clemens et al., 2001; Cornish et al., 1999; Cornish et al., 1997; De Miguel et al., 1999; Goltzman, 1999; Goomer et al., 2000; Hastings et al., 2003; Lanske et al., 1999; Maioli and Fortino, 2004; Nissenson, 2000; Strewler, 2000; Strid et al., 2002). These studies implicate the existence of receptors to non-amino terminal peptides of PTHrP that have been demonstrated but not yet cloned.

Using affinity chromatography, 2-D gel electrophoresis, and mass spectroscopy, we have recently identified cell surface-expressed heat shock protein-70 (HSP70) as the major PTHrP-binding protein from cancer cell lines, including pancreatic, prostate, and osteosarcoma (Grzesiak et al., 2006; Grzesiak et al., 2005c) (Figure 3). HSP70 antibody inhibition studies resulted in increased PTHrP secretion, decreased total cell protein, and differentially regulated proliferation of these cancer cell lines (Figure 4). These studies indicate a novel interaction between PTHrP and surface-expressed HSP70 in cancer cells with cytoprotective consequences.

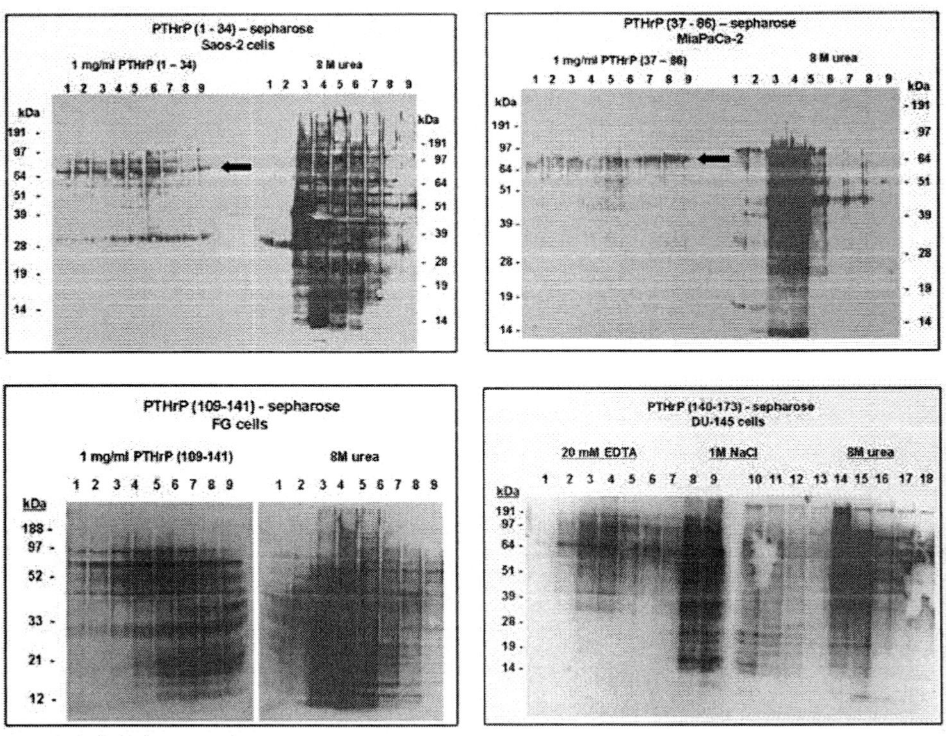

Figure 3. Interaction of cell-surface biotinylated proteins from cancer cell extracts on PTHrP peptide–sepharose by affinity chromatography. Extracts of cell-surface biotinylated proteins from osteosarcoma, pancreatic cancer, and prostate cancer cells were applied onto PTHrP (1-34), (37-86), (109-141), and (140-173) – Sepharose 4B, the columns were washed and eluted with either 1 mg/ml PTHrP peptide as indicated, followed by 8 M urea, or with EDTA and NaCl at the indicated concentrations, followed by 8 M urea. The eluted fractions were analyzed on a 12% Bis/Tris NuPAGE gel in MOPS buffer under reducing conditions, transferred to nitrocellulose, incubated with streptavidin-HRP and proteins were visualized using chemiluminescence and autoradiography. Arrows indicate HSP70. Molecular mass markers are indicated (Grzesiak et al., 2005c).

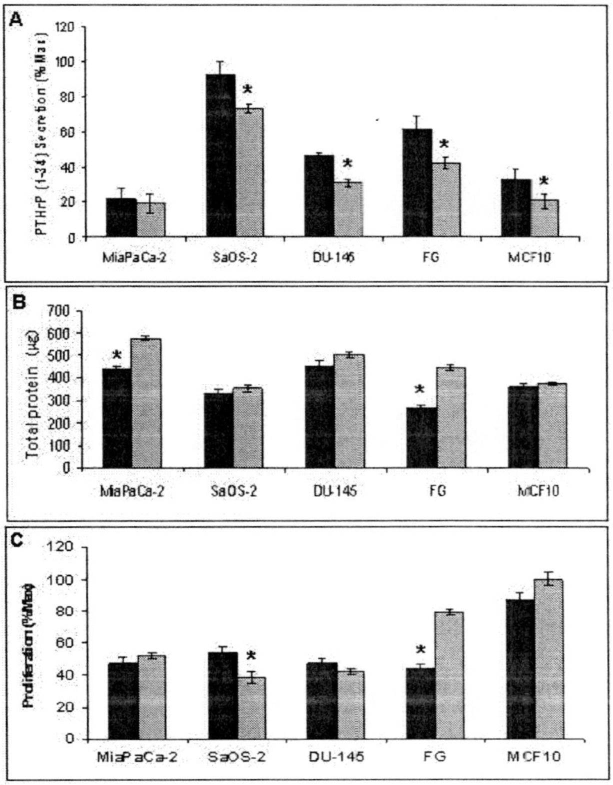

Figure 4. The effect of anti-HSP70 polyclonal antibody on PTHrP secretion, total protein and proliferation of cancer and normal cells after 72h in culture in the presence of 5% serum. 2.5 x 10^5 cells/well of 6-well tissue culture plates were cultured in the presence of polyclonal anti-HSP70 antibody at 25 μg/ml (black bars) or an irrelevant rabbit IgG at 25 μg/ml (gray bars) for 72h. (A) Media from triplicate wells were harvested and assayed for PTHrP (1-34) by radioimmunoassay to assess secretion. Data presented represent the mean ± SEM from three independent experiments. 100% = 2.4 pg/μg protein. P values were derived from two-tailed Student's t-test. * $p<0.05$ (B) Cell lysates were prepared from the experiments described in (A) and assayed for total protein using BioRad protein assay according to manufacture's instructions. Black bars – anti-HSP70. Grey bars – irrelevant rabbit IgG. Data presented represent the mean ± SEM from three independent experiments. *$p<0.05$. (C) Proliferation assays were conducted in the presence of polyclonal anti-HSP70 antibody at 25 μg/ml or irrelevant rabbit IgG at 25 μg/ml using the CellTiter 96 Aqueous One Solution Cell Proliferation Assay according to manufacture's instructions (Promega, Madison, WI). The absorbance at 450 nm at T=0 is subtracted from the absorbance at 450 nm at 72 hours and expressed as % Max considering all five cell lines. Data presented represent the mean ± SEM from three independent experiments *$p<0.05$. (Grzesiak et al., 2005c).

HSP70 has recently been shown in a number of studies to be among a set of chaperone proteins expressed on the surface of many types of cancer cells, including neuroblastoma, lung, and colon adenocarcinoma, acute lymphoblastic leukemia, and ovarian tumor cell lines (Botzler et al., 1998; Multhoff et al., 1995; Okazaki et al., 2000; Shin et al., 2003; White et al., 1995; Xiao et al., 1999), as well as freshly isolated human biopsy material of colorectal, lung, neuronal, and pancreatic carcinomas, liver metastases, and leukemic blasts of patients with acute myelogenous leukemia (Hantschel et al., 2000). These observations were extended by our recent studies, where cell surface-expressed HSP70 from DU-145 prostate cancer cells was also demonstrated (Grzesiak et al., 2006; Grzesiak et al., 2005c).

The functions of HSP70 inside of normal cells and at the cancer cell surface in particular, include productive substrate or "client" protein folding to the native state, membrane translocation, multiprotein complex maintenance in activation-competent states, and direction of misfolded and short-lived proteins to proteosomal degradation pathways (Mosser and Morimoto, 2004). The PTH/PTHrP receptor shares in the membrane translocation function of HSP70 in that PTHrP binding to its receptor triggers internalization of the whole complex (Maioli and Fortino, 2004). These intriguing results suggest that HSP70 expressed at the cell surface may be the PTHrP "receptor", and is itself involved in the internalization of PTHrP peptides, which results in overall growth-promoting or cytoprotective effects in cancer. It is worth noting that all the PTHrP peptides used in these studies, including amino acids (1-34), (37-86), (109-141), and (140-173), bound HSP70 by affinity chromatography. Besides the suggestion that HSP70 may be the receptor for non-amino terminal peptides of PTHrP, these data also suggest a second and cancer cell-specific pathway for the internalization of the N-terminal peptide of PTHrP (amino acids 1-34) in addition to the classical PTH/PTHrP receptor in cancer.

HSP70 present at the cell surface may also act in the presentation of PTHrP to its cognate receptor. In either case, mechanisms are obviously in place to traffic HSP70 to the cell surface. It seems reasonable to posit that the same mechanisms could work in reverse, transporting HSP70 and its bound peptides into the cell as well. A relationship between PTHrP and stress-related genes, including the co-chaperone HSP90, has precedent in studies demonstrating that PTHrP (67–86) regulates the expression of stress proteins in breast cancer cells, inducing modifications in urokinase-plasminogen activator and matrix metalloproteinase-1 expression, and results in increased tumor cell invasiveness (Luparello et al., 2003). HSP90 is more specialized to capture and hold client proteins in intermediate conformations with refolding of denatured substrates requiring transfer to the HSP70/HSP40 chaperone machine (Mosser and Morimoto, 2004). Interestingly, HSP90, which is found bound to PTHrP (140-173) in affinity chromatography experiments with DU-145 prostate cancer cells, appears to have selective capacities to associate with client proteins involved in cell signaling, including nuclear hormone receptors and protein kinases (Mosser and Morimoto, 2004).

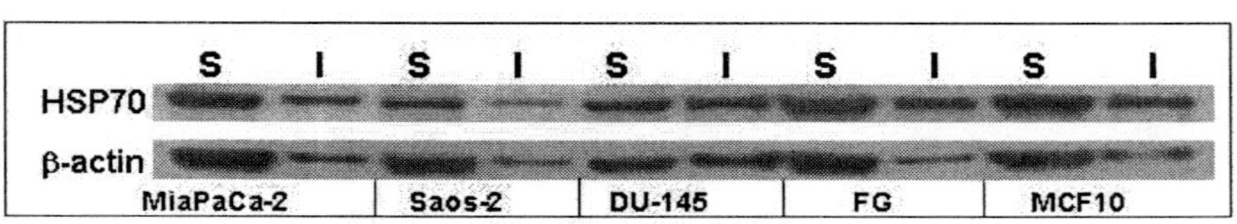

Figure 5. HSP70 is expressed in both the soluble and insoluble fractions of cancer cell lysates. Whole cell lysates were prepared for each cell line, and the soluble (S) and insoluble (I) fractions (5 μg protein/lane) were analyzed by immunoblotting for HSP70 and β-actin expression (Grzesiak et al., 2005c).

HSP70 has been shown previously to exist in two forms within epithelial cells; a major detergent soluble form and a minor detergent insoluble form associated with detergent-resistant microdomains (DRMs) where lipid rafts are localized and where HSP70 is thought to function in the plasma membrane (Broquet et al., 2003). We have demonstrated that cell surface-expressed HSP70 is present in both fractions in cancer cells (Grzesiak et al., 2005c) (Figure 5). As stated earlier in this chapter, G-protein coupled receptors, of which the PTH/PTHrP receptor is a member, also localize to lipid rafts where their trafficking is modulated (Chini and Parenti, 2004). Lipid raft theory suggests that cholesterol and sphingolipids partition away from other membrane lipids and that these lipid rafts are important in processes such as signaling and vesicle traffic (Foster et al., 2003). With that in mind, it is well established that HSP70 has the capacity for multiple protein binding. Some of the proteins identified by mass spectroscopy in vivo that bind to HSP70 include keratin, actin, HSP60, and elongation factors 1 and 2 (Grossmann et al., 2004). Although not differentiating between cell surface and intracellular expression, it is notable that mass spectroscopy analyses of eluates from PTHrP (140–173)-Sepharose affinity chromatography of DU-145 prostate cancer cell extracts identified a complex mixture of proteins, including keratin, actin, elongation factors 1 and 2, and HSP60 and HSP90 as well as other proteins (Tables 2 and 3). Additionally, proteins involved in membrane trafficking and cytoskeletal rearrangement with cytoprotective consequences were also found bound to PTHrP (140–173). These included heat shock proteins 84 and 90, actin, tubulin, myosin alkali light chain, and profilin-2 (Witke, 2004). Taken together, these novel protein–protein interactions further support the hypothesis that the C-terminus of PTHrP plays a role in cancer cell survival, and suggest that HSP70 present on the surface of cancer cells is involved in the mechanism regulating the biological function of PTHrP peptides.

Table 2. Identification of proteins bound to PTHrP (140-173)-Sepharose from DU-145 prostate cancer cell extracts by mass spectroscopy using MALDI/MS methodology

Protein	MW	p value
actin	41.33	1.9×10^{-3}
40S ribosomal protein S12	14.90	0.086
peroxiredoxin 1	22.32	0.024
PKC inhibitor protein-1	28.46	0.014
ATP synthase beta subunit	51.18	6.1×10^{-6}.
beta-tubulin	50.25	0.018
HSP84	83.59	0.014
HSP90	85.04	2.6×10^{-9}
elongation factor 2b	58.17	3.4×10^{-5}

Fractions eluted with 8 M urea from affinity chromatography experiments using DU-145 prostate cancer cells and PTHrP (140-173) – Sepharose-4B were pooled, concentrated, and electrophoresed. Gels were Coomassie blue-stained, the visible bands were excised, digested with trypsin, and the peptides analyzed by matrix-assisted laser desorption ionization mass spectrometry (MALDI/MS). p values<0.05 were considered significant (Grzesiak et al., 2006).

As described earlier in this chapter, PTHrP increases the integrin-mediated adhesion of pancreatic and other cancer cells to the extracellular matrix (ECM) (Grzesiak et al., 2004;

Grzesiak et al., 2005a; Grzesiak et al., 2005b; Luparello et al., 1999; Shen and Falzon, 2003; Shen and Falzon, 2005; Shen et al., 2004) through as yet unknown mechanisms. In particular, we have shown that growth on Fn increases PTHrP expression relative to type I collagen (Figure 2) (Grzesiak et al., 2004; Grzesiak et al., 2005a; Grzesiak et al., 2005b). This increased PTHrP expression on Fn is associated with strong cell-ECM and cell-cell adhesion and decreased migration relative to type I collagen. Recent studies demonstrate that HSP70 prevents the caspase-3-mediated cleavage of focal adhesion kinase (FAK) at the plasma membrane by binding FAK (Mao et al., 2003). FAK is a non-receptor tyrosine kinase recruited to focal adhesion complexes upon integrin ligation (Juliano, 2002). FAK plays important roles in cell motility and in the control of apoptosis. It is intriguing to speculate that if HSP70 is the "receptor" or part of the cancer cell machinery that binds PTHrP peptides at the cell surface, it is possible that PTHrP could be involved in the complex with HSP70 and FAK at the plasma membrane, providing a potential mechanism for the observed effects of the ECM on PTHrP expression in pancreatic cancer, and perhaps, other desmoplastic cancers as well.

Table 3. Identification of DU-145 prostate cancer cell proteins bound to PTHrP (140-173)-Sepharose by mass spectroscopy using Nano LC/MS/MS

Protein	MW	Mascot score
40S ribosomal protein S12	14.90	153
60S ribosomal protein L30	13.11	137
profilin-2	15.42	101
myosin alkali light chain	17.70	95
peroxiredoxin 1	22.32	405
peroxiredoxin 3	27.71	182
DJ-1 protein	19.83	106
S3 ribosomal protein	26.87	206
14-3-3-pro	28.46	448
ribosomal protein SA	32.99	107
elongation factor 1-alpha 1	50.47	411
elongation factor 1 gamma	50.46	278

Fractions were prepared as described for Table 2 and analyzed by nano-liquid chromatography/tandem mass spectrometry (Nano-LC/MS/MS). Mascot search results yielding scores >69 are considered significant at the >95% confidence level (Grzesiak et al., 2006).

Parathyroid Hormone-Related Protein as a Survival Factor in Lung Cancer

PTHrP has been studied extensively in lung cancer because of its relation to humoral hypercalcemia of malignancy. PTHrP is expressed in more advanced, aggressive tumors, and has effects on apoptosis in many malignant and nonmalignant cells. Thus, it also may play an active role in cancer progression. We recently investigated the effects of PTHrP on apoptosis in BEN cells, a human squamous lung carcinoma cell line (Hastings et al., 2003). Cells were treated for 24 h with 100 nmol/L PTHrP (1–34), (38–64), (67–86), (107–139), or (140–173). Cells were then exposed for 30 min to 50 mJ/cm^2 ultraviolet (UV)-B light. The activities of caspases 3, 8, and 9 increased five-fold 24 h after UV exposure in the absence of PTHrP peptides. PTHrP (1–34) and (140–173) reduced caspase 3 activity after UV exposure (mean ± SEM reduction, 19 ± 4% and 29 ± 7%, respectively), with similar effects on caspases 8 and 9. The two peptides increased cell protein levels, and PTHrP (140–173) augmented clonal survival after UV exposure. Other PTHrP peptides had no effects. PTHrP (140–173) also reduced the activation of all three caspases after the ligation of Fas by neutralizing antibody, but neither peptide ameliorated the activation of caspases 3 and 9 after staurosporine administration, which elicited a solely mitochondria-dependent apoptotic pathway. UV light exposure causes Fas clustering, indicating that it initiates a death receptor pathway in BEN cells. Collectively, these data indicate that PTHrP (1–34) and (140–173) protect against apoptosis in lung cancer cells, as evidenced by reduced caspase activity and increased cell survival. The effects appear to be mediated at or upstream of caspase 8.

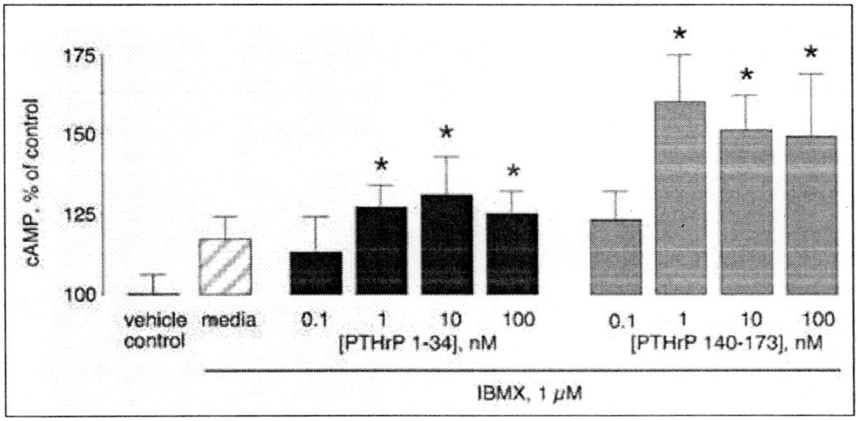

Figure 6. In BEN lung cancer cells, 10-min stimulation with PTHrP-(1–34) and PTHrP-(140–173) augmented cAMP content in a dose-dependent manner. Between the lowest and highest doses of PTHrP-(1–34), the increase in cAMP was 15% of basal levels whereas the levels for PTHrP-(140–173) increased about 35%. Data represent results from 3–6 cell-containing wells/group from 3 independent experiments (* $p < 0.05$ vs. 0.1 nM PTHrP peptide) (Hastings et al., 2004).

Signaling studies indicated further that PTHrP (1-34) and PTHrP (140-173) increased cAMP levels in BEN lung cancer cells by 15-35% in a dose-dependent manner, suggesting signaling through protein kinase A (PKA) (Figure 6) (Hastings et al., 2004). In support of this hypothesis, the PKA inhibitor H89 abrogated the protective effects of both peptides against caspase activation and DNA loss (Figure 7). In BEN cells, PKA activation by forskolin, 3-isobutyl-1-methylxanthine (IBMX), or 8-(4-chlorophenylthio)adenosine 3',5'-cyclic monophosphate mimicked the effects of PTHrP peptides in attenuating apoptosis. In addition, H89 augmented apoptosis after UV exposure as indicated by caspase-3 activation, cell DNA loss, and morphological criteria. Studies with IBMX and varying doses of forskolin indicated that small increases in cAMP, on the order of those generated by IBMX alone and the PTHrP peptides were sufficient to protect lung cancer cells from apoptosis. These data indicate that PTHrP (1-34) and PTHrP (140-173) stimulate PKA in lung carcinoma cells and protect cells against UV-induced caspase-3 activation and DNA fragmentation. PKA activation by other means has also been shown to induce resistance to apoptosis, and the protective effect of the PTHrP peptides are blocked by PKA inhibition. Thus PKA appears to play a role in the mechanism of PTHrP-mediated lung cancer cell survival. The induction of a cAMP response also suggests that PTHrP (140-173) could engage a G protein coupled receptor, although the identity of such a receptor remains unresolved.

As described earlier in this chapter, HSP70 binding to FAK protects cells from caspase-3-mediated FAK cleavage. Furthermore, HSP70 has been localized to the cell membrane by binding to HSP70-associated scaffolding complexes with G protein-coupled receptors and a host of other structural and signaling proteins. Though speculative, the reduced activities of caspases, including caspase-3, by PTHrP (1-34) and (140-173) add further support to the hypothesis that PTHrP may directly or indirectly, through association with HSP70 and/or FAK, protect cancer cells against apoptosis. These PTHrP-mediated protective effects against apoptosis may contribute to lung cancer cell survival and promote cancer progression.

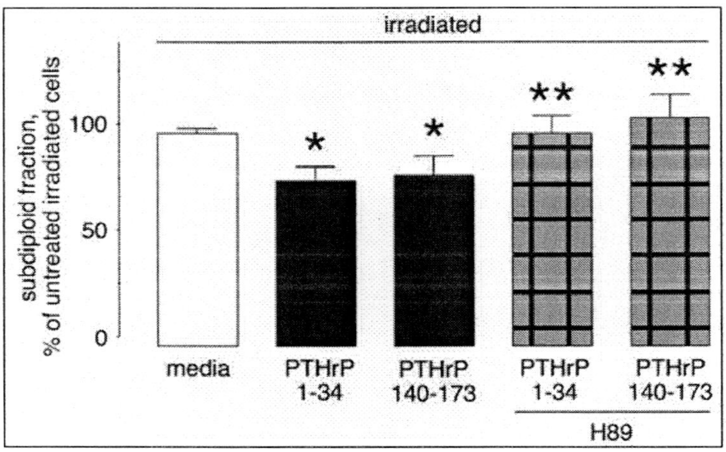

Figure 7. PKA inhibition abrogates the protective effect of PTHrP peptides against DNA loss after UV. DNA distributions were measured by flow cytometry to assess apoptosis. PTHrP (1-34) and (140-173) treatment reduced the percentage of UV-irradiated cells with subdiploid DNA content from 27.3 ± 0.5% to 21.0 ± 1.3% and 23.4 ± 2.4%, respectively (*$p<0.05$ vs. cells with no peptide treatment). However, in the presence of H89, a PKA inhibitor, the levels of apoptosis were not significantly different from levels in control irradiated cells (**$p<0.05$ vs. corresponding group without H89) (Hastings et al., 2004).

Parathyroid Hormone-Related Protein Effects in Prostate Cancer

PTHrP levels are greater in malignant prostate tissue than in hyperplastic and normal prostate (Asadi et al., 1996; Deftos, 2000; Iwamura et al., 1993; Wu et al., 1998). Furthermore, mRNA levels and intensity of PTHrP immunostaining correlate with increasing tumor grade (Iwamura et al., 1993; Iwamura et al., 1995; Perez-Martinez et al., 2006; Wu et al., 1998). PTHrP expression in malignant prostate cell lines also correlates with tumor invasiveness and metastatic potential: PC-3 cells, derived from a prostatic bone metastasis, produce greater levels of PTHrP than LNCaP or DU-145 cells, derived from lymph node and brain metastases, respectively (Deftos et al., 2005; Iwamura et al., 1994). PTHrP acts as a growth regulator of many different cell types and studies by us and our colleagues have demonstrated that PTHrP expression promotes prostate tumor development, growth, progression and metastasis (Deftos et al., 2005; Dougherty et al., 1999; Iddon et al., 2000; Iwamura et al., 1994; Rabbani et al., 1999; Tovar Sepulveda and Falzon, 2002).

In the prostate, as in other tissues, PTHrP is processed into distinct peptides that have unique biological effects (Cramer et al., 1996; Deftos, 2000; Deftos et al., 2001; Iwamura et al., 1996). Our own studies, along with those of other investigators, have also demonstrated novel growth regulatory effects of PTHrP through its derived peptides (Asadi and Kukreja, 2005; Tovar Sepulveda and Falzon, 2002). We, like other investigators, have observed that PTHrP transfection (intracrine) and treatment (endocrine) of cancer cells have different effects on the expression of cytokines that regulate cancer cell growth (Gujral et al., 2001). Furthermore, we found that these differences are due to the intracrine effects of PTHrP, independent of the classical N-terminal moieties of the oncoprotein and dependent on novel non-amino terminal forms (Gujral et al., 2001).

Sizing studies indicate that PC-3 and LNCaP cells process PTHrP to smaller forms, likely those that respectively stimulate and inhibit osteoclast activity (Hook et al., 2001; Iwamura et al., 1996). Prostatic expression of PTHrP is associated with regulatory effects and interactions (e.g., with cytokines and oncoproteins) that are important in the development and progression of prostate cancer (Asadi and Kukreja, 2005; Deftos, 2000; Gujral et al., 2001). However, the molecular mechanisms of these interactions have not been elucidated. Several studies indicate further that PTHrP measurements might have diagnostic and prognostic value for the tumor (Iddon et al., 2000; Imamura et al., 1991; Perez-Martinez et al., 2006).

Prostate cancer metastasis to bone is associated with increased osteoblast activity (Asadi and Kukreja, 2005; Deftos et al., 2005; Iddon et al., 2000; Philbrick, 2001; Rabbani et al., 1999). The osteoblastic phenotype of metastatic prostate cancer lesions results largely from the actions of several stimulatory factors produced by prostate cancer cells, such as ornithine decarboxylase (ODC) which catalyzes the decarboxylation of ornithine producing, as a result, diamine putrescine. This is the first and rate-limiting step in humans for the production of polyamines, compounds required for cell division (Asadi et al., 2001). The identification of the receptor activator of nuclear factor kappa B ligand (RANKL), its cognate receptor RANK, and its decoy receptor, osteoprotegerin (OPG) has led to a new molecular perspective on osteoclast biology and bone homeostasis (Hofbauer et al., 2000). Most prostate cancer cells express these proteins and we hypothesized that metastatic prostate carcinomas utilize the OPG/RANK/RANKL pathway to localize to the bone (Chen et al., 2006). Our studies indicate that OPG expression is increased by treatment of prostate cancer cells in vitro with PTHrP (1-34) and (38-64), and was decreased by PTHrP (109-138). PTHrP (140-173) stimulated OPG levels in PC-3 and PPC-1 cells but inhibited OPG levels in Dupro-1 cells (Ahmadpour et al., 2002). RANKL expression was inhibited by PTHrP (140-173) in most of the prostate cancer cell lines. PTHrP (140-173) treatment increased IL-6 expression in 267B1 cells, but decreased the IL-8 levels in 267B1 and LNCaP cells (Ahmadpour et al., 2002). We also examined the intracrine effects of PTHrP by transfecting DU-145 cells with full-length PTHrP and mutant (without the 1-32 amino acid region) expression plasmids. Deletion of the

Table 4. Genes regulated by PTHrP 33-173 in DU-145 prostate cancer cells (Tsigelny et al., 2005)

Upregulated genes	Expression with PTHrP 33-173 transfection* (%)	Downregulated genes	Expression with PTHrP 33-173 transfection* (%)
Class 1 major histocompatibility complex proteins		**Cell-Matrix/Cytoskeleton-related proteins**	
HLA-A	224	Sterile alpha motif domain containing 4, SAMD4	22
HLA-B	200	Dual-specificity tyrosine-(Y)-phosphorylation-regulated kinase 4	33
HLA-C	201	Myosin light polypeptide kinase, MYLK	10
HLA-F	180	Transmembrane 4 superfamily member 2, TM4SF2	34
HLA-G	242	Lysyl oxidase-like 2, LOXL2	37
Proteasome-related proteins		Dicer1, Dcr-1 homolog, DICER1	34
Proteasome (prosome, macropain) subunit, beta type, 8	358		
Proteasome (prosome, macropain) subunit, beta type, 9	318		
Ring finger protein 1, RING1	249		
Arachidonic acid pathway proteins			
Glutathione peroxidase 1, GPX1	200		
Glutathione peroxidase 3, GPX3	718		
Proteins mediating cell-cell interactions			
E-cadherin, CDH1	334		
P-cadherin, CDH3	229		
Nuclear proteins			
Basic leucine nuclear zipper factor Jem-1, BLZF1	221		
Kruppel-like factor 3, KLF3	197		
Zinc finger protein 305, ZNF305	229		

*Expression is presented as a % of the expression by the vector-only transfected control cells.

(1-32) region from the PTHrP plasmids prevented the decrease in RANK expression levels, indicating that the (1-32) region was critical for these changes (Figure 8). Conversely, deletion of the (1-32) region from the PTHrP expression plasmids had no significant effects on the increased ODC levels compared to controls, indicating that a non-amino terminal PTHrP region was responsible for the increase. There were also differences in the expression of IL-8 and OPG/RANK/RANKL levels in the PTHrP (1-173)-transfected cells compared to the PTHrP (1-139)- and (1-141)-transfected cells, indicating a biological function for the 140-173 region (Ahmadpour et al., 2002; Gujral et al., 2001). It is evident from these studies that

PTHrP and the peptides derived from its processing can have multiple and varying biological effects in different tissues and in different preparations of the same tissue.

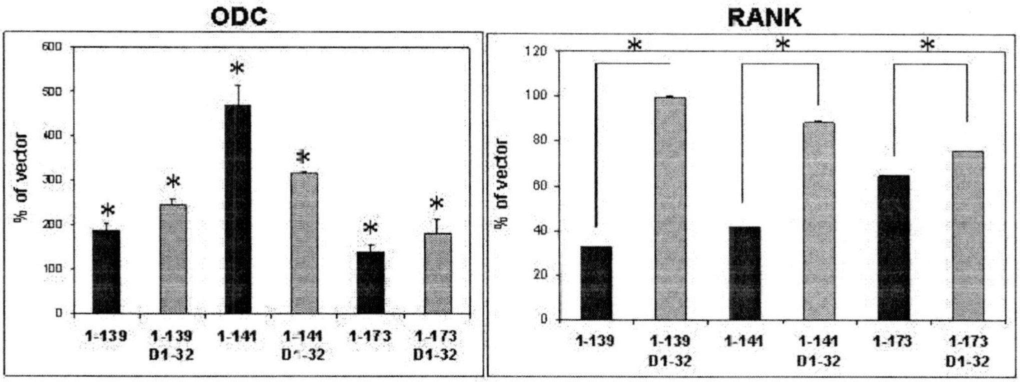

Figure 8. PTHrP increases ornithine decarboxylase (left panel) and decreases RANK (right panel) expression in prostate cancer cells. DU-145 cells transformed with PTHrP expression plasmids (n = 2-3 independent clones/group) were analyzed for ODC (left panel) and RANK (right panel) mRNA levels by qPCR and compared to vector control levels. A non-amino terminal PTHrP peptide (33-141) appears to be responsible for the robust increase in ODC expression, and the PTHrP (1-32) moiety causes the decrease in RANK mRNA levels. * $p<0.05$ based on two-tailed Student t-tests (Ahmadpour et al., 2002).

In a related study using microarray technology to identify genes regulated by PTHrP in the human prostate carcinoma cell line DU-145, we compared gene expression profiles between cells transfected with vector-only control, PTHrP (1-173), and (33-173) (Tsigelny et al., 2005). This strategy provided a means to distinguish between the effects of N-terminal PTHrP and the rest of the molecule. For example, a gene that was upregulated only by PTHrP (1-32) would be upregulated by PTHrP (1-173) and not by (33-173), while one that was under the control of a region within PTHrP (33-173) would be upregulated by both constructs. Analysis of these cDNA expression profiles in DU-145 prostate cancer cells demonstrated non-overlapping groups of differentially expressed genes (Table 4). N-terminal PTHrP generally affected groups of genes involved in apoptosis, prostaglandin and sex steroid metabolism, cell-matrix interactions, and cell differentiation, while PTHrP (33-173) caused substantial increases in MHC class I antigen expression.

We also examined DU-145 cells prostate cancer cells genetically transformed to stably express various PTHrP peptides as well as wild-type control cells for their effect on apoptosis (Maheshwari et al., 2003). Apoptosis was induced using gamma radiation and PTHrP's effect was evaluated using clonogenic-cell survival assays. Multiple clones of DU-145 PTHrP (1-173)-expressing cells demonstrated a 2-10 fold increase in colony formation after receiving a 4 Gy radiation dose compared to the vector transformed cells ($p < 0.01$). Conversely, DU-145 PTHrP (1-87)- and (1-141)-expressing cells demonstrated a 30-50% decrease in colony formation after gamma radiation (4 Gy) compared to the vector-only control cells (Figure 9) (Maheshwari et al., 2003) We also evaluated staurosporine-induced apoptosis on the same cells and evaluated PTHrP's effect on nuclear condensation and caspase-3 and -9 activities. The DU-145 PTHrP (1-173)-expressing cells showed reductions in nuclear condensation and caspase-3 and -9 activities ($p < 0.01$ and $p < 0.05$, respectively) compared to the vector-only control cells. DU-145 PTHrP (1-87)- and (1-141)- expressing cells increased caspase-3 and -9 activities compared to vehicle-only control cells. The effect of PTHrP on staurosporine-induced apoptosis was further studied using exogenous PTHrP peptides in wild-type DU-145 cells. PTHrP (140-173) peptide treatment decreased caspase-3 and -9 activities and nuclear condensation compared to vehicle treated cells. No significant effects on nuclear condensation and caspase-3 or -9 were observed with treatment using PTHrP (1-34) or scrambled PTHrP (140-173) peptide. Since no protective effects were observed for PTHrP (1-34), (1-87), or (1-141), these results indicate that the human-specific (140-173) region is responsible for the anti-apoptotic properties of PTHrP in prostate cancer cells. These data are seemingly at odds with the microarray studies, where the (1-32) region of PTHrP up-regulated genes involved with apoptosis in DU-145 cells, and with the lung cancer cell studies, where both PTHrP (1-32) and (140-173) were protective against apoptosis. It is important to note that the microarray studies utilized PTHrP-transfected cells, while the staurosporine and lung cancer studies both used exogenous PTHrP. This is an excellent example of the differential and often confounding effects that transfection (intracrine) versus exogenous (paracrine) expression of PTHrP and its processed peptides may have on the same cell line and in cells from different tissues.

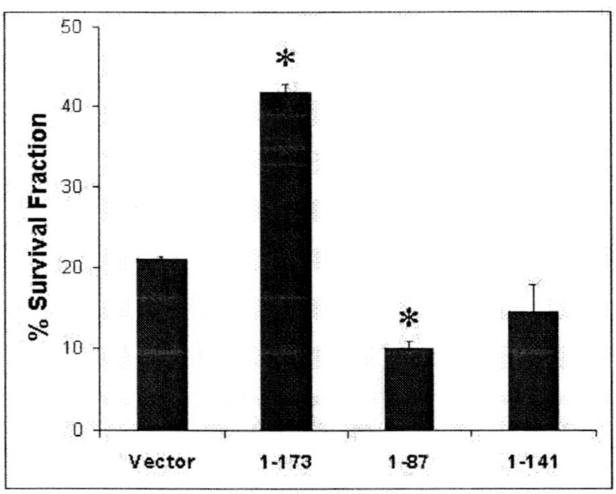

Figure 9. PTHrP (1-173) is anti-apoptotic in gamma irradiated prostate cancer cells. The DU-145/PTHrP stable cell lines were gamma irradiated with 4 Gy and replated into 60-mm dishes. After 14 days in culture, colonies (>50 cells) were counted. Two independent clones were used for each group. (*$p<0.05$ vs. vector control) (Maheshwari et al., 2003).

Parathyroid Hormone-Related Protein and Androgens

Further analysis of the expression profiles generated from DU-145 prostate cancer cells by microarray described above also demonstrated substantial differences between the effects of PTHrP (1-173) and the vector-transfected DU-145 cells on the expression of the aldo-keto reductase family. Three members of the aldo-keto reductase family, AKR1C1, AKR1C2, and

AKR1C3, were increased 8-14 fold in DU-145 cells transfected with PTHrP (1-173) compared to vector-only control cells (Table 5). This finding is notable because only 9 of the genes probed by the U133A chip (Affymetrix, Inc.), approximately 0.04% of the total, code for proteins with aldo-keto reductase activity, yet 18% of the genes with Gene Ontology (GO) terms upregulated by PTHrP (1-173) fall into that category. The three aldo-keto reductase genes are all located on chromosome 10p15 (Tsigelny et al., 2005). Since prostate tissue utilizes AKR1C3 predominantly (Penning et al., 2000), we focused further studies on this isoform.

Table 5. Genes regulated by PTHrP 1-173 but unaffected by PTHrP 33-173 in DU-145 prostate cancer cells (Tsigelny et al., 2005)

Upregulated genes	Expression with PTHrP 1-173 transfection*(%)	Downregulated genes	Expression with PTHrP 1-173 transfection*(%)
Transforming growth factor, beta 2	265	Tumor necrosis factor receptor superfamily, member 25	20
Interferon, gamma-inducible protein 16	264	Pre-B-cell leukemia transcription factor 1	23
ALL1-fused gene from chromosome 1q	271	Kinesin family member 5C	39
Interferon-induced protein 44	344	Butyrylcholinesterase	21
Caspase 10, apoptosis-related cysteine protease	255	Somatostatin	31
Zinc finger protein 288	281	Hypothetical protein FLJ23235	34
Cysteine-rich with EGF-like domains 1	253	Hypothetical protein FLJ23548	39
I factor (complement)	494	Hypothetical protein DKFZp434N1235	12
Rab coupling protein	292	Potassium intermediate/small conductance	
Syndecan 2	253	Calcium-activated channel, subfamily N, member 2	16
Aldo-keto reductase family 1, member C1	991	Lysyl oxidase	32
Aldo-keto reductase family 1, member C2	1328	Diphtheria toxin receptor	36
Aldo-keto reductase family 1, member C3	785	Intestinal cell kinase	37
Hypothetical protein FLJ12616	260	Connexin 43	29
Nebulette	277	Connective tissue growth factor	33
p8 protein (candidate of metastasis 1)	263	Adipose differentiation-related protein	34
Junction plakoglobin	298	Myotubularin-related protein 2	38

*Expression is presented as a % of the expression by the vector-only transfected control cells.

AKRs, also known as hydroxysteroid dehydrogenases, play pivotal roles in cellular differentiation of prostate cells by regulating prostaglandin metabolism and the biosynthesis and inactivation of the potent androgen, 5α-dihydrotestosterone (Asadi et al., 2001; Bauman et al., 2004; Fung et al., 2006; Ji et al., 2003; Penning et al., 2000; Penning et al., 2001; Penning et al., 2004; Penning et al., 2006; Yuan et al., 2006). Using PTHrP (1-139), (1-141), and (1-173) expression plasmids in quantitative PCR and immunoblotting studies, we confirmed the gene chip results described above (Tsigelny et al., 2005), and showed that transfected PTHrP increased AKR1C3 expression 3-15 fold in LNCaP and DU-145 cells (Figure 10). Deletion of the amino-terminal (1-32) or the nuclear localization sequence (NLS) (87-106) regions of PTHrP prevented the increase in AKR1C3 expression compared to vector-only control cells. These data indicate that the N-terminal (1-32) and the NLS (87-106) regions of PTHrP are both required for the upregulation of AKR1C3, and indicate that PTHrP has an important role in AKR regulation. The AKR pathway reveals a novel mechanism whereby PTHrP can regulate prostate tissue progression from normal to benign prostate hyperplasia (BPH) or adenocarcinoma by modulating steroid levels. Further definition of the molecular interactions between PTHrP and the AKR family will lead to an improved knowledge of the growth regulatory effects of PTHrP as well as an initial step towards the identification of potential diagnostic and therapeutic targets for prostate cancer.

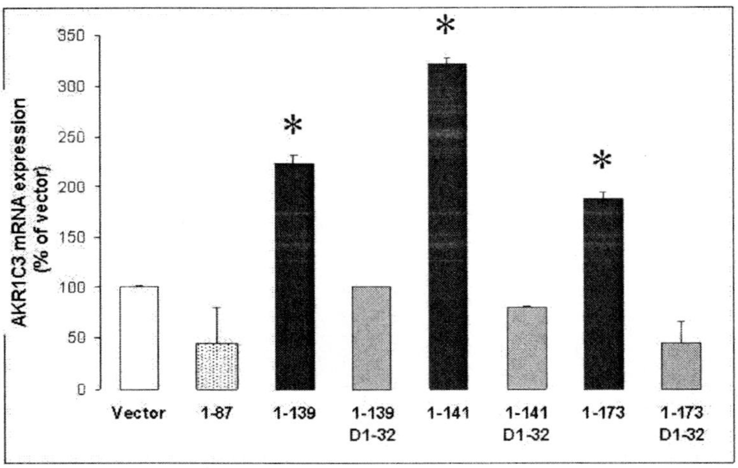

Figure 10. AKR1C3 mRNA is upregulated by PTHrP (1-139), (1-141), and (1-173) but not by PTHrP (1-87) or the amino terminal deletion (D1-32) PTHrP mutants. These results are based on qPCR using DU-145 prostate cancer cells stably transformed with the various PTHrP expression plasmids. The asterisks indicate significant differences ($p<0.05$) compared to vector. The results are derived from 4 independent experiments (Ahmadpour et al., 2002).

The Nuclear Export of Parathyroid Hormone-Related Protein

As discussed earlier in this chapter for lung and prostate cancer cells, PTHrP has distinct proliferative and anti-apoptotic roles that are affected by nucleocytoplasmic shuttling (Henderson et al., 1995; Massfelder et al., 1997). The protein's nuclear export is sensitive to leptomycin B, consistent with a chromosome region maintenance protein 1(CRM1)-dependent pathway (Fornerod et al., 1997). We recently determined that the 109-139 region of PTHrP was involved in its nuclear export by demonstrating that a C-terminal truncation mutant, residues 1-108, exports at a reduced rate, compared with the wild-type 139 amino acid isoform (Pache et al., 2006). We searched for potential nuclear export sequences within the 109-139 region, which is leucine rich. Comparisons with established nuclear export sequences identified a putative consensus signal at residues 126-136. Deletion of this region resulted in nuclear export characteristics that closely matched those of the C-terminal truncation mutant. Confocal microscopic analyses of transfected 293, COS-1, and HeLa cells showed that steady-state nuclear levels of the truncated and deletion mutants were significantly greater than levels of wild-type PTHrP and were unaffected by leptomycin B (LMB), unlike the wild-type protein (Figure 11). In addition, both mutants demonstrated greatly reduced nuclear export with assays using nuclear preparations and intact cells. Based on these results, we conclude that the 126-136 amino acid sequence closely approximates the structure of a CRM1-dependent leucine-rich nuclear export signal and is critical for nuclear export of PTHrP.

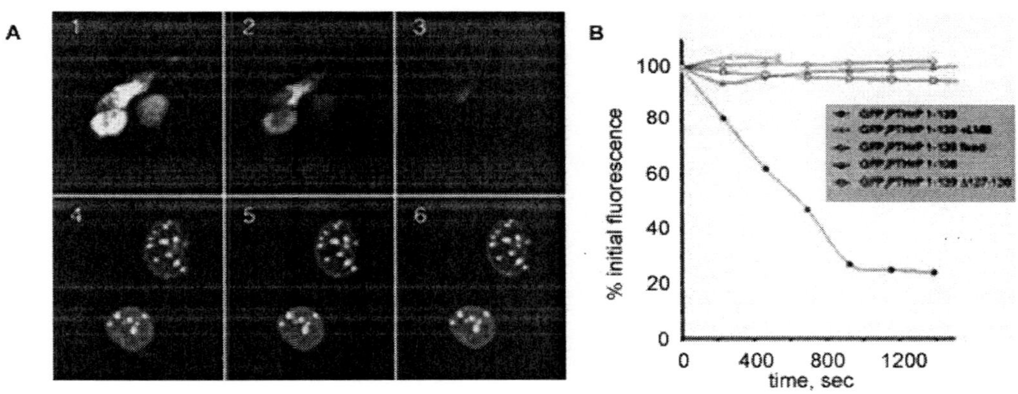

Figure 11. Time course for nuclear export of GFP_3-PTHrP constructs using *in vitro* assays. (A) Permeabilized COS-1 cells transiently transfected with GFP-PTHrP (1–139) (panels 1, 2, and 3) or GFP-PTHrP 1–139 Δ127–136 (panels 4, 5, and 6) demonstrate nuclear fluorescence. Export of the chimeric protein from the nucleus was initiated by adding RanGTP, a small co-factor necessary for CRM1-mediated export, at time 0 (panels 1 and 4). Nuclear fluorescence from the wild-type protein progressively decreased after 700 sec (panel 2) and 1400 sec (panel 3), indicating nuclear export. Fluorescence was virtually unchanged over the same periods (panels 5 and 6) for the deletion mutant. (B) Nuclear fluorescence as a percentage of the initial value is plotted vs. time beginning at the point of adding RanGTP to the transport buffer. The group of untreated, non-fixed cells transfected with wild-type GFP_3-PTHrP (1–139) was the only one in which nuclear fluorescence declined appreciably with time over 1200 sec. Fixing the cells in 3.7% paraformaldehyde to prevent export physically, treatment with LMB, truncation of the PTHrP sequence at residue 108, or deletion of pNES3 in GFP_3-PTHrP (1–139 Δ127–136) construct abrogated the decrease in nuclear fluorescence completely. The curves are representative of assays from three to five cells per experimental group (Pache et al., 2006).

Parathyroid Hormone-Related Protein Processing

The earliest studies of PTHrP processing were based on biochemical analyses and were limited to the identification of multiple size forms of the polypeptide (Brandt et al., 1994; Deftos et al., 2001; Deftos, 1993; Hook et al., 2001). The application of immunochemical procedures allowed tentative identification of some of these multiple forms (Brandt et al., 1991; Ratcliffe et al., 1990). However, the persistent limitations of these studies, discussed subsequently, have not permitted the documentation of PTHrP processing with scientific methodology that is up to the standards set by comparable studies of other precursor polypeptides that are processed into peptide hormones (Dey et al., 2005; Orloff et al., 1994; Paterson et al., 2004; Raffin-Sanson et al., 2003).

Several investigators have shown indirectly that PTHrP can be processed. Ratcliffe, et al., were among the first to attempt PTHrP processing studies (Emly et al., 1992; Ratcliffe et al., 1990). They assessed PTHrP forms in biological fluids by radioimmunoassay, gel filtration chromatography, and immunoblotting; and they identified several peaks with mobility's similar to those of PTHrP and some of its synthetic fragments. While confirming the presence of immuno- and bio-active PTHrP forms, post-translational processing of the polypeptide was revealed to be complex and variable. The same group studied PTHrP forms in conditioned media from human and rat cell lines by gel-filtration chromatography, immunoassays, and bioassays (Emly et al., 1992). They showed evidence of N-terminal species in the molecular mass ranges of 10-18 kDa and 24-25 kDa, suggesting that processing occurs at the C-terminus and within the mid-region to form N-terminal fragments.

We have examined the production of PTHrP to determine the predominant species produced by human cells. Guanidine hydrochloride extracts analyzed by HPLC estimated molecular sizes ranging from 3.5-11.7 kDa (Brandt et al., 1991; Deftos et al., 1989). Furthermore, we observed PTHrP heterogeneity among these different cell types, which we hypothesize to be tissue-specific processing (Brandt et al., 1991; Deftos et al., 2001; Deftos, 1993; Deftos et al., 1989; Hook et al., 2001; Tsigelny et al., 2005).

Other investigators also conducted experiments aimed at characterizing PTHrP peptides (Soifer et al., 1992; Wu et al., 1991; Wu et al., 1996; Yang et al., 1994). Using an anti-PTHrP (1-36) antibody column, they affinity purified human PTHrP secreted under conditions of protease protection and showed that human keratinocyte-conditioned medium contained a single 18 kDa form of the peptide. In contrast to recombinant and synthetic PTHrP's, which migrated as distinct, well-focused bands on SDS-PAGE, this PTHrP 18 kDa peptide displayed the broad electrophoretic profile of a glycoprotein.

This group also harvested media from human renal cells (SKRC-1), human keratinocytes, and rat insulinoma cells stably transfected with cDNA for PTHrP (1-141) (RIN-141 cells) (Soifer et al., 1992). Immunopurified N-terminal and mid-region species were further resolved by RP-HPLC and region-specific immunoassays. The cells secreted three distinct N-terminal species and a then novel, non-amino terminal, mid-region fragment. Sequence and SDS-PAGE analysis indicated that the RIN-141 cell mid-region fragment begins at amino acid 38 of the cDNA-predicted sequence and is approximately 70 amino acids in length. The authors concluded that multiple PTHrP species are secreted, including a novel mid-region fragment, that Arg37 serves as a cleavage site, that PTHrP (1-36) is likely to be a secretory form of PTHrP, and tentatively identified a C-terminal fragment that reacted with PTHrP (109-138) antiserum (Wu et al., 1996; Yang et al., 1994). They postulated three distinct mid-region PTHrP species: PTHrP (38-94) amide, PTHrP (38-95), and less conclusively, PTHrP (38-101) (Soifer et al., 1992; Wu et al., 1996; Yang et al., 1994). Recent studies by our laboratory have demonstrated that processing likely applies to the human specific PTHrP (1-173), and generates a functional (140-173) peptide (Goomer et al., 2000).

Early pulse-chase studies by Rabbani, et al., examined the processing of endogenous PTHrP in cultured rat H-500 Leydig cells pulse-labeled with [^{3}H]-Ile and analyzed by affinity chromatography employing an antibody directed against PTHrP (1-34) followed by gel-filtration or RP-HPLC (Rabbani et al., 1993). Although they tentatively identified three molecular forms of PTHrP co-migrating with (1-36), (1-86), and (1-141) standards; the identification was indirect and compromised by the low-specific activity of radiolabled PTHrP.

Notwithstanding these studies by productive investigators, it is important to note that most have been by immunochemical and limited biochemical procedures and have not been well represented by complementary metabolic labeling and pulse-chase studies necessary for cellular confirmation of in vitro studies. Thus, many controversies still exist about the identification of PTHrP–derived peptides in biological fluids and tissues (Chorev, 2001; Deftos, 2005). For example, the N-terminal form of PTHrP is presumed to be generated by cleavage at Arg37, but most biological studies have been conducted on the shorter PTHrP (1-34) peptide (Soifer et al., 1992; Wu et al., 1996). This difference of just a few amino acids is not trivial as has been shown for PTH and is likely to apply to PTHrP as well. The deletion of just one N-terminal amino acid can destroy its biological activity (Chorev, 2001; Fiaschi-Taesch and Stewart, 2003; Gao and D'Amour, 2005). Similar considerations apply to the mid-region of PTHrP, which stimulates intracellular calcium translocation in several cell types, affects the viability and growth of several cell lines, and promotes transplacental calcium transport from the maternal to the fetal circulation (Care et al., 1990; Gao and D'Amour, 2005; Strewler, 2000).

Like the N-terminus, there remains controversy about the exact structure of the mid-region peptide as well; early studies identified it as (67-86) (Wu et al., 1996), cell culture studies identify it as (38-94), and in vivo studies suggest a mid-molecule of (37-67) (Emly et al., 1992; Strid et al., 2002; Yang et al., 1994). Our own studies indicate that the mid-molecule can generate several sub-peptides (Deftos et al., 2001; Hook et al., 2001; Tsigelny et al., 2005). And Luparello, et al., showed opposing effects of PTHrP (38-94) and (67-86) in breast cancer cells (Luparello et al., 2001; Luparello et al., 2003). Furthermore, some of the studies are cross-species despite the lack of exact homology among PTHrP forms (Diefenbach-Jagger et al., 1995; Meerovitch et al., 1997). And there are no published studies of the processing of 1-173, although in vitro studies demonstrate biological action for its far-C-terminal region (Ditmer et al., 1996; Goomer et al., 2000; Tsigelny et al., 2005).

At this time, a critical assessment of the processed forms commonly recognized for PTHrP includes only PTHrP (1-34/37), (38-94), a sub-peptide of 107-139 (likely 107-111), and, based on our studies, (140-173), even though the structure of PTHrP predicts over 90 possible peptides (Deftos, 2001; Philbrick, 2001; Strewler, 2000). While these and other PTHrP forms have been identified, most of these characterizations have been based only on immunochemical procedures. Most important, the vast majority of the peptides that can be predicted for PTHrP have yet to be identified in any manner.

A full appreciation of the cellular and molecular biology, as well as physiology and pathobiology of PTHrP requires conclusive identification of its processed peptides. To address the hurdle for metabolic labeling studies imposed by PTHrP's scarcity of methionines that can be labeled with ^{35}S for classical pulse-chase studies, we have genetically engineered a methionine-rich PTHrP expression plasmid (Figure 12) that retains the naturally occurring methionine residues at positions -36, 159, and 162, and has mutations of leucine to methionine residues at positions -32, 8, 68, 83, and 126. We demonstrated in immunochemical studies that expressed PTHrP (1-173) (5L-M) is indistinguishable from native PTHrP and can be transfected and metabolically labeled with high specific activity. Using classical protocols (Eskeland et al., 1996), we demonstrated in preliminary studies of the processing of these methionine-rich mutants that PTHrP activity can be immunoprecipitated with antibodies to PTHrP (Figure 13). This metabolic labeling method can be complemented by the attendant biochemical and immunochemical procedures discussed earlier. Also as discussed earlier, we expect that different cell types will yield different profiles of processed PTHrP peptides. We should thus be able to compare the processing signatures for the different cell types. In concert with biological studies of PTHrP-derived peptides, these profiles should yield basic and much-needed information about the effects of PTHrP moieties on cell function in different cell types.

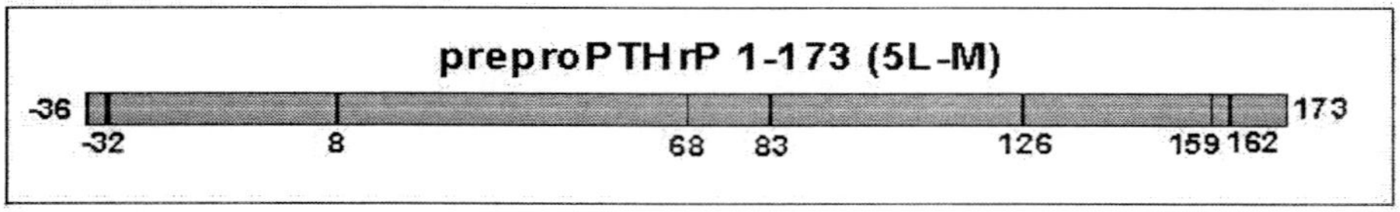

Figure 12. Diagram of the preproPTHrP (1-173)(5L-M) mutant showing the mutated methionine residues. The naturally occurring methionine residues are at positions -36, 159, and 162. The mutated leucine to methionine residues are at positions -32, 8, 68, 83, and 126.

Some of the PTHrP peptides seemingly derived from native forms have been studied for their biological effects (Fenton et al., 1991; Iwamura et al., 1996; Meerovitch et al., 1997). The N-terminus of PTHrP is well-studied as PTHrP (1-34), even though it is presumed to be generated by processing at Arg37 (Emly et al., 1992; Soifer et al., 1992; Wu et al., 1991). Studies of other PTHrP-derived peptides have corresponding limitations. While some studies have shown PTHrP (107-139) to be a potent direct inhibitor of osteoclastic bone resorption, the biological relevance of the identification of a unique and non-amino-terminal functional domain for PTHrP remains controversial (Fenton et al., 1991; Strewler, 2000). In functional mutation studies of PTHrP (1-173), we identified the C-terminal sequences as responsible for the intracellular degradation of this polypeptide, which may regulate the amount of processed and secreted PTHrP (Goomer et al., 2000; Tsigelny et al., 2005). In transfection studies, we demonstrated that PTHrP (140-173) is growth regulating and that the tetrabasic (147-150) motif determines how PTHrP (1-173) regulates collagen synthesis and levels of extracellular inorganic pyrophosphate (Ppi) (Goomer et al., 2000). Synthetic PTHrP (38-94) markedly inhibited cell proliferation and accelerated cell death in breast cancer cells, whereas (67-86) had opposing actions; in addition, the nucleus appears to be a destination for PTHrP (38-94) (Jans et al., 2003; Luparello et al., 2001; Luparello et al., 2003). Curiously, in rat hippocampal slices, PTH (1-34) induced cell toxicity while PTHrP (1-34) did not (Hirasawa et al., 2000). As stated earlier, the often inconclusive and sometimes contradictory nature of these studies support the need for definitive identification of the amino acid structures of PTHrP-derived peptides and for functional studies that evaluate the biological activities of PTHrP-derived peptides produced by different cell types.

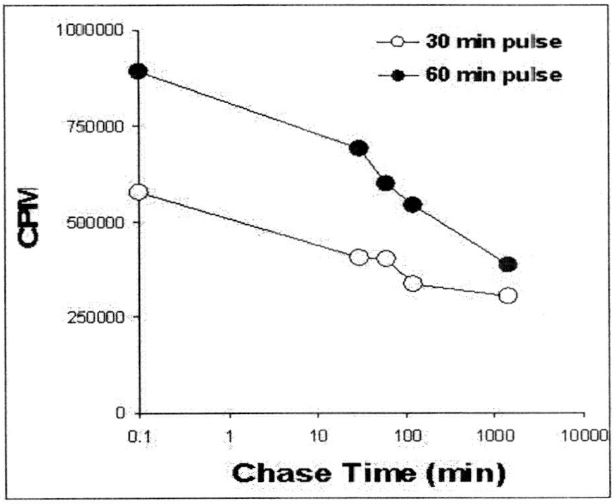

Figure 13. Pulse-chase study of cells stably transfected with PTHrP (1-173)(5L-M). COS-1/PTHrP (1-173)(5L-M) cells were plated at 70% confluency and pulse-labeled with ^{35}S-methionine for the indicated times in methionine-deficient DMEM with 5% FBS. After removing the labeling media and washing the cells, normal growth medium was added for the indicated times (chase). The conditioned media and cell extracts were collected and the labeled PTHrP proteins were immunoprecipitated with anti-PTHrP (1-34) antibody. After washing, the pellets were counted using a beta scintillation counter. These results demonstrate the incorporation of radiolabel in an amino-terminal antibody precipitable form of PTHrP that declines with time, consistent with the processing of this species. Additional analyses can be accomplished by the appropriate immunochemical and biochemical procedures, notably SDS-PAGE.

Conclusion

In conclusion, our studies of PTHrP pathobiology in various cancers demonstrate novel mechanisms involved in the regulation of PTHrP gene expression and peptide processing as well as novel functions for PTHrP independent of its N-terminus. These include regulatory interactions with the ECM in pancreatic cancer, where PTHrP appears to be part of a set of "survival factor" proteins preferentially expressed in pancreatic cancer cells grown on ECM substrates that yield a relatively slower growing, non-migratory phenotype such as Fn. The up-regulated expression of PTHrP on Fn is associated with well defined cell-cell adhesion architecture, and activation of downstream signaling effectors like β-catenin and GSK3 that are associated with Lef/Tcf target gene expression. Future studies will be aimed at the definitive determination of PTHrP as a Lef/Tcf target gene and the signaling effectors mediating this regulatory pathway. Additionally, the specific regions of PTHrP involved in the regulatory loop with the ECM axis will also be explored.

In multiple cancer cell types, including pancreatic, prostate, and osteosarcoma, we also demonstrate a novel and cancer cell-specific interaction between cell surface-expressed HSP70 and peptides of PTHrP spanning the human protein sequence, absent the NLS, with apparent cytoprotective consequences. These data suggest that HSP70 may be the elusive "receptor" or part of the cell surface mechanism regulating the functional effects of non-amino terminal PTHrP peptides. These data also indicate the potential for an additional and cancer cell-specific pathway for function of the N-terminal PTHrP peptide apart from the classical PTH/PTHrP receptor. Future studies include the elucidation of the precise mechanism and functional significance of these potentially exploitable cancer cell-specific interactions between PTHrP and HSP70 at the cell surface.

A role for PTHrP (1-34) and PTHrP (140-173) in the protection of UV-induced caspase activation and apoptosis in lung carcinoma cells has also been demonstrated. This cytoprotective effect against apoptosis appears to be mediated upstream of the caspases by PKA, indicating that PKA plays a role in the mechanism of PTHrP-mediated lung cancer cell survival. Future studies include investigation of the hypothesis that PTHrP peptides inhibit the activation of death receptor pathways, and determination of upstream intermediates and targets of PKA involved in the mechanism of PTHrP-mediated protection from apoptosis in lung cancer cells.

In prostate cancer, we have demonstrated various effects of PTHrP and its processed peptides. These include inhibition of apoptosis and regulation of IL-8 and OPG/RANK/RANKL, as well as the AKR family. As discussed earlier for lung cancer, further definition of the mechanisms regulating the anti-apoptotic effects of PTHrP and its processed peptides, both N- and C-terminal, in prostate cancer, as well as the novel molecular interactions between PTHrP and the AKR family should lead to an improved knowledge of the growth regulatory effects of PTHrP.

We also demonstrated that PTHrP exports from the nucleus via the CRM1 pathway via a leucine-rich NES and that the PTHrP (126-139) region is critical for this function. The physiological relevance of this NES-mediated PTHrP export is the subject of current studies.

And finally, we discussed the current standing of vital research relating to PTHrP processing. While PTHrP forms have been identified, most of these characterizations have been immunochemical in nature. Conclusive identification of the amino acid structures of PTHrP-derived peptides and functional studies that evaluate the biological activities of these peptides in different cell types remains a difficult hurdle that must be overcome for a complete understanding of the functions of PTHrP in vivo.

Ultimately, the PTHrP-related research efforts in different cancers discussed in this chapter should result in the identification of potential diagnostic and therapeutic targets for the treatment of, not only these, but other cancers as well.

Acknowledgements

The authors would like to acknowledge the contributions of Drs. Tracy Downs, Igor Tsigelny, and Jared Pache, as well as the Bouvet, Deftos, and Hastings laboratories in the conduct of this research. This work was funded by VA Merit grants from the Department of

Veterans Affairs (M.B., R.H.H., and L.J.D.), National Institutes of Health grants DK60588 and AR47347 (L.J.D.), CA109949-01 (M.B.), National Cancer Institute grant 5P30 CA14089-24 (L.J.D.), Robert E. and Mary R. Wright Foundation, USC Research Center for Liver Disease grant DK98-016 (LJD), State of California Cancer Research Program grant 1PF0263 (LJD), the Flight Attendants Medical Research Institute (R.H.H.), the University of California Tobacco-Related Disease Research Program (R.H.H.), American Cancer Society grant RSG-05-137-01-CCE (M.B.), and a National Pancreas Foundation grant (M.B.).

REFERENCES

Ahmadpour, O.A., D.W. Burton, S. Tu, and L.J. Deftos. 2002. Regulation of OPG/RANK/RANKL by PTHrP peptides in human protstate cancer cells. *J Bone Min Res. 17(S)*:286.

Asadi, F., M. Faraj, S. Malakouti, and S.C. Kukreja. 2001. Effect of parathyroid hormone related protein, and dihydrotestosterone on proliferation and ornithine decarboxylase mRNA in human prostate cancer cell lines. *Int Urol Nephrol. 33*:417-22.

Asadi, F., M. Farraj, R. Sharifi, S. Malakouti, S. Antar, and S. Kukreja. 1996. Enhanced expression of parathyroid hormone-related protein in prostate cancer as compared with benign prostatic hyperplasia. *Hum Pathol. 27*:1319-23.

Asadi, F., and S. Kukreja. 2005. Parathyroid hormone-related protein in prostate cancer. *Crit Rev Eukaryot Gene Expr. 15*:15-28.

Bardeesy, N., and R.A. DePinho. 2002. Pancreatic cancer biology and genetics. *Nat Rev Cancer*. 2:897-909.

Bauman, D.R., S. Steckelbroeck, and T.M. Penning. 2004. The roles of aldo-keto reductases in steroid hormone action. *Drug News Perspect. 17*:563-78.

Binkley, C.E., L. Zhang, J.K. Greenson, T.J. Giordano, R. Kuick, D. Misek, S. Hanash, C.D. Logsdon, and D.M. Simeone. 2004. The molecular basis of pancreatic fibrosis: common stromal gene expression in chronic pancreatitis and pancreatic adenocarcinoma. *Pancreas. 29*:254-63.

Botzler, C., J. Schmidt, A. Luz, L. Jennen, R. Issels, and G. Multhoff. 1998. Differential Hsp70 plasma-membrane expression on primary human tumors and metastases in mice with severe combined immunodeficiency. *Int J Cancer. 77*:942-8.

Bouvet, M., S.R. Nardin, D.W. Burton, C. Behling, J.M. Carethers, A.R. Moossa, and L.J. Deftos. 2001. Human pancreatic adenocarcinomas express parathyroid hormone-related protein. *J Clin Endocrinol Metab. 86*:310-6.

Bouvet, M., S.R. Nardin, D.W. Burton, N.C. Lee, M. Yang, X. Wang, E. Baranov, C. Behling, A.R. Moossa, R.M. Hoffman, and L.J. Deftos. 2002. Parathyroid hormone-related protein as a novel tumor marker in pancreatic adenocarcinoma. *Pancreas. 24*:284-90.

Brandt, D.W., D.W. Burton, A.F. Gazdar, H.E. Oie, and L.J. Deftos. 1991. All major lung cancer cell types produce parathyroid hormone-like protein: heterogeneity assessed by high performance liquid chromatography. *Endocrinology. 129*:2466-70.

Brandt, D.W., W. Wachsman, and L.J. Deftos. 1994. Parathyroid hormone-like protein: alternative messenger RNA splicing pathways in human cancer cell lines. *Cancer Res. 54*:850-3.

Brantjes, H., N. Barker, J. van Es, and H. Clevers. 2002. TCF: Lady Justice casting the final verdict on the outcome of Wnt signalling. *Biol Chem. 383*:255-61.

Broquet, A.H., G. Thomas, J. Masliah, G. Trugnan, and M. Bachelet. 2003. Expression of the molecular chaperone Hsp70 in detergent-resistant microdomains correlates with its membrane delivery and release. *J Biol Chem. 278*:21601-6.

Care, A.D., S.K. Abbas, D.W. Pickard, M. Barri, M. Drinkhill, J.B. Findlay, I.R. White, and I.W. Caple. 1990. Stimulation of ovine placental transport of calcium and magnesium by mid-molecule fragments of human parathyroid hormone-related protein. *Exp Physiol. 75*:605-8.

Chen, G., K. Sircar, A. Aprikian, A. Potti, D. Goltzman, and S.A. Rabbani. 2006. Expression of RANKL/RANK/OPG in primary and metastatic human prostate cancer as markers of disease stage and functional regulation. *Cancer. 107*:289-98.

Chini, B., and M. Parenti. 2004. G-protein coupled receptors in lipid rafts and caveolae: how, when and why do they go there? *J Mol Endocrinol. 32*:325-38.

Chorev, M.J., and M. Rosenblatt. 2001. Interactions of parathyroid hormone and parathyroid hormone-related protein with their receptors. *In The Parathyroids*. Vol. Chapter 4. R.M. JP Bilezikian, and A Levine, editor. Academic Press, San Diego, CA. pp. 53-92.

Clemens, T.L., S. Cormier, A. Eichinger, K. Endlich, N. Fiaschi-Taesch, E. Fischer, P.A. Friedman, A.C. Karaplis, T. Massfelder, J. Rossert, K.D. Schluter, C. Silve, A.F. Stewart, K. Takane, and J.J. Helwig. 2001. Parathyroid hormone-related protein and its receptors: nuclear functions and roles in the renal and cardiovascular systems, the placental trophoblasts and the pancreatic islets. *Br J Pharmacol. 134*:1113-36.

Cornish, J., K.E. Callon, C. Lin, C. Xiao, J.M. Moseley, and I.R. Reid. 1999. Stimulation of osteoblast proliferation by C-terminal fragments of parathyroid hormone-related protein. *J Bone Miner Res. 14*:915-22.

Cornish, J., K.E. Callon, G.C. Nicholson, and I.R. Reid. 1997. Parathyroid hormone-related protein-(107-139) inhibits bone resorption in vivo. *Endocrinology. 138*:1299-304.

Cramer, S.D., Z. Chen, and D.M. Peehl. 1996. Prostate specific antigen cleaves parathyroid hormone-related protein in the PTH-like domain: inactivation of PTHrP-stimulated cAMP accumulation in mouse osteoblasts. *J Urol. 156*:526-31.

De Miguel, F., P. Martinez-Fernandez, C. Guillen, A. Valin, A. Rodrigo, M.E. Martinez, and P. Esbrit. 1999. Parathyroid hormone-related protein (107-139) stimulates interleukin-6 expression in human osteoblastic cells. *J Am Soc Nephrol. 10*:796-803.

Deftos, L.J. 2000. Prostate carcinoma: production of bioactive factors. *Cancer*. 88:3002-8.

Deftos, L.J. 2001. Immunoassays for PTH and PTHrP. In: *The Parathyroids*, Second Edition, JP Bilezikian, R. Marcus, and A Levine (eds.), Chapter 9, pp. 143-165.

Deftos, L.J., I. Barken, D.W. Burton, R.M. Hoffman, and J. Geller. 2005. Direct evidence that PTHrP expression promotes prostate cancer progression in bone. *Biochem Biophys Res Commun. 327*:468-72.

Deftos, L.J., D. Burton, R.H. Hastings, R. Terkeltaub, and V.Y. Hook. 2001. Comparative tissue distribution of the processing enzymes "prohormone thiol protease," and prohormone convertases 1 and 2, in human PTHrP-producing cell lines and mammalian neuroendocrine tissues. *Endocrine*. *15*:217-24.

Deftos, L.J., Burton, D.W., Hastings, R.J. 2005. PTHrP and cancer: prostate and lung. *In* Bone metastasis: experimental and clinical therapeutics. Vol. Chapter 10. S.A.R. G. Singh, editor. Humana Press, Totowa, N.J. p. 147.

Deftos, L.J., Fieck, A., Burton, D.W., Tu, S., Ditmer, L.S., Petrin, E.M., Bohoun, C., Smeekins, S.P., and Brandt, D.W. 1993. Expression of the endoproteolytic convertases by endocrine and neuroendocrine tumors. *Endocrine Journal*. *1*:285-289.

Deftos, L.J., A.F. Gazdar, K. Ikeda, and A.E. Broadus. 1989. The parathyroid hormone-related protein associated with malignancy is secreted by neuroendocrine tumors. *Mol Endocrinol*. *3*:503-8.

Dey, A., G.M. Lipkind, Y. Rouille, C. Norrbom, J. Stein, C. Zhang, R. Carroll, and D.F. Steiner. 2005. Significance of prohormone convertase 2, PC2, mediated initial cleavage at the proglucagon interdomain site, Lys70-Arg71, to generate glucagon. *Endocrinology*. *146*:713-27.

Diefenbach-Jagger, H., C. Brenner, B.E. Kemp, W. Baron, J. McLean, T.J. Martin, and J.M. Moseley. 1995. Arg21 is the preferred kexin cleavage site in parathyroid-hormone-related protein. *Eur J Biochem*. *229*:91-8.

Ditmer, L.S., D.W. Burton, and L.J. Deftos. 1996. Elimination of the carboxy-terminal sequences of parathyroid hormone-related protein 1-173 increases production and secretion of the truncated forms. *Endocrinology*. *137*:1608-17.

Doble, B.W., and J.R. Woodgett. 2003. GSK-3: tricks of the trade for a multi-tasking kinase. *J Cell Sci*. *116*:1175-86.

Dougherty, K.M., E.A. Blomme, A.J. Koh, J.E. Henderson, K.J. Pienta, T.J. Rosol, and L.K. McCauley. 1999. Parathyroid hormone-related protein as a growth regulator of prostate carcinoma. *Cancer Res*. *59*:6015-22.

Emly, J.F., W.A. Ratcliffe, E. Green, S.J. Bowden, D.A. Heath, A. Blight, S. Hughes, and J.G. Ratcliffe. 1992. Immunochemical characterisation of parathyroid hormone-related protein from tumour and non-tumour cells. *Biochim Biophys Acta*. *1180*:58-64.

Eskeland, N.L., A. Zhou, T.Q. Dinh, H. Wu, R.J. Parmer, R.E. Mains, and D.T. O'Connor. 1996. Chromogranin A processing and secretion: specific role of endogenous and exogenous prohormone convertases in the regulated secretory pathway. *J Clin Invest*. *98*:148-56.

Fenton, A.J., B.E. Kemp, G.N. Kent, J.M. Moseley, M.H. Zheng, D.J. Rowe, J.M. Britto, T.J. Martin, and G.C. Nicholson. 1991. A carboxyl-terminal peptide from the parathyroid hormone-related protein inhibits bone resorption by osteoclasts. *Endocrinology*. *129*:1762-8.

Fiaschi-Taesch, N.M., and A.F. Stewart. 2003. Minireview: parathyroid hormone-related protein as an intracrine factor--trafficking mechanisms and functional consequences. *Endocrinology*. *144*:407-11.

Foley, J., P. Dann, J. Hong, J. Cosgrove, B. Dreyer, D. Rimm, M. Dunbar, W. Philbrick, and J. Wysolmerski. 2001. Parathyroid hormone-related protein maintains mammary epithelial fate and triggers nipple skin differentiation during embryonic breast development. *Development*. *128*:513-25.

Fornerod, M., M. Ohno, M. Yoshida, and I.W. Mattaj. 1997. CRM1 is an export receptor for leucine-rich nuclear export signals. *Cell. 90*:1051-60.

Foster, L.J., C.L. De Hoog, and M. Mann. 2003. Unbiased quantitative proteomics of lipid rafts reveals high specificity for signaling factors. *Proc Natl Acad Sci U S A. 100*:5813-8.

Fung, K.M., E.N. Samara, C. Wong, A. Metwalli, R. Krlin, B. Bane, C.Z. Liu, J.T. Yang, J.V. Pitha, D.J. Culkin, B.P. Kropp, T.M. Penning, and H.K. Lin. 2006. Increased expression of type 2 3alpha-hydroxysteroid dehydrogenase/type 5 17beta-hydroxysteroid dehydrogenase (AKR1C3) and its relationship with androgen receptor in prostate carcinoma. *Endocr Relat Cancer. 13:*169-80.

Gao, P., and P. D'Amour. 2005. Evolution of the parathyroid hormone (PTH) assay--importance of circulating PTH immunoheterogeneity and of its regulation. *Clin Lab. 51*:21-9.

Goltzman, D. 1999. Interactions of PTH and PTHrP with the PTH/PTHrP receptor and with downstream signaling pathways: exceptions that provide the rules. *J Bone Miner Res. 14*:173-7.

Goomer, R.S., K.A. Johnson, D.W. Burton, D. Amiel, T.M. Maris, A. Gurjal, L.J. Deftos, and R. Terkeltaub. 2000. The tetrabasic KKKK(147-150) motif determines intracrine regulatory effects of PthrP 1-173 on chondrocyte PPi metabolism and matrix synthesis. *Endocrinology. 141*:4613-22.

Gradl, D., M. Kuhl, and D. Wedlich. 1999. The Wnt/Wg signal transducer beta-catenin controls fibronectin expression. *Mol Cell Biol. 19*:5576-87.

Grossmann, M.E., B.J. Madden, F. Gao, Y.P. Pang, J.E. Carpenter, D. McCormick, and C.Y. Young. 2004. Proteomics shows Hsp70 does not bind peptide sequences indiscriminately in vivo. *Exp Cell Res. 297*:108-17.

Grzesiak, J.J., and M. Bouvet. 2006. The alpha2beta1 integrin mediates the malignant phenotype on type I collagen in pancreatic cancer cell lines. *Br J Cancer. 94*:1311-9.

Grzesiak, J.J., D.W. Burton, L.J. Deftos, and M. Bouvet. 2006. Identification of DU 145 prostate cancer cell proteins that bind to the carboxy-terminal peptide of human PTHrP in vitro. *Peptides. 27*:1898-901.

Grzesiak, J.J., P. Clopton, C. Chalberg, K. Smith, D.W. Burton, S. Silletti, A.R. Moossa, L.J. Deftos, and M. Bouvet. 2004. The extracellular matrix differentially regulates the expression of PTHrP and the PTH/PTHrP receptor in FG pancreatic cancer cells. *Pancreas. 29*:85-92.

Grzesiak, J.J., K.C. Smith, D.W. Burton, L.J. Deftos, and M. Bouvet. 2005a. GSK3 and PKB/Akt are associated with integrin-mediated regulation of PTHrP, IL-6 and IL-8 expression in FG pancreatic cancer cells. *Int J Cancer. 114*:522-530.

Grzesiak, J.J., K.C. Smith, C. Chalberg, D.W. Burton, L.J. Deftos, and M. Bouvet. 2005b. Type I Collagen and Divalent Cation Shifts Disrupt Cell-Cell Adhesion, Increase Migration, and Decrease PTHrP, IL-6, and IL-8 Expression in Pancreatic Cancer Cells. *Int J Gastrointest Cancer. 36*:131-46.

Grzesiak, J.J., K.C. Smith, C. Chalberg, C. Truong, D.W. Burton, L.J. Deftos, and M. Bouvet. 2005c. Heat shock protein-70 expressed on the surface of cancer cells binds parathyroid hormone-related protein in vitro. *Endocrinology. 146*:3567-76.

Gujral, A., D.W. Burton, R. Terkeltaub, and L.J. Deftos. 2001. Parathyroid hormone-related protein induces interleukin 8 production by prostate cancer cells via a novel intracrine mechanism not mediated by its classical nuclear localization sequence. *Cancer Res. 61*:2282-8.

Hantschel, M., K. Pfister, A. Jordan, R. Scholz, R. Andreesen, G. Schmitz, H. Schmetzer, W. Hiddemann, and G. Multhoff. 2000. Hsp70 plasma membrane expression on primary tumor biopsy material and bone marrow of leukemic patients. *Cell Stress Chaperones. 5*:438-42.

Hastings, R.H., F. Araiza, D.W. Burton, M. Bedley, and L.J. Deftos. 2004. Parathyroid hormone-related protein regulates apoptosis in lung cancer cells through protein kinase A. *Am J Physiol Cell Physiol. 287*:C1616-22.

Hastings, R.H., F. Araiza, D.W. Burton, L. Zhang, M. Bedley, and L.J. Deftos. 2003. Parathyroid hormone-related protein ameliorates death receptor-mediated apoptosis in lung cancer cells. *Am J Physiol Cell Physiol. 285*:C1429-36.

Henderson, J.E., N. Amizuka, H. Warshawsky, D. Biasotto, B.M. Lanske, D. Goltzman, and A.C. Karaplis. 1995. Nucleolar localization of parathyroid hormone-related peptide enhances survival of chondrocytes under conditions that promote apoptotic cell death. *Mol Cell Biol. 15*:4064-75.

Hirasawa, T., T. Nakamura, A. Mizushima, M. Morita, I. Ezawa, H. Miyakawa, and Y. Kudo. 2000. Adverse effects of an active fragment of parathyroid hormone on rat hippocampal organotypic cultures. *Br J Pharmacol. 129*:21-8.

Hofbauer, L.C., S. Khosla, C.R. Dunstan, D.L. Lacey, W.J. Boyle, and B.L. Riggs. 2000. The roles of osteoprotegerin and osteoprotegerin ligand in the paracrine regulation of bone resorption. *J Bone Miner Res. 15*:2-12.

Hook, V.Y., D. Burton, S. Yasothornsrikul, R.H. Hastings, and L.J. Deftos. 2001. Proteolysis of ProPTHrP(1-141) by "prohormone thiol protease" at multibasic residues generates PTHrP-related peptides: implications for PTHrP peptide production in lung cancer cells. *Biochem Biophys Res Commun. 285*:932-8.

Huber, O., R. Korn, J. McLaughlin, M. Ohsugi, B.G. Herrmann, and R. Kemler. 1996. Nuclear localization of beta-catenin by interaction with transcription factor LEF-1. *Mech Dev. 59*:3-10.

Hynes, R.O. 2002. Integrins: bidirectional, allosteric signaling machines. *Cell. 110*:673-87.

Iacobuzio-Donahue, C.A., R. Ashfaq, A. Maitra, N.V. Adsay, G.L. Shen-Ong, K. Berg, M.A. Hollingsworth, J.L. Cameron, C.J. Yeo, S.E. Kern, M. Goggins, and R.H. Hruban. 2003a. Highly expressed genes in pancreatic ductal adenocarcinomas: a comprehensive characterization and comparison of the transcription profiles obtained from three major technologies. *Cancer Res. 63*:8614-22.

Iacobuzio-Donahue, C.A., A. Maitra, M. Olsen, A.W. Lowe, N.T. van Heek, C. Rosty, K. Walter, N. Sato, A. Parker, R. Ashfaq, E. Jaffee, B. Ryu, J. Jones, J.R. Eshleman, C.J. Yeo, J.L. Cameron, S.E. Kern, R.H. Hruban, P.O. Brown, and M. Goggins. 2003b. Exploration of global gene expression patterns in pancreatic adenocarcinoma using cDNA microarrays. *Am J Pathol. 162*:1151-62.

Iddon, J., N.J. Bundred, J. Hoyland, S.E. Downey, P. Baird, D. Salter, R. McMahon, and A.J. Freemont. 2000. Expression of parathyroid hormone-related protein and its receptor in bone metastases from prostate cancer. *J Pathol. 191*:170-4.

Imamura, H., K. Sato, K. Shizume, T. Satoh, K. Kasono, M. Ozawa, E. Ohmura, T. Tsushima, and H. Demura. 1991. Urinary excretion of parathyroid hormone-related protein fragments in patients with humoral hypercalcemia of malignancy and hypercalcemic tumor-bearing nude mice. *J Bone Miner Res. 6*:77-84.

Iwamura, M., P.A. Abrahamsson, K.A. Foss, G. Wu, A.T. Cockett, and L.J. Deftos. 1994. Parathyroid hormone-related protein: a potential autocrine growth regulator in human prostate cancer cell lines. *Urology. 43*:675-9.

Iwamura, M., P.A. di Sant'Agnese, G. Wu, C.M. Benning, A.T. Cockett, L.J. Deftos, and P.A. Abrahamsson. 1993. Immunohistochemical localization of parathyroid hormone-related protein in human prostate cancer. *Cancer Res. 53*:1724-6.

Iwamura, M., S. Gershagen, O. Lapets, R. Moynes, P.A. Abrahamsson, A.T. Cockett, L.J. Deftos, and P.A. di Sant'Agnese. 1995. Immunohistochemical localization of parathyroid hormone-related protein in prostatic intraepithelial neoplasia. *Hum Pathol. 26*:797-801.

Iwamura, M., J. Hellman, A.T. Cockett, H. Lilja, and S. Gershagen. 1996. Alteration of the hormonal bioactivity of parathyroid hormone-related protein (PTHrP) as a result of limited proteolysis by prostate-specific antigen. *Urology. 48*:317-25.

Jan, Y., M. Matter, J.T. Pai, Y.L. Chen, J. Pilch, M. Komatsu, E. Ong, M. Fukuda, and E. Ruoslahti. 2004. A mitochondrial protein, Bit1, mediates apoptosis regulated by integrins and Groucho/TLE corepressors. *Cell. 116*:751-62.

Jans, D.A., R.J. Thomas, and M.T. Gillespie. 2003. Parathyroid hormone-related protein (PTHrP): a nucleocytoplasmic shuttling protein with distinct paracrine and intracrine roles. *Vitam Horm. 66:*345-84.

Ji, Q., L. Chang, D. VanDenBerg, F.Z. Stanczyk, and A. Stolz. 2003. Selective reduction of AKR1C2 in prostate cancer and its role in DHT metabolism. *Prostate. 54*:275-89.

Juliano, R.L. 2002. Signal transduction by cell adhesion receptors and the cytoskeleton: functions of integrins, cadherins, selectins, and immunoglobulin-superfamily members. *Annu Rev Pharmacol Toxicol. 42*:283-323.

Lanske, B., M. Amling, L. Neff, J. Guiducci, R. Baron, and H.M. Kronenberg. 1999. Ablation of the PTHrP gene or the PTH/PTHrP receptor gene leads to distinct abnormalities in bone development. *J Clin Invest. 104*:399-407.

Lee, B.H., and E. Ruoslahti. 2005. alpha(5)beta(1) integrin stimulates Bcl-2 expression and cell survival through Akt, focal adhesion kinase, and Ca(2+)/calmodulin-dependent protein kinase IV. *J Cell Biochem. 95*:1214-23.

Levy, L., C. Neuveut, C.A. Renard, P. Charneau, S. Branchereau, F. Gauthier, J.T. Van Nhieu, D. Cherqui, A.F. Petit-Bertron, D. Mathieu, and M.A. Buendia. 2002. Transcriptional activation of interleukin-8 by beta-catenin-Tcf4. *J Biol Chem. 277*:42386-93.

Linder, S., E. Castanos-Velez, A. von Rosen, and P. Biberfeld. 2001. Immunohistochemical expression of extracellular matrix proteins and adhesion molecules in pancreatic carcinoma. *Hepatogastroenterology. 48*:1321-7.

Luparello, C., R. Romanotto, A. Tipa, R. Sirchia, N. Olmo, I. Lopez de Silanes, J. Turnay, M.A. Lizarbe, and A.F. Stewart. 2001. Midregion parathyroid hormone-related protein inhibits growth and invasion in vitro and tumorigenesis in vivo of human breast cancer cells. *J Bone Miner Res. 16*:2173-81.

Luparello, C., T. Schilling, R. Cirincione, and I. Pucci-Minafra. 1999. Extracellular matrix regulation of PTHrP and PTH/PTHrP receptor in a human breast cancer cell line. *FEBS Lett. 463*:265-9.

Luparello, C., R. Sirchia, and D. Pupello. 2003. PTHrP [67-86] regulates the expression of stress proteins in breast cancer cells inducing modifications in urokinase-plasminogen activator and MMP-1 expression. *J Cell Sci. 116*:2421-30.

Maheshwari, V.V., D.W. Burton, R.H. Hastings, J.A. Aguilera, F.S. Pardo, and L.J. Deftos. 2003. Apoptotic effects of parathyroid hormone related protein in prostate cancer cells. *J Bone Min Res. 18(S)*:119.

Maioli, E., and V. Fortino. 2004. The complexity of parathyroid hormone-related protein signalling. *Cell Mol Life Sci. 61*:257-62.

Mangin, M., K. Ikeda, B.E. Dreyer, and A.E. Broadus. 1990. Identification of an up-stream promoter of the human parathyroid hormone-related peptide gene. *Mol Endocrinol. 4*:851-8.

Mao, H., F. Li, K. Ruchalski, D.D. Mosser, J.H. Schwartz, Y. Wang, and S.C. Borkan. 2003. hsp72 inhibits focal adhesion kinase degradation in ATP-depleted renal epithelial cells. *J Biol Chem. 278*:18214-20.

Massfelder, T., P. Dann, T.L. Wu, R. Vasavada, J.J. Helwig, and A.F. Stewart. 1997. Opposing mitogenic and anti-mitogenic actions of parathyroid hormone-related protein in vascular smooth muscle cells: a critical role for nuclear targeting. *Proc Natl Acad Sci U S A. 94*:13630-5.

Meerovitch, K., S. Wing, and D. Goltzman. 1997. Preproparathyroid hormone-related protein, a secreted peptide, is a substrate for the ubiquitin proteolytic system. *J Biol Chem. 272*:6706-13.

Mollenhauer, J., I. Roether, and H.F. Kern. 1987. Distribution of extracellular matrix proteins in pancreatic ductal adenocarcinoma and its influence on tumor cell proliferation in vitro. *Pancreas. 2*:14-24.

Mosser, D.D., and R.I. Morimoto. 2004. Molecular chaperones and the stress of oncogenesis. *Oncogene*. 23:2907-18.

Multhoff, G., C. Botzler, M. Wiesnet, E. Muller, T. Meier, W. Wilmanns, and R.D. Issels. 1995. A stress-inducible 72-kDa heat-shock protein (HSP72) is expressed on the surface of human tumor cells, but not on normal cells. *Int J Cancer. 61*:272-9.

Nissenson, R.A. 2000. Parathyroid hormone-related protein. *Rev Endocr Metab Disord. 1*:343-52.

Okazaki, Y., H. Ohno, K. Takase, T. Ochiai, and T. Saito. 2000. Cell surface expression of calnexin, a molecular chaperone in the endoplasmic reticulum. *J Biol Chem. 275*:35751-8.

Orloff, J.J., D. Reddy, A.E. de Papp, K.H. Yang, N.E. Soifer, and A.F. Stewart. 1994. Parathyroid hormone-related protein as a prohormone: posttranslational processing and receptor interactions. *Endocr Rev. 15*:40-60.

Pache, J.C., D.W. Burton, L.J. Deftos, and R.H. Hastings. 2006. A carboxyl leucine-rich region of parathyroid hormone-related protein is critical for nuclear export. *Endocrinology*. *147*:990-8.

Paterson, A.C., S.M. Lockhart, J. Baker, G. Neumann, G.S. Baldwin, and A. Shulkes. 2004. Identity and regulation of stored and secreted progastrin-derived peptides in sheep. *Endocrinology*. *145*:5129-40.

Penning, T.M., M.E. Burczynski, J.M. Jez, C.F. Hung, H.K. Lin, H. Ma, M. Moore, N. Palackal, and K. Ratnam. 2000. Human 3alpha-hydroxysteroid dehydrogenase isoforms (AKR1C1-AKR1C4) of the aldo-keto reductase superfamily: functional plasticity and tissue distribution reveals roles in the inactivation and formation of male and female sex hormones. *Biochem J*. *351*:67-77.

Penning, T.M., M.E. Burczynski, J.M. Jez, H.K. Lin, H. Ma, M. Moore, K. Ratnam, and N. Palackal. 2001. Structure-function aspects and inhibitor design of type 5 17beta-hydroxysteroid dehydrogenase (AKR1C3). *Mol Cell Endocrinol*. *171*:137-49.

Penning, T.M., Y. Jin, S. Steckelbroeck, T. Lanisnik Rizner, and M. Lewis. 2004. Structure-function of human 3 alpha-hydroxysteroid dehydrogenases: genes and proteins. *Mol Cell Endocrinol*. *215*:63-72.

Penning, T.M., S. Steckelbroeck, D.R. Bauman, M.W. Miller, Y. Jin, D.M. Peehl, K.M. Fung, and H.K. Lin. 2006. Aldo-keto reductase (AKR) 1C3: role in prostate disease and the development of specific inhibitors. *Mol Cell Endocrinol*. *248*:182-91.

Perez-Martinez, F.C., V. Alonso, J.L. Sarasa, S.G. Nam-Cha, R. Vela-Navarrete, F. Manzarbeitia, F.J. Calahorra, and P. Esbrit. 2007. Immunohistochemical analysis of low-grade and high-grade prostate carcinoma: relative changes of pthrp and its pth1 receptor, osteoprotegerin and receptor activator of nuclear factor-kb ligand. *J Clin Pathol*. *60*:290-4.

Philbrick, W. 2001. Parathyroid hormone-related protein: gene structure, biosynthesis, metabolism and regulation. *In The Parathyroids*. R.M. JP Bilezikian, and A Levine, editor. Academic Press, San Diego, CA. pp. 93-105.

Rabbani, S.A., J. Gladu, P. Harakidas, B. Jamison, and D. Goltzman. 1999. Over-production of parathyroid hormone-related peptide results in increased osteolytic skeletal metastasis by prostate cancer cells in vivo. *Int J Cancer*. *80*:257-64.

Rabbani, S.A., M. Haq, and D. Goltzman. 1993. Biosynthesis and processing of endogenous parathyroid hormone related peptide (PTHRP) by rat Leydig cell tumor H-500. *Biochemistry*. *32*:4931-7.

Raffin-Sanson, M.L., Y. de Keyzer, and X. Bertagna. 2003. Proopiomelanocortin, a polypeptide precursor with multiple functions: from physiology to pathological conditions. *Eur J Endocrinol*. *149*:79-90.

Ratcliffe, W.A., E. Green, J. Emly, S. Norbury, M. Lindsay, D.A. Heath, and J.G. Ratcliffe. 1990. Identification and partial characterization of parathyroid hormone-related protein in human and bovine milk. *J Endocrinol*. *127*:167-76.

Ruoslahti, E. 1991. Integrins. *J Clin Invest*. *87*:1-5.

Ruoslahti, E. 1996. RGD and other recognition sequences for integrins. *Annu Rev Cell Dev Biol*. *12*:697-715.

Ruoslahti, E., N.A. Noble, S. Kagami, and W.A. Border. 1994. Integrins. *Kidney Int Suppl. 44*:S17-22.

Shen, X., and M. Falzon. 2003. PTH-related protein modulates PC-3 prostate cancer cell adhesion and integrin subunit profile. *Mol Cell Endocrinol. 199*:165-77.

Shen, X., and M. Falzon. 2005. PTH-related protein enhances LoVo colon cancer cell proliferation, adhesion, and integrin expression. *Regul Pept. 125*:17-27.

Shen, X., L. Qian, and M. Falzon. 2004. PTH-related protein enhances MCF-7 breast cancer cell adhesion, migration, and invasion via an intracrine pathway. *Exp Cell Res. 294*:420-33.

Shimoyama, S., F. Gansauge, S. Gansauge, T. Oohara, and H.G. Beger. 1995. Altered expression of extracellular matrix molecules and their receptors in chronic pancreatitis and pancreatic adenocarcinoma in comparison with normal pancreas. *Int J Pancreatol. 18*:227-34.

Shin, B.K., H. Wang, A.M. Yim, F. Le Naour, F. Brichory, J.H. Jang, R. Zhao, E. Puravs, J. Tra, C.W. Michael, D.E. Misek, and S.M. Hanash. 2003. Global profiling of the cell surface proteome of cancer cells uncovers an abundance of proteins with chaperone function. *J Biol Chem. 278*:7607-16.

Soifer, N.E., K.E. Dee, K.L. Insogna, W.J. Burtis, L.M. Matovcik, T.L. Wu, L.M. Milstone, A.E. Broadus, W.M. Philbrick, and A.F. Stewart. 1992. Parathyroid hormone-related protein. Evidence for secretion of a novel mid-region fragment by three different cell types. *J Biol Chem. 267*:18236-43.

Stein, W.D., T. Litman, T. Fojo, and S.E. Bates. 2004. A Serial Analysis of Gene Expression (SAGE) database analysis of chemosensitivity: comparing solid tumors with cell lines and comparing solid tumors from different tissue origins. *Cancer Res. 64*:2805-16.

Strewler, G.J. 2000. The physiology of parathyroid hormone-related protein. *N Engl J Med. 342*:177-85.

Strid, H., A. Care, T. Jansson, and T. Powell. 2002. Parathyroid hormone-related peptide (38-94) amide stimulates ATP-dependent calcium transport in the Basal plasma membrane of the human syncytiotrophoblast. *J Endocrinol. 175*:517-24.

Takeichi, M. 1991. Cadherin cell adhesion receptors as a morphogenetic regulator. *Science. 251*:1451-5.

Tovar Sepulveda, V.A., and M. Falzon. 2002. Parathyroid hormone-related protein enhances PC-3 prostate cancer cell growth via both autocrine/paracrine and intracrine pathways. *Regul Pept. 105*:109-20.

Tsigelny, I., D.W. Burton, Y. Sharikov, R.H. Hastings, and L.J. Deftos. 2005. Coherent expression chromosome cluster analysis reveals differential regulatory functions of amino-terminal and distal parathyroid hormone-related protein domains in prostate carcinoma. *J Biomed Biotechnol.* 2005:353-63.

White, T.K., Q. Zhu, and M.L. Tanzer. 1995. Cell surface calreticulin is a putative mannoside lectin which triggers mouse melanoma cell spreading. *J Biol Chem. 270*:15926-9.

Witke, W. 2004. The role of profilin complexes in cell motility and other cellular processes. *Trends Cell Biol. 14*:451-9.

Wong, N.A., and M. Pignatelli. 2002. Beta-catenin--a linchpin in colorectal carcinogenesis? *Am J Pathol. 160*:389-401.

Wu, G., M. Iwamura, P.A. di Sant'Agnese, L.J. Deftos, A.T. Cockett, and S. Gershagen. 1998. Characterization of the cell-specific expression of parathyroid hormone-related protein in normal and neoplastic prostate tissue. *Urology*. *51*:110-20.

Wu, T.L., N.E. Soifer, W.J. Burtis, L.M. Milstone, and A.F. Stewart. 1991. Glycosylation of parathyroid hormone-related peptide secreted by human epidermal keratinocytes. *J Clin Endocrinol Metab*. *73*:1002-7.

Wu, T.L., R.C. Vasavada, K. Yang, T. Massfelder, M. Ganz, S.K. Abbas, A.D. Care, and A.F. Stewart. 1996. Structural and physiologic characterization of the mid-region secretory species of parathyroid hormone-related protein. *J Biol Chem*. *271*:24371-81.

Xiao, G., T.F. Chung, R.E. Fine, and R.J. Johnson. 1999. Calreticulin is transported to the surface of NG108-15 cells where it forms surface patches and is partially degraded in an acidic compartment. *J Neurosci Res*. *58*:652-62.

Yang, K.H., A.E. dePapp, N.E. Soifer, B.E. Dreyer, T.L. Wu, S.E. Porter, M. Bellantoni, W.J. Burtis, K.L. Insogna, A.E. Broadus, and et al. 1994. Parathyroid hormone-related protein: evidence for isoform- and tissue-specific posttranslational processing. *Biochemistry*. *33*:7460-9.

Yuan, T.C., S. Veeramani, F.F. Lin, D. Kondrikou, S. Zelivianski, T. Igawa, D. Karan, S.K. Batra, and M.F. Lin. 2006. Androgen deprivation induces human prostate epithelial neuroendocrine differentiation of androgen-sensitive LNCaP cells. *Endocr Relat Cancer*. *13*:151-67.

In: Novel Aspects of PTHrP Physiopathology
Editor: Claudio Luparello, pp. 305-319
ISBN: 978-1-60021-857-6

Chapter XII

GENOMEWIDE HYPOMETHYLATION AND *PTHRP* GENE HYPERMETHYLATION AS A MODEL FOR THE PREDICTION OF CANCER RISK IN RHEUMATOID ARTHRITIS

Fabio Caradonna**, *Giusi Barbata, Giulia Sciandrello
Dipartimento di Biologia Cellulare e dello Sviluppo, Università di Palermo, Italy.

ABSTRACT

Rheumatoid arthritis (RA) is a chronic multisystem inflammatory disease characterized by high recurrence of lymphomas as well as hypercalcemia, the latter based upon *PTHrP* overexpression. Since DNA methylation plays a critical role in development of neoplasias, we determined in RA patients the global DNA methylation status and local methylation pattern of the CpG island of one of the three promoters of *PTHrP* gene, utilizing cytogenetic and molecular techniques.

Chromosomal DNA methylation pattern analysis, performed by indirect immunofluorescence technique with anti 5-methylcytosine antibody, showed that all peripheral lymphocyte metaphases from RA patients exhibited weakly fluorescent chromosomes without discrete grains; instead, chromosomes of control subjects were almost uniformly decorated by brilliant grains. Similarly, investigations performed on DNA from peripheral blood of patients and healthy donors, amplified by Methylation-Sensitive Arbitrarily-Primed Polymerase Chain Reaction (MeSAP-PCR), indicated that RA is strongly associated with global DNA hypomethylation.

Studies on methylation of *PTHrP* gene promoter II, performed on five CpG island internal sites using the MeSAP-PCR showed that one of the sites, i.e. the closest to the

* Correspondence concerning this article should be addressed to: Fabio Caradonna, Dipartimento di Biologia Cellulare e dello Sviluppo, Università di Palermo, Viale delle Scienze, Edificio 16 – 90128 PALERMO – Italy. Fax. N. 0039-91-6577347; E-mail: Fabio.Caradonna@unipa.it.

transcription starting point, is heavy methylated in a significantly high number of RA patients.

Thus, RA seems to be characterized by genomewide hypomethylation associated with local DNA hypermethylation, as in the majority of tumors. This result raises the possibility that susceptibility to lymphomas is related to abnormal DNA methylation levels and suggests the opportunity to evaluate the DNA methylation status in RA patients; in fact, the demethylating therapies together with diet and life style can act towards an increase of tumor risk.

INTRODUCTION

Rheumatoid arthritis (RA), a chronic autoimmune disease, is often associated with the development of malignant lymphomas: RA patients have the risk of developing this tumor twofold than expected in a gender and age-matched population, due to both the therapy which they are submitted to and an intrinsec correlation, independent of the treatment, with potentially-carcinogenic chemicals (Ekbom, 2005).

It has been well-documented that RA is also associated with hypercalcemy (Kohno et al., 1997; Kartsogiannis et al., 1998), one of the characteristics of malignancies in relation with the production of parathyroid hormone-related protein (PTHrP) (Solimando, 2001). In particular, overexpression of *PTHrP* has been found in fibroblasts and epithelial cells as well as very high concentrations of PTHrP have been detected in synovial fluids from RA patients (Funk et a., 2001; Kohno et al., 1997).

The etiology of RA is unknown but its genesis is believed to be multifactorial; genetic factors can contribute for approximately 60% of the variation in the liability to disease (MacGregor et al., 2000). The involvement of HLA system and of T lymphocytes receptorial repertory is one of the "genetic media" predisposing to RA.

Today it is well-known that deregulation of gene expression may be also due to epigenetic alterations (Jones and Laird, 1999) and the methylation of some cytosines into promoter sites of genes may affect their expression (Breivik and Gandernak, 1999). Methylation, moreover, plays a critical role in the development of malignant diseases, since genomic DNA methylation patterns are often aberrant in tumor cells (McCabe and Caudill, 2005).

This study aimed to evaluate the DNA methylation status in RA patients with cytogenetic and molecular techniques in order to ascertain a possible correlation between methylation levels and RA; careful investigations were performed on *PTHrP* that is epigenetically controlled and, in RA, deregulated.

METERIALS AND METHODS

Patients and Donors

We examined 19 RA patients (Table I) and 17 healthy donors (9 women and 8 men ranging in age from 22 to 71).

Table I. RA patients main clinical data

Patient	Age/Sex	RA phase	Therapy		
			CSA	PQL	MTX
RA 1	64/F	4°	+		+
RA 2	57/F	1°			+
RA 3	48/F	3°	+		
RA 4	56/F	3°		+	+
RA 5	52/F	3°	+	+	
RA 6	72/F	3°	+		
RA 7	61/F	3°		+	
RA 9	47/M	2°			+
RA 10	56/F	2°			+
RA 12	30/F	1°			+
RA 13	62/F	1°		+	
RA 14	52/F	1°		+	
RA 15	51/F	1°		+	
RA 16	57/F	1°			+
RA 17	56/F	4°		+	
RA 18	50/M	1°		+	
RA 19	54/M	1°		+	
RA 20	47/F	1°		+	
RA 21	52/F	2°			+

CSA: Cyclosporin A; PQL: Plaquenil; MTX: Methothrexate.

Chromosomal Methylation Analysis

In Situ 5-Methylcytosine (5MeC) Detection by Indirect Immunofluorescence

In order to observe chromosomal DNA methylation patterns, indirect immunofluorescence technique with anti-5MeC antibody was performed on metaphase chromosomes of peripheral lymphocytes from 6 patients (RA1, 2, 3, 4, 15, 20) and 2 control subjects (C33, 34). To this purpose, cytogenetic preparations were obtained according to Carbone et al. (1984) and subsequently stained according to Bensaada et al. (1998) with some modifications (Sciandrello et al., 2004).

Genomic Methylation Analysis

DNA Extraction

Genomic DNA from peripheral blood lymphocyte was obtained using a conventional silica column kit (GenElute, Sigma), according to the manufacturer's suggestions.

Methylation-Sensitive Arbitrarily-Primed Polymerase Chain Reaction (MeSAP-PCR)

The technique was carried out according to Liang et al. (2002) with some modifications. Briefly, DNA was digested for at least 16h at 37°C with 10 U of *Rsa*I restrictrion endonuclease (single-digested DNA). Then, half of the amount of single-digested DNA was further treated with 10 U of *Hpa*II, a methylation-sensitive restriction endonuclease unable to cut DNA if methylated cytosine is present in its recognition site (CC*GG) (double-digested DNA). Single and double-digested DNA were heat inactivated for 20 min at 65°C and separately amplified by Arbitrarily-Primed Polymerase Chain Reaction using two subsequent amplification cycles, called AP1-M e AP2-M.

In AP1-M (low stringency cycle), a permissive annealing temperature was set to allow arbitrary primer annealing to the best matches in the template, supported by high concentration of the primer itself and divalent ions. Cycle profile was 94°C for 5 min, 4 cycles at 94°C for 30 sec, 40°C for 60 sec and 72°C for 90 sec; the reaction mixture was: 250 ng template DNA, 10 μM 21-mer arbitrary primer [sequence: 5'-AAC TGA AGC AGT GGC CTC GCG –3'], 200 μM dNTPs and 0.8 U Taq DNA polymerase (Roche) in Tris-HCl 10 mM, pH 8.3, containing 1,5 mM $MgCl_2$ and 50 mM KCl, (total volume: 25 μl).

AP2-M (high stringency cycle), run immediately after AP1-M, was a conventional PCR reaction aimed to increase the amount of DNA fragments previously produced. Cycle profile was 94°C for 60 sec, and 29 cycles at 60°C for 60 sec and 72°C for 120 sec; for the reaction mixture, 75μl of Tris-HCl 10 mM, pH 8.3, containing 1.5 mM $MgCl_2$, 50mM KCl, 200μM dNTPs and 2.5 U Taq DNA polymerase were added to the 25μl of AP1-M mix. Amplified DNA was resolved by a non-denaturing 6% acrylamide-bisacrylamide (29:1 ratio) gel electrophoresis.

Chemiluminescent Detection

The visualization of DNA fingerprinting was obtained by chemiluminescent detection of digoxigenin according to a novel protocol developed in our laboratory, allowing to obtain a very high resolution. Brieflly, DNA fragments were blotted from gel onto positively-charged nylon membranes (Roche) and detected by hybridization with the same primer used in MeSAP-PCR, 5'-labelled with digoxigenin (Roche), as a probe. Blots were washed with 0.4 X SSC-0.1% SDS for 15 min at room temperature and subjected to chemiluminescent detection as recommended by the manufacturer (Roche).

Densitometric Scanning and Image Analysis

The lumigraphs were submitted to densitometric scanning and subsequently analysed by SigmaGel image analysis software (Jandel Scientific) which allowed us to obtain a graph representing fragments intensity and position for each lane, and to overlap the densitometry originating from single- and double-digested DNA. By comparison of the pairs of densitometric profiles, it was possible to estimate the two following differences: (i) the presence or the absence of peaks representing the appearing or the disappearing of amplified DNA fragments in DNA fingerprinting, (ii) the higher or shorter peak height corresponding to intensification or attenuation of bands containing several fragments with the same molecular weight but with different sequence. All the profiles were calculated referring to standard molecular weight densitometric scanning.

PTHrP Gene Methylation Analysis

DNA Extraction

Genomic DNA from peripheral blood lymphocytes was obtained using Fassst DNA Releaser kit (Celbio-Euroclone) according to the manufacturer's suggestions; due to thermal treatment, randomly-fragmented DNA, more suitable to PCR reactions on GC-rich difficult templates, is obtained.

Methylation-SensitiveRestriction Endonucleases Multiplex-Polymerase Chain Reaction (MSREM-PCR)

In order to analyze the CpG island of *PTHrP* promoter II, genomic DNA was digested with excess (5 U/μg DNA) *Hha*I or *Hpa*II or *Msp*I methylation-sensitive restriction endonucleases (MSRE), for at least 16h at 37°C, according to the manufacturer's suggestions (Invitrogen). Afterwards, every parallel sample of genomic and MSRE-digested DNA was amplified by Multiplex-PCR (M-PCR) in the presence of oligos flanking five sites located within the CpG island of *PTHrP* promoter II as primers (see Figure 4). M-PCR of MSRE-digested DNA will give a product only when MSRE do not cut DNA, leaving the template intact and suitable for amplification. Three out of five sites were studied using two isoschizomers (*Hpa*II and *Msp*I) with different methylation sensitivity; the other two were analyzed only with *Hha*I since no corresponding isoschizomer with different methylation sensitivity is available.

Reaction mixture of M-PCR reactions contained approximatively 200 ng genomic DNA, 0.2 mM of each dNTP, 0.2μM of each primer (see table II), 1.2-1.25 mM $MgCl_2$ and 2.5 U Taq polymerase in 1X buffer provided by the manufacturer (Invitrogen). Amplification was carried out in a total volume of 100μl using a Biometra "T-Personal" thermocycler. Cycle profile was 94°C for 5 min, 30 cycles of 94 °C for 2 min, 55 °C for 2 min, and 72 °C for 2 min, and a final extension at 72 °C for 10 min.

Table II. Amplification primers for the five sites of the CpG island in *PTHrP* promoter II

CpG Island site	Primer	5'-3' sequence
S-1	SU1/5	CGTCGACTCGATCAGCTTC
S-5	SL1/5	GTCTAAACTCTCCGGCAGG
S-2	SU2	GGTTCATGTGGGGAACTGG
	SL2	CCCAGTCCTGATCTCCTGG
S-3	SU3	TGTGGCCTCGTACAAGTCC
	SL3	CTGGAGGAACTGCCTCAGG
S-4	SU4	CAGGAGACTCCAGAGAAGG

Co-amplification of *IL-4* internal region (998 bp) was concurrently carried out as a control (primers: IL4-1A: 5'-GGTAAGACTGTAGCTCTTTTTCC-3'; IL4-1B: 5'-ACACCAGATTGTCAGTCACTTGG-3'). This pair of primers, in fact, gives always a product using either genomic or MSRE-digested DNA, since the sequence to be amplified has no recognition site for all the enzymes used.

All the M-PCR products were resolved by non-denaturing 6% acrylamide-bisacrylamide (29:1, ratio) gel electrophoresis, stained with ethidium bromide, and the fluorescent images acquired by a Kodak image analysis equipment.

Results and Discussion

Chromosomal Methylation Patterns

In situ 5-MeC Detection by Indirect Immunofluorescence

Metaphases from control subjects showed a strong chromosomal decoration with fluorescent stain appearing as brilliant grains localized into pericentromeric regions of chromosome 1, 9 and 16, and into R-band (euchromatic regions) (Figure 1, a-b); on the contrary, chromosomes from RA patients showed a faint fluorescence (Figure 1, c-h).

In particular, binding sites of anti-5MeC antibody resulted to be not much evident for the patients RA 4 (Figure 1f) and RA 15 (Figure 1g). Sometimes, it was possibile to observe the labelling of telomeric (RA 20, Figure 1h) and pericentromeric regions (RA 1, Figure 1c), but they appeared with weak fluorescence intensity and without discrete decorations in R-band regions.

Genomic Methylation Levels

MeSAP-PCR

First of all, it is opportune to remark that banding patterns obtained after amplification of DNA digested with both *Rsa*I and *Hpa*II restriction enzymes and of DNA digested with *Rsa*I enzyme only are the same only when CpG-rich sequences are hypermethylated; on the contrary, banding patterns result to be different when these sequences are hypomethylated since *Hpa*II recognizes its restriction site producing additional fragments suitable for MeSAP-PCR amplification. As the amplification obtained with the use of this methodology is quantitative, i.e. the intensity of amplified bands results to be proportional to the concentration of the corresponding target sequences (Micheli & Bova, 1997), the electrophoretograms of the amplification products of double-digested DNA (RH lanes, figures 2 and 3) if compared with those of single-digested DNA (R lanes, figures 2 and 3) can show either the presence of additional bands representing other fragments with different molecular weight or variations in the intensity of pre-existing bands, depending on the comigration of several fragments with the same molecular weight but with different sequence.

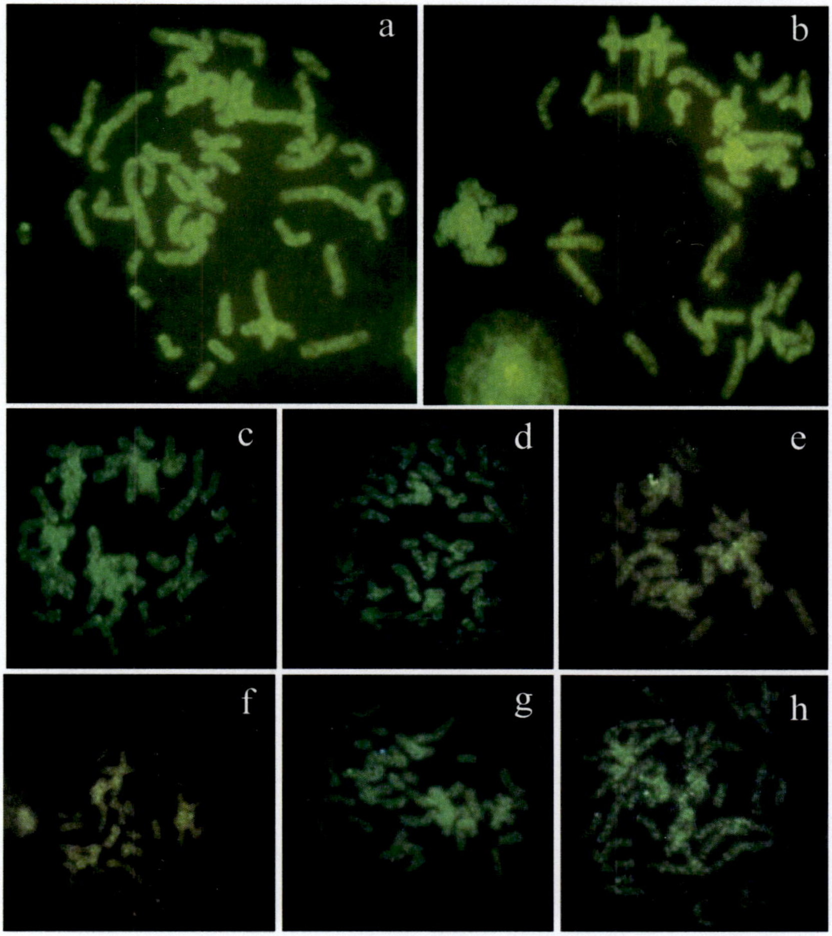

Figure 1. Metaphase chromosomes from control subjects (a,b) and RA patients (c-h) visualized by indirect immuno-fluorescence with anti-5-Methylcytosine antibody.

For each individual densitometric profile, double-digested DNA (blu line, figures 2 and 3) was compared with single-digested DNA (red line, figures 2 and 3), considered as the "standard lane".

DNA-fingerprinting of control subjects (Figure 2) showed that the banding pattern of single-digested and double-digested DNA was equivalent, thereby demonstrating that the methylation-sensitive restriction enzyme did not find other different cutting sites. This is the expected result for DNA from differentiated cells, namely peripheral lymphocytes of healthy subjects.

The same investigation was performed on DNA from peripheral lymphocytes of RA patients which, being cells that belong to the tissue implicated in the immune response, are involved in the onset of the pathology. DNA-fingerprinting (Figure 3) showed a very different banding pattern between the two preparations of digested DNA, thereby demonstrating that *Hpa*II had found a larger number of available cutting sites.

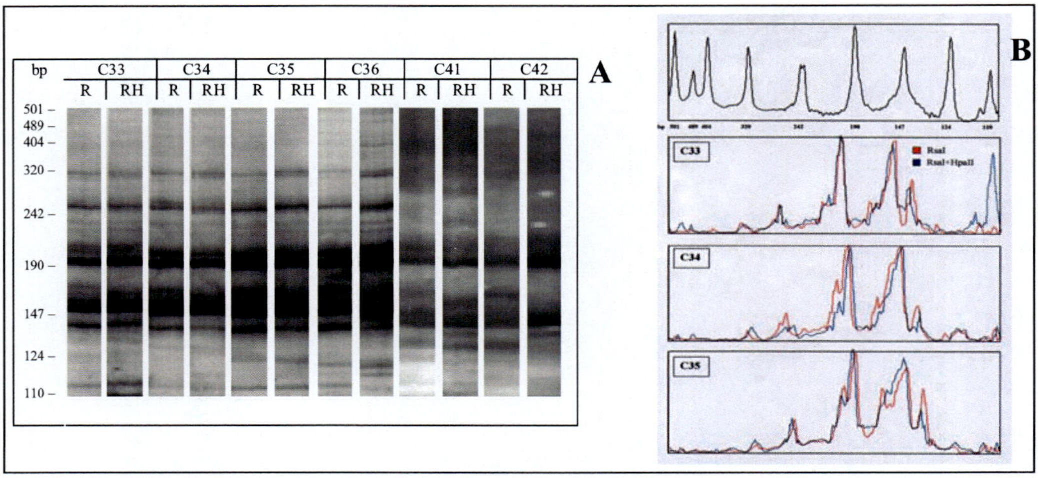

Figure 2. DNA fingerprinting (A) and corresponding densitometric scanning (B) of some control subjects.

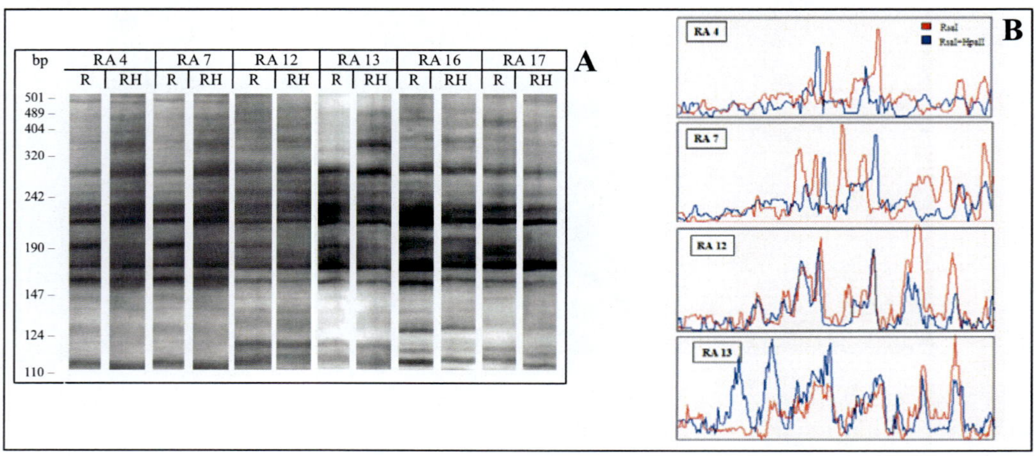

Figure 3. DNA fingerprinting (A) and corresponding densitometric scanning (B) of some RA patients.

Tables III and IV report fragment pattern variation number from DNA fingerprintings of control subjects and RA patients; the number of variations noticed for each patient was high and significantly greater in the average than that of control subjects.

The differences in both chromosomal and genomic methylation status demonstrated that the DNA from RA patients was strongly hypomethylated; this finding is in agreement with the reports of other authors (Corvetta et al., 1991; Kim et al., 1996).

It is well known that DNA hypomethylation promote oncogenesis, as it is a peculiarity of both highly- and moderately-repeated DNA sequences from several cancer cell types (Ehrlich, 2002). On this matter, cancer can be considered an epigenetic as well as genetic disease; in fact, epigenetic changes, and in particular DNA methylation, are strictly correlated with the effect of some environmental factors, exposure to which can increase the cancer risk (Esteller and Herman, 2002).

One of these factors is definitely represented by the therapy to which RA patients are submitted; several perspective studies reported in the literature have highlighted the relationship between RA and increased risk of haematological tumours, namely leukemia and lymphomas, in patients treated with antiblastic and/or immunosuppressant chemotherapy (Mariette et al., 2002; Wing-Yan Au et al., 2006). Noteworthy, the anti-folate property of methothrexate (MTX) was proven to indirectly promote DNA hypomethylation (Morgan et al., 1990); on the other hand, so far no evidence has been provided in the literature about a similar effect of cyclosporin or plaquenil.

Table III. Fragment pattern variation number in control subjects DNA fingerprintings

Healthy donor	Appearing or disappearing	Attenuation or intensification	Total
C33	1	1	2
C34	0	0	0
C35	0	0	0
C36	2	2	4
C41	1	0	1
C42	1	0	1
C43	1	0	1
C44	0	2	2
C45	1	0	1
C46	1	0	1
C47	1	1	2
C48	1	2	3
C49	2	3	5
C50	2	3	5
C51	0	0	0
Total:15	14	14	28
Average	**0.93**	**0.93**	**1.87**

In order to ascertain if therapeutic treatment could have affected the DNA methylation level, data reported in Table IV were grouped according to the kind of utilized drug. As shown in Table V, the DNA methylation level was found to be always very lower in patients than in control subjects as demonstrated by the high number of fragment pattern variations, independently of the therapies; moreover, in disagreement with other authors (Kim et al.,1996), MTX treatment of this autoimmune disease seemed to have not reverted the DNA hypomethylation.

Thus, RA patients here examined, having a very low level of genomic DNA methylation, appeared to be in a condition of high tumour risk; however, it is necessary to specify that, although some of them were affected by RA since a long time, at the moment of analysis they had not developed any malignancy.

Table IV. Fragment pattern variation number in RA patients DNA fingerprintings

Patient	Appearing or disappearing	Attenuation or intensification	Total
RA1	5	4	9[b]
RA2	1	4	5[d]
RA3	3	5	8[b]
RA4	16	2	18[b]
RA5	5	5	10[b]
RA6	1	8	9[b]
RA7	13	4	17[b]
RA9	8	1	9[b]
RA10	4	4	8[b]
RA12	8	8	16[b]
RA13	3	8	11[b]
RA14	3	2	5[d]
RA15	5	6	11[b]
RA16	6	6	12[b]
RA17	7	5	12[b]
RA18	5	4	9[b]
RA19	2	4	6[c]
RA20	3	3	6[c]
RA21	5	4	9[b]
Total: 19	103	87	190
Average	**5.42[a]**	**4.58[a]**	**10.00**

[a], $p < 0.0001$; [b], $p < 0.001$; [c], $0.001 < p < 0.005$, according to *t* Student's test; [d], $0.02 < p < 0.025$, according to χ^2 test.

Table V. Fragment pattern variation number in RA patients pooled by therapy

Therapy	Patients (*)	Fragment pattern variation number
MTX	6	9.83
Cyclosporin	1	8
Plaquenil	9	9.55

(*) Three patients submitted to combined treatment (see Tab. I) were excluded from this table.

Nevertheless, to assess a possible relationship between severity of disease and DNA methylation status, data reported in Table IV were grouped according to 4 classes corresponding to RA clinical phases; the results shown in Table VI demonstrated that patients in advanced phases presented a fragment pattern variation number slightly greater than patients in early phases. The observed trend suggested an association between DNA hypomethylation and the course of disease.

Table VI. Fragment pattern variation number in patients pooled by RA phase

RA phase	Patients	Fragment pattern variation number
First	9	9
Second	3	8.66
Third	5	12,4
Fourth	2	10.5

PTHrP Gene Methylation Status

Investigations were performed on five sites located into CpG island of *PTHrP* promoter II (Figure 4). All these M-PCR products resulted particularly difficult to be obtained since GC-rich sequences and secondary structures in DNA template interfere with complete denaturation of DNA during the melting step and in DNA polymerase-slipping during the extension phase.

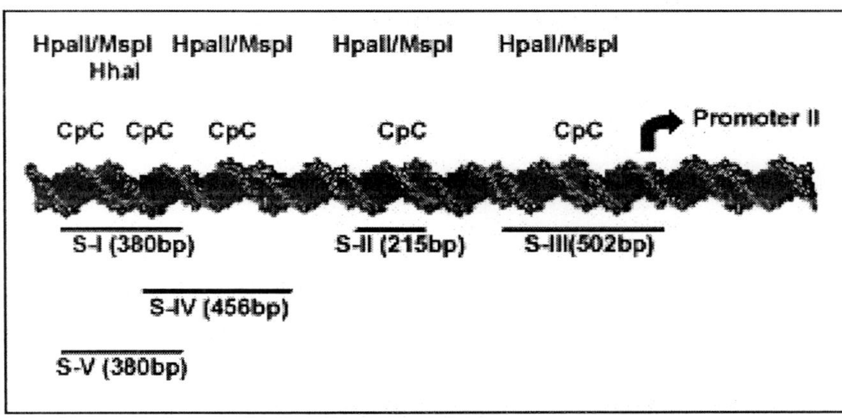

Figure 4. Localization of the MSRE sites into CpG island of *PTHrP* promoter II.

Three out of five sites were analysed by utilizing two isoschizomers (*Hpa*II e *Msp*I) with different sensitivity to methylation: the sites unavailable for cutting by both enzymes were considered as "strongly methylated", on the contrary, the sites available for cutting by both MSRE were recorded as "unmethylated". Moreover, as regards sites cleaved by *Hha*I (S-4 and S-5), analysis could supply only generic informations about the presence and/or the absence of methyl groups into the restriction site.

Some results obtained from the analysis of methylation status of CpG island S-1 site are reported in Figure 5; the amplification product was present only for undigested DNA (380 bp fragment); this demonstrated that S-1 site was "unmethylated", since *Hpa*II and *Msp*I enzymes did cut DNA thereby making the amplification impossible. Regarding S-3 site (Figure 6), it was possible to find a 502 bp band in almost all the examined subjects; this allowed us to state that the site was "strongly methylated", since both MSRE did not found their site available for cutting.

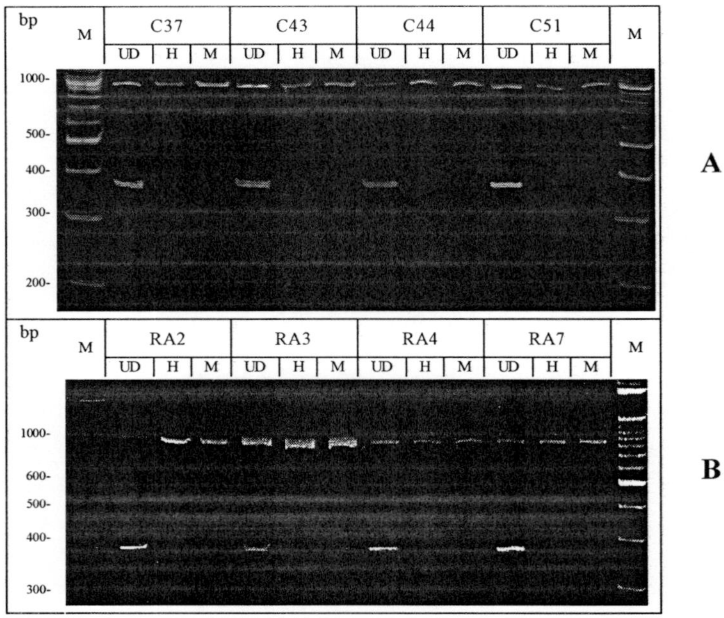

Figure 5. Methylation analysis of S-1 site (380 bp) into *PTHrP* promoter II. All sites were "unmethylated". A: control subjects; B: RA patients; UD = undigested; H=digested with *Hpa*II; M=digested with *Msp*I.

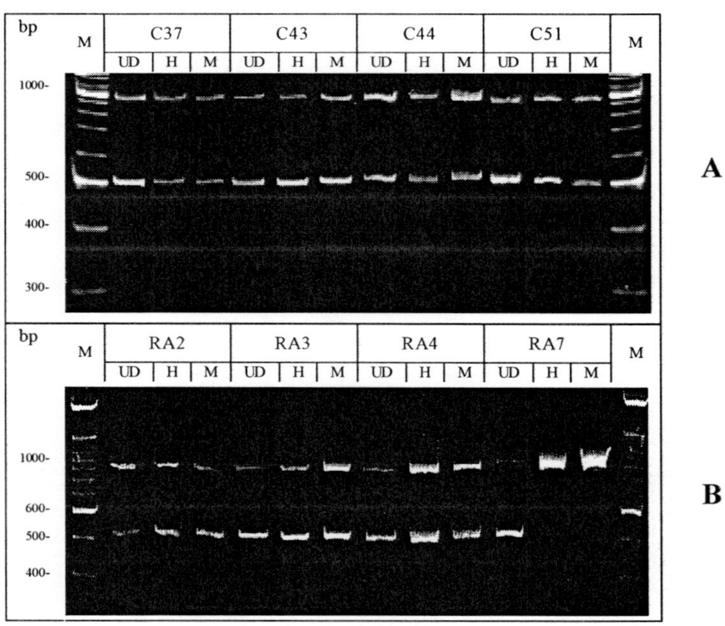

Figure 6. Methylation analysis of S-3 site (502 bp) into *PTHrP* promoter II. All but one (RA7 patient) sites were "strongly methylated". A: control subjects; B: RA patients; UD = undigested; H=digested with *Hpa*II; M=digested with *Msp*I.

Comprehensive results of methylation status analysis of CpG island into *PTHrP* promoter II in RA patients and in control subjects are reported in Table VII. Two sites, S-1 and S-5, resulted to be not informative as they were "unmethylated" both in patients and in controls; also S-2 site gave no information because it was either "methylated" or "strongly methylated" with a similar frequency in two groups of individuals. Instead, S-3 site was found to be "strongly methylated" in most patients (81.80% *vs* 47.06%, $p < 0.001$, according to the χ^2 test) and S-4 site was more generically methylated in RA patients than in control subjects (90.90% *vs* 70.59%, $0.01 < p < 0.02$).

Table VII. PTHrP promotor II sites methylation status in healthy donors and RA patients (%).

	PTHrP promotor II sites					
	S - I		S - 2		S - 3	
	Controls	Patients	Controls	Patients	Controls	Patients
Unmethylated	94.11	100	0	9.10	0	9.10
Methylated	0	0	35.29	27.27	35.29	9.10**
Highly Methylated	0	0	64.71	63.63	47.06	81.80**
Generically Methylated	-	-	-	-	-	-
Not determined	5.89	0	0	0	17.65	0
TOTAL	100	100	100	100	100	100

	PTHrP promotor II sites			
	S - 4		S -5	
	Controls	Patients	Controls	Patients
Unmethylated	0	9.10	76.47	72.73
Methylated	-	-	-	-
Highly Methylated	-	-	-	-
Generically Methylated	70.59	90.90*	0	0
Not determined	29.41	0	23.53	27.27
TOTAL	100	100	100	100

* $0.01 < p < 0.02$; ** $p < 0.001$; according to χ^2 test.

Conclusion

Our results indicate that RA is strongly associated with global DNA hypomethylation, in agreement with other reports (Kim et al., 1996), and also with region-specific hypermethylation, similarly to the situation of tumour cells (Robertson e Jones, 2000). As RA patients have a quite high risk of developing cancer, particularly leukemias and lymphomas, (Thomas et al., 2000), it is reasonable to think that the increased susceptibility to lymphomas is correlated with the abnormal DNA methylation levels.

The long-time exposure to risk factors, such as demethylating chemotherapies, diet or life-style are considered "sustained stress environment" capable of epigenetically-reprogramming the genome (Karpinets and Foy, 2005), Thus, RA patients are noticeably exposed to cancer risk; within this context, the evaluation of DNA methylation status could be a promising "biomarker" during the clinical course of this disease.

Acknowledgments

This work is supported by a grant from the University of Palermo (R.S. "ex 60%") to G.B.

Reeferences

Breivik, J & Gaudernack, G. Genomic instability, DNA methylation, and natural selection in colorectal carcinogenesis. *Cancer Biology*, 1999, 9, 245-254.

Carbone, P; Barbata, G; Mirto, S; Marceno, R; Leone, S; Granata, G. Cytogenetic studies in five patients with myelofibrosis and myeloid metaplasia. *Cancer Genet Cytogenet*, 1984, 12(3), 209-15.

Corvetta, A; Della Bitta, R; Luchetti, MM; Pomponio, G. 5-Methylcytosine content of DNA in blood, synovial mononuclear cells and synovial tissue from patients affected by autoimmune rheumatic diseases. *J Chromatogr*, 1991, 566 (2), 481-91.

Ehrlich, M. DNA methylation in cancer: too much, but also too little. *Oncogene*, 2002, 21(35), 5400-5413.

Ekbom, A. Epidemiology of lymphoma development in patients with rheumatoid arthritis. *Semin Arthritis Rheum*, 2005, 34 (5 Suppl. 1), 28-30.

Esteller, M & Herman, JG. Cancer as an epigenetic disease: DNA methylation and chromatin alterations in human tumours. *J Pathol*, 2002, 196 (1), 1-7.

Funk, JL.: A role for parathyroid hormone-related protein in the pathogenesis of inflammatory/autoimmune diseases. *Int Immunopharmacol*, 2001, 1(6),1101-1121.

Jones, PA & Laird, PW. Cancer epigenetics comes of age. Nature Genet, 1999, 98, 163-167.

Karpinets, TV & Foy, BD. Tumorigenesis: the adaptation of mammalian cells to sustained stress environment by epigenetic alterations and succeeding matched mutations. *Carcinogenesis*, 2005, 26(8), 1323-34.

Kartsogiannis, V; Udagawa, N; Ng, KW; Martin, TJ; Moseley, JM; Zhou, H. Localization of parathyroid hormone-related protein in osteoclasts by in situ hybridization and immunohistochemistry. *Bone*, 1998, 22, 189-194.

Kim, Young-In; Logan, JW; Mason, JB; Roubenoff R. DNA hypomethylation in infiammatory arthritis: reversal with methotrexate. *J Lab Clin Med*, 1996, 128, 2.

Kohno, H; Shigeno, C; Kasai, R; Akiyama, H; Iida, H; Tsuboyama, T; et al. Synovial fluids from patients with osteoarthritis and rheumatoid arthritis contain high levels of parathyroid hormone-related peptide. *J bone Miner Res*, 1997, 12, 847-54.

Liang, G; Gonzalgo, ML; Salem, C; Jones PA. Identification of DNA methylation differences during tumorigenesis by Methylation-sensitive arbitrarily primed polymerase chain reaction. *Methods*, 2002, 27, 150-155.

MacGregor, AJ; Snieder, H; Rigby, AS; Koskenvuo, M; Kaprio, J; Aho, K; Silman, AJ. Characterizing the quantitative genetic contribution to rheumatoid arthritis using data from twins. *Arthritis Rheum*, 2000, 43(1), 30-37.

McCabe, DC & Caudill, MA. DNA methylation, genomic silencing, and links to nutrition and cancer. *Nutr Rev*, 2005, 63 (6 Pt 1), 183-95.

Mariette, X; Cazals-Hatem, D; Warszawki, J; Liote, F; Balandraud, N; Sibilia, J. et al. Lymphomas in rheumatoid arthritis patients treated with methotrexate: a 3-year prospective study in France. *Blood*, 2002, 99 (11), 3909-3915.

Micheli, MR; & Bova, R. *Fingerprinting methods based on arbitrarily primed PCR.* Springer-Verlag Berlin Heidelberg, 1997.

Morgan, SL ; Baggott, JE ; Vaughn, WH; et al. The effect of folic acid supplementation on the toxicity of low-dose methotrexate treatment of rheumatoid arthritis. A double bind, placebo-controlled trial. *Ann Intern Med*, 1994, 121, 833-841.

Robertson, K.D & Jones, PA. DNA methylation: past, present and future directions. *Carcinogenesis*, 2000, 21 (3), 461-467.

Sciandrello, G; Caradonna, F; Mauro, M; Barbata, G. Arsenic-induced DNA hypomethylation affects chromosomal instability in mammalian cells. *Carcinogenesis*, 2004, 25(3), 413-417.

Solimando, DA. Overview of hypercalcemia of malignancy. *Am J Health Syst Pharm*, 2001, 58 (3), 4-7.

Wing-Yan, Au; Edmond, SK Ma; Carolyn, Choy; Lap-Ping, Chung; Tsz-Kin, Fung; Raymond, Liang; Yok-Lam, Kwong. Therapy-related lymphomas in patients with autoimmune diseases after treatment with disease-modifying anti-rheumatic drugs. *Am J Hematol*, 2006, 81, 5-11.

In: Novel Aspects of PTHrP Physiopathology
Editor: Claudio Luparello, pp. 321-340
ISBN: 978-1-60021-857-6

Chapter XIII

ASPECTS OF THE CYTOTOXIC ACTIVITY OF PTHRP [38-94]-AMIDE ON HUMAN BREAST CANCER CELLS

Rosalia Sirchia, Arianna Gullo and Claudio Luparello
Dipartimento di Biologia Cellulare e dello Sviluppo, Università di Palermo, Italy.

ABSTRACT

It was previously reported that the midregion PTHrP domain [38-94]-amide restrains growth and invasion "in vitro", causes striking toxicity and accelerates the death of some breast cancer cell lines, the most responsive being MDA-MB231 whose tumorigenesis was also attenuated "in vivo". In addition, more recent data has demonstrated that midregion PTHrP is imported in the nucleoplasm of cultured MDA-MB231 cells, and that "in vitro" it can bind chromatin of metaphase spread preparations, as well as an isolated 20-mer oligonucleotide, thereby appearing endowed with a putative transcription factor-like DNA-binding ability. In this chapter we will collectively discuss both precedent and more updated data from our lab. The latter studies arising from preliminary assays on DNA status, and gene and protein expression patterns of treated cells, aimed to check whether the cytotoxicity of the peptide may result from a reprogramming of gene expression towards apoptotic death or, instead, is to be ascribed to an unprogrammed perturbation of cell functions.

INTRODUCTION

The human breast is a modified sweat gland that originates from the epidermal mammary ridge, whose epithelial component in the post-pubertal age consists of a monolayer of polarized luminal cells organized into branching ducts terminating in multiple acini. The epithelial and myoepithelial component of the gland, leaning onto the basal lamina, is embedded in an abundant interstitial stroma composed of fat tissue, fibrous and loose connective tissue, and blood vessels. It is generally acknowledged that cancer development by breast luminal epithelium, apart from multistep genetic alterations, is strongly influenced by the complex interactions occurring between cancer cells and the novel microenvironment originating within the tissue structure. It is in this microenvironment that newly-synthesized soluble factors providing additional and different biological stimuli, and macromolecular polymers of the stromal matrix exposed after the dissolution of the basal lamina, are now available for epithelial cell attachment and signalization (e.g. Byers et al., 1994; Ethier, 1995; Weaver et al., 1996; Shekhar et al., 2003, for reviews).

Substantial evidence indicates that one of those microenvironmental factors strongly involved in breast tumor progression is PTHrP, a protein whose involvement in ductal branching morphogenesis of the developing breast and in the physiology of lactation has been widely documented (Budayr et al., 1989; Ratcliffe, 1992; Wysolmerski et al., 1995, 1998; Dunbar et al., 1999; Hens and Wysolmerski, 2005). It must be remembered that one of the original tumours from which PTHrP was purified and sequenced, because of the elevated concentration of its circulating form, was breast cancer (Stewart et al., 1987, Ikeda et al., 1988). It is now well-known that PTHrP is centrally involved in both the osteotropism of breast cancer and in the onset of the tumor-associated humoral hypercalcemic syndrome resulting from systemic overproduction of the protein and its local release at skeletal metastasis sites with the following activation of bone resorption (Guise et al., 1996; 2002). Indeed, immunohistochemical and "in situ" hybridization studies indicated that PTHrP expression was higher and more frequent in breast tumor skeletal metastases than in the parental primary tumor (Southby et al., 1990; Powell et al., 1991; Vargas et al., 1992). Auto- and intracrine regulation of breast tumor cells by PTHrP has been supported by experimental data in both "in vivo" and "in vitro" model systems (e.g. Birch et al., 1995; Iezzoni et al., 1998; Falzon and Du, 2000; Tovar Sepulveda et al., 2002; Hoey et al., 2003; Torricelli et al., 2006). In addition, breast stromal cells, both embryonic and neoplastic, and myoepithelial cells have been proven to synthesize and secrete PTHrP, thus critically contributing to the maintenance of epithelial/mesenchymal signalling paracrine circuits in mammary tissue (Dunbar et al., 1998; Sopel and Lis, 2000; Cros et al., 2002).

An aspect of PTHrP which attracted attention by several laboratories, including ours, is that its biological effects are actually exerted by discrete fragments, originating by its post-translational processing and which can mediate opposing functions, whose properties have been investigated in different "in vitro" model system (e.g. Clemens et al., 2001 for review). Within this context, dealing with breast cancer we have previously demonstrated that: i) PTHrP expression was restricted to subpopulations of the heterogeneous 8701-BC cell line, derived from a biopsy fragment of a primary neoplasm, endowed with a more "aggressive" phenotype (Luparello et al.,1993), ii) its expression in parental 8701-BC cells could be drastically modulated by modifications of the "in vitro" microenvironment, such as addition of either stromal components, growth factors, hormones or chemicals (Luparello et al., 1999, 2000), and, iii) [1-34], [67-86] and [107-138], but not [38-64], PTHrP domains actively controlled the proliferative and invasive behaviour as well as the expression of genes encoding for stress response proteins and extracellular lytic enzymes in both parental cell line and selected sublines (Luparello et al., 1995, 1997, 2003a).

In the following chapters, we will discuss our findings obtained about the cytotoxic activity exerted on breast cancer cells by PTHrP [38-94]-amide, a fragment that has potentially important therapeutic implications for anti-neoplastic molecular modelling.

PTHrP is Biologically-Active on Breast Tumor Cells

A number of literature reports were focussed on the evaluation of the biological properties of different midregion PTHrP domains, such as [38-64] able to promote growth of type II pneumocytes (Hastings et al., 2002), and [67-86] whose activation of phospholipase C-dependent pathways in SqCC/Y1 cells and sensitization of pneumocytes to apoptosis was recognized (Orloff et al., 1997; Hastings et al., 2003), apart from results coming from our lab, cited in the previous paragraph. Subsequent to the collective data of Soifer et al. (1992), Yang et al. (1994), and Wu et al. (1996), which demonstrated that the actual mid-region physiologic secretory form was PTHrP [38-94]-amide, the first experimental data on the effect exerted by this specific fragment was enclosed in the same paper by Wu and coworkers (Wu et al., 1996), being related to its ability in stimulating transients in cytosolic calcium in rat insulinoma RIN and human cervix carcinoma YCC cultured cells, and transplacental calcium transport "in vivo". Successive studies on PTHrP [38-94] and calcium fluxes were also performed by Strid et al. (2002), who found that the peptide was able to selectively stimulate the ATP-dependent transport of the ion by syncytiotrophoblast basal membrane vesicles through the IP_3–DAG–PKC second messenger pathway. In 2001, some of us published a paper exploring the effect of PTHrP [38-94]-amide on viability, proliferation, invasiveness and growth in nude mice of six different breast cancer cell lines (Hs578T, MDA-MB231, T47-D, 8701-BC and its clonal lines BC-3A and BC-61), representing the spectrum of breast tumors encountered in medical practice and spanning the range of histochemical subtypes, estrogen receptor status, vimentin expression, activity in chemotaxis and chemoinvasion assays and invasive behaviour in nude mice. We demonstrated that, differently from the other PTHrP fragments tested, (i.e. [1-34], [38-64], [67-86] and [107-138]), PTHrP [38-94]-amide, administered at 1 nM concentration, was able to restrain growth and invasion "in vitro" as well as to cause striking toxicity and accelerate death of the panel of cells assayed, the most responsive being MDA-MB231 whose tumorigenesis in immunocompromised mice was markedly restrained by daily intratumoral inoculation of the peptide (Luparello et al., 2001).

These results prompted a more detailed study on tumor cell-PTHrP interactions and the molecular pathway(s) through which midregion peptide may accomplish its powerful effects on the phenotypic modulation of mammary carcinoma cells.

PTHrP [38-94] Possesses Potential Transcription Factor-Like Properties

It is known that PTHrP contains a nuclear localization sequence (NLS) mediating importin β-driven nuclear import, and that nucleo-cytoplasmatic fluxes of the protein are cell cycle dependent (e.g. Lam et al., 2000; Fiaschi-Taesch and Stewart, 2003); PTHrP NLS has been localized in the sequence spanning aminoacids 87 to 106, with the preceding sequence, i.e. [71-82], likely required to guarantee a more stable importin binding (Lam et al., 2001). This implies that NLS possessing-fragments once gained access to nucleoplasm could play potential transcription factor-like roles. As a support to this hypothesis, intracrine role for PTHrP in cell growth, adhesion, migration, invasion, and integrin expression regulation has been documented for MCF-7 breast tumor cells over-expressing wild type *vs.* NLS-mutated protein (Tovar Sepulveda et al., 2002; Shen et al., 2004), and mobilization of intracellular calcium has been observed in different breast cancer cell lines treated with PTHrP-[67-101], whose ability to translocate to the nucleus was reported in the same paper by Kumari et al. (2006). Noteworthy, intracrine effects of midregion PTHrP domains have been described also in other experimental models (e.g. Aarts et al., 1999; Shen and Falzon, 2003; Fiaschi-Taesch et al., 2004) .

One of the questions remained unsolved was whether PTHrP could be allowed to interact directly with nuclear chromatin or it would bind other nuclear components thereby participating to the formation of putative supra-molecular regulatory complexes.

Some of us have recently produced data demonstrating that midregion PTHrP applied to the exterior of living breast cancer MDA-MB231 cells accumulates in their nucleoplasm at interphase (Sirchia et al., in press). Moreover, although so far lacking of "in vivo" counterparts, we have also obtained "in vitro" results confirming the direct chromatin binding by PTHrP [38-94]-amide, which was shown to "decorate" MDA-MB231 chromosomes of metaphase spread preparations in a selective and stable manner, with a conspicuous number of evenly-distributed discrete intense fluorescent spots that display no accumulation at specific chromosomal sites. Interestingly, the "decoration" pattern appears to be cell type-specific, since in preliminary studies using immortalized non-malignant mammary epithelial cells we have observed smaller number of hybridization signals per genome (manuscript in preparation). In the same paper, we have also identified the sequence recognized by the protein, i.e. 5'-GAGTAGAATTCTAATATCTC-3, and the specific requirements for optimal binding employing a combination of "whole genome"/conventional PCR, EMSA and DNAse footprinting techniques. In particular, the collective data indicated that the binding i) was selective, ii) required double-stranded DNA, iii) was effectively competed by pre-incubation of mid-region PTHrP with the anti-PTHrP [34-53] antibody, iv) was undetectable when either PTHrP [38-64]-amide or [67-86]-amide were submitted to EMSAs in the place of the intact [38-94]-amide fragment, v) critically needed the presence of the GA/GAG terminal motifs albeit repetitive GA and GAG modules were insufficient to create binding sites, and therefore, vi) was somehow sequence context-dependent. Interestingly, also literature data support the concept that this sequence is involved in protein recognition; in fact, PATCH software analysis (available on-line at http://www.gene-regulation.com/cgi-bin/pub/programs/patch/bin/patch.cgi) indicated that portions of this 20-mer oligonucleotide were targets for transcriptional modulators of various species, including human GATA-1 and POU2F1; on the other hand, the existence of factors able to bind the GA-rich sequences present in several gene promoters in a context-dependent way, i.e. under the selective control of local sequence characteristics, has been documented in various model systems (e.g. Van Steensel et al., 2003).

In light of our and other researchers' observations strongly suggesting a nuclear activity for midregion PTHrP endowed with a likely transcription factor-like DNA-binding ability, we have performed a set of pilot assays aimed to check whether the cytotoxic activity of midregion peptide resulted from a reprogramming of gene expression towards apoptotic death or, instead, was to be ascribed to an unprogrammed perturbation of cell physiology, by analyzing DNA status, and gene and protein expression patterns in treated cells.

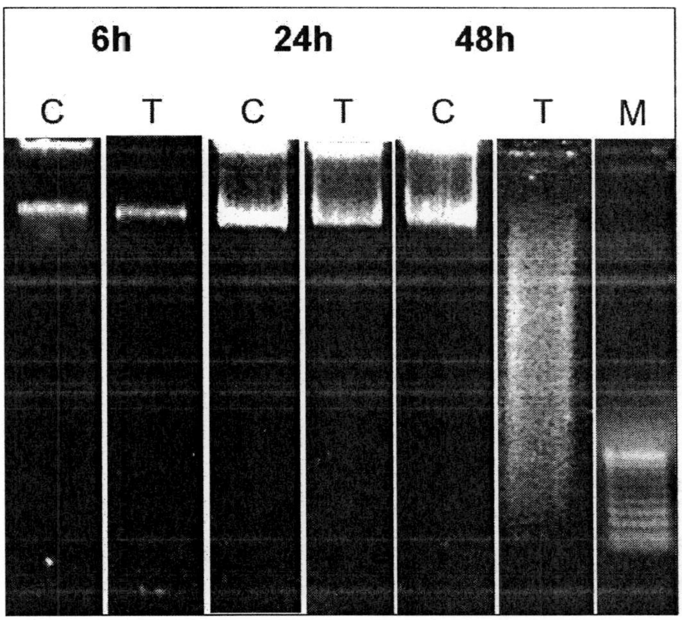

Figure 1. Representative VGGE of the DNA isolated from MDA-MB231 cells, cultured in control conditions (C) and in the presence of 1nM PTHrP [38-94]-amide (T) for 6, 24 and 48 h. M = size marker (100 bp ladder).

PTHrP [38-94] Treatment Induces Random DNA Fragmentation in MDA-MB231 Breast Cancer Cells

We planned to check whether MDA-MB231 cell treatment with 1 nM PTHrP [38-94]-amide (Luparello et al., 2001) was accompanied by oligonucleosomal DNA fragmentation, a hallmark of apoptosis, by a combination of electrophoretic and cytochemical assays. To this purpose, in a first set of experiments DNA was extracted from control and treated cell lysates and submitted to voltage gradient gel electophoresis (VGGE, see Izzo et al., 2000), as reported by Luparello et al. (2003b); secondly, control and treated cell cultures were assayed using the ApopTag Peroxidase In Situ Oligo Ligation kit (Serologicals Co., Norcross GA/USA), as reported by Luparello and Sirchia (2005). Figure 1 shows the DNA status after 6, 24 and 48 h of treatment: DNA obtained from cells treated for 6 and 24 h appeared to be in an intact high molecular weight-form, but when DNA was extracted at 48 h from incubation and assayed, an electrophoretic smear, due to random digestion characteristic of "non-apoptotic" death response (at least in a "conventional" conception) could be observed. No "ladder-like" pattern of DNA fragmentation was evident in all the experiments performed.

A similar result was obtained by cytochemical analysis. We used the apoptosis-discriminating Apoptag technique, that is based upon "in situ" ligation in the presence of either biotinylated oligo A, which contains a 3'-dA overhang, or biotinylated oligo B, which is blunt-ended, the first oligo being more selective for the detection of "classical" apoptosis than other types of cell death; labelled DNA is then reacted with streptavidin-horseradish peroxidase and detected with diaminobenzidine substrate. As shown in figure 2, more cells stained positively using the "necrosis-related" oligo B *vs.* the "apoptosis-related" oligo A.

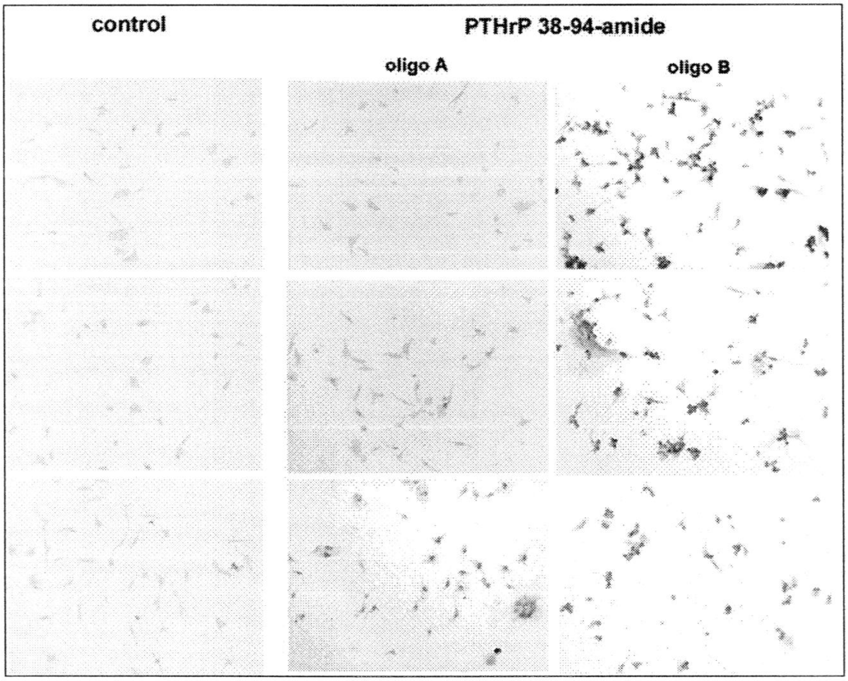

Figure 2. Panel of micrographs of MDA-MB231 cells cultured in control conditions and in the presence of 1nM PTHrP [38-94]-amide, and submitted to Apoptag labeling using oligo A (one-base 30-dT overhang-end detection) and oligo B (blunt-end detection). Original magnification: 20x.

Thus, in light of the cumulative data obtained it appeared plausible that PTHrP [38-94]-driven cytotoxic effect on MDA-MB231 breast cancer cells was not to be ascribed to activation of mechanisms of "classical" programmed cell death. On the other hand, comparison analysis of PTHrP-binding sequence, described in the preceding paragraph, with non-human DNA sequences deposited in on-line data banks indicated that this sequence was also contained in a 183 bp-DNA fragment from *M. musculus* (acc. nr. AJ403155), which is recognized by vimentin through specific Y and/or F amino acidic residues of its N-terminal head domain which allows it to participate in the control of both chromatin architecture and DNA recombination/repair events (Tolstonog et al., 2000; Wang et al., 2001). We consider these data intriguing within the context of our work for the two following reasons: 1) they represent the second documented case in which this specific DNA sequence is involved in protein binding, and. more importantly, 2) the interaction of vimentin with DNA occurs in segments containing inverted repeats and forming cruciform structures, thereby eliciting helix-destabilizing configurational changes which render the zone more accessible to the action of T7 endonuclease I (Li et al., 2003). Therefore, in light of our data on extensive chromatin cleavage following cell incubation with midregion PTHrP, the binding sites detected on the different chromosomes could seemingly represent selective start-points for chromatin degradation by some still-unidentified endonuclease. Further experiments will be necessary to validate this fascinating hypothesis.

PTHrP [38-94] Treatment Induces Selective Changes in the Expression Levels of Genes Coding for Apoptosis Factors and Stress Response Proteins

In a following set of experiments, we examined whether midregion PTHrP could actively control gene expression. Firstly, we focused our attention on the cytogenetic sites where the 20-mer sequence recognized by mid-region PTHrP "in vitro" was localized, thereby selecting some genes for evaluation of their expression levels in control and treated cell samples. In particular, we tested *PCP4/PEP19* since the sequence is located between two of its exons in the 21q22.3 cytogenetic band, and other genes involved in the control of cell life/death and carcinogenesis, mapping into 8q23 cytogenetic band (*COX6C, OXR1, FZD6, RRM2B, EIF3S6, EBAG9*); in addition, we included in our experiments also *HOX7/MSX1* and WT1, whose promoters are rich in GA sequences, due to the documented mid-region PTHrP affinity to GAG and GA motifs (Sirchia et al., in press). Also, we submitted cDNA samples, obtained from enriched mRNA preparations of both control and treated MDA-MB231 cells, to differential display (DD)-PCR assays to further supplement the catalogue of mid-region PTHrP-dependent genes. The data obtained by a combination of conventional- and semiquantitative multiplex (SM)-PCR techniques (Sirchia and Luparello, 2007) indicated that four genes implicated in cell survival, mitochondrial respiration and protection from injury, i.e. *OXR1 (Oxidation Resistance 1), FZD6 (Frizzled Homologue 6), COX6C* (*Cytochrome c Oxidase, subunit VIc)* and *HOX7/MSX1* (*Homeobox 7/Muscle Segment Homeobox, Drosophila, Homolog 1)* were down-regulated by PTHrP treatment, thereby being potentially involved in PTHrP-mediated cytotoxic effect. This result also provided further support to the hypothesis of the intrinsic transcriptional modulation capability owned by midregion PTHrP. Moreover, DD-PCR experiments identified other genes whose expression levels were affected by incubation with PTHrP [38-94]-amide and whose biological implications are still to be determined.

In light of this first group of data demonstrating that treatment with midregion PTHrP actually induced transcriptional alterations in MDA-MB231 cells, secondly we wanted to test whether modifications in the expression levels of genes coding for stress factors and for proteins involved in the onset of apoptosis could also occur following incubation of cells with the peptide. To this purpose, cDNA preparations from control and PTHrP-treated MDA-MB231 cells were submitted to conventional- and (SM)-PCR in the presence of primers specific for the cDNAs of various genes encoding for heat shock proteins (hsp), i.e. *hsp60, hsc70, hsp70, mthsp75, hsp90α* and *β*-(e.g. Garrido et al., 2001, for a review), and for some apoptosis-agonist and –antagonist factors, i.e. *Bcl-2, Bcl-xL, Bcl-xS, Bad, Bax-α, p53, Tiar, Rip-1, Dap-kinase* (*Dap-k*), *Cellular Apoptosis Susceptibility* (*Cas*) and *Waf-1* (e.g. Wang et al., 1999, for a review), as reported by Luparello et al. (2003a,b) and Luparello and Sirchia (2005). The panel in figure 3, representative of three independent experiments, shows that in conventional PCR assays a positive signal was found for all the cDNA tested and obtained from cell samples with or without exposition to PTHrP [38-94], indicating that gene expressions are switched-on in both experimental conditions.

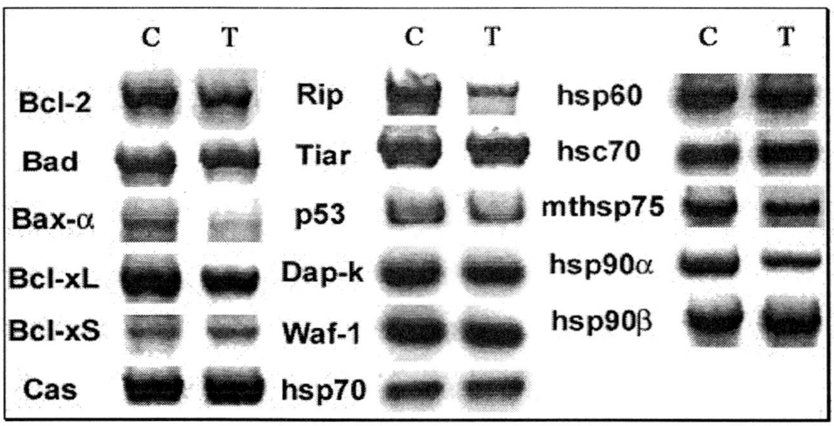

Figure 3. PCR analysis of expression of genes coding for stress response proteins and apoptosis-related factors by control (C) and midregion PTHrP-treated (T) MDA-MB231 cells.

The cDNA preparations were then submitted to triplicate SM-PCR (Spencer and Christensen, 1999) to compare the expression levels of the selected genes. Essentially, the cDNA species of interest was co-amplified with β-actin cDNA, as "housekeeping" gene, over a range of cycles, followed by 2% agarose electrophoresis and ethidium bromide stain. The intensities of the bands of interest, evaluated with SigmaScan software (SPSS, USA), were normalized for those of β-actin, and plotted as a function of cycle number. Exponential regression equations fitted to the curves were used to calculate the number of cycles necessary to reach a normalized intensity threshold value = 1 for each sample. The relative difference in abundance between two samples was taken as 2^n where n is the difference between the numbers of cycles required by the samples to reach the threshold. As shown in the panels in figures 4 and 5, we found that incubation of MDA-MB231 cells with PTHrP [38-94]-amide was able to modulate the expression levels of only *hsc70* (+3.9 folds), *hsp70* (+2 folds) and *hsp90α* (-2.6 folds) among the stress protein genes, and of only *Bcl-xS* (+ 2.2

folds), *Bad* (+2.7 folds) and, more prominently, *Rip-1* (+4.26 folds) among the apoptosis factor genes. All the standard errors of the mean (s.e.m) were less than 0.05. No significant difference was found for the expression levels of the other tested genes between control and treated breast tumor cells (not shown).

Although the data obtained put in evidence a certain stability of the expression levels for most of the genes coding for apoptosis modulators, nonetheless the cytotoxic effect triggered by midregion PTHrP on MDA-MB231 could see the involvement of some pro-apoptotic factors, such as Bad and Bcl-xS, whose up-regulation was found to promote cell death in different breast cancer cell lines, including MDA-MB231 (Sumantran et al., 1995; Lim et al., 2001; Majumder et al., 2002; Zhang et al., 2003; Luparello and Sirchia, 2005). According to Tudor et al. (2000), alteration of *Bad* transcription or mRNA stability is an early cellular response to stress or drug-induced injury, and a potentially-critic regulation point of downstream steps, susceptible to be restrained by survival mechanisms, which cumulatively govern the ultimate predisposition to apoptosis. Particularly interesting appears to be the over-expression of *Rip-1*, a gene encoding for a member of receptor-interacting protein (Rip) family kinases which function as integrators of extracellular and intracellular stresses and crucial regulators of cell survival (Meylan and Tschopp, 2005). In light of our observation that *Rip-1* is the gene undergoing the most significant change of expression level among those tested, and that Rip-1 has been reported to trigger pro-survival responses as well as opposite death-inducing mechanisms, the identification of the specific effect exerted by such up-regulation in our model system will deserve further and more detailed investigations.

Concerning the expression of hsps, the up-regulation of *hsp70* and *hsc70* may be interpreted as a typical stress response. Ciocca et al. (1992) have produced evidence that *hsp70* over-expression in MDA-MB231 cells is associated with acquisition of resistance to anticancer drug doxorubicin; it is also worth-mentioning that Grzesiak et al. (2005) have recently reported interaction between various PTHrP fragment, including midregion [37-86], and hsp70 expressed on the surface of cancer cells, thereby being somehow involved in the internalization of extracellular PTHrP. On the other hand, up-regulation of *hsc70* (i.e. cognate of hsp70), encoding for another cytosolic molecular chaperone important for the folding of newly-synthesized polypeptides, has been correlated to apoptosis-resistance in ovarian cancer cells (Sugimura et al., 2004). Noteworthy, hsc70 is reported to be involved in the so-called "chaperone-mediated autophagy", in that it stimulates an intracellular pathway of proteolysis that is selective for particular cytosolic proteins which are bound and targeted to the lysosomes for destruction (e.g. Agarraberes and Dice, 2001); thus, up-regulation of *hsc70* could be seemingly related to the enhanced protein degradation identified by electrophoretic analysis in preparations from PTHrP [38-94]-treated breast cancer cells (see following paragraph). Moreover, also *hsp90α* expression level appears to be correlated to cell growth behaviour, since its decrease has been reported to determine the switching-off of proliferation in osteoblasts (Shakoori et al., 1992), whilst its increase seems to be involved in the enhanced proliferation of pancreatic carcinomas (Ogata et al., 2000).

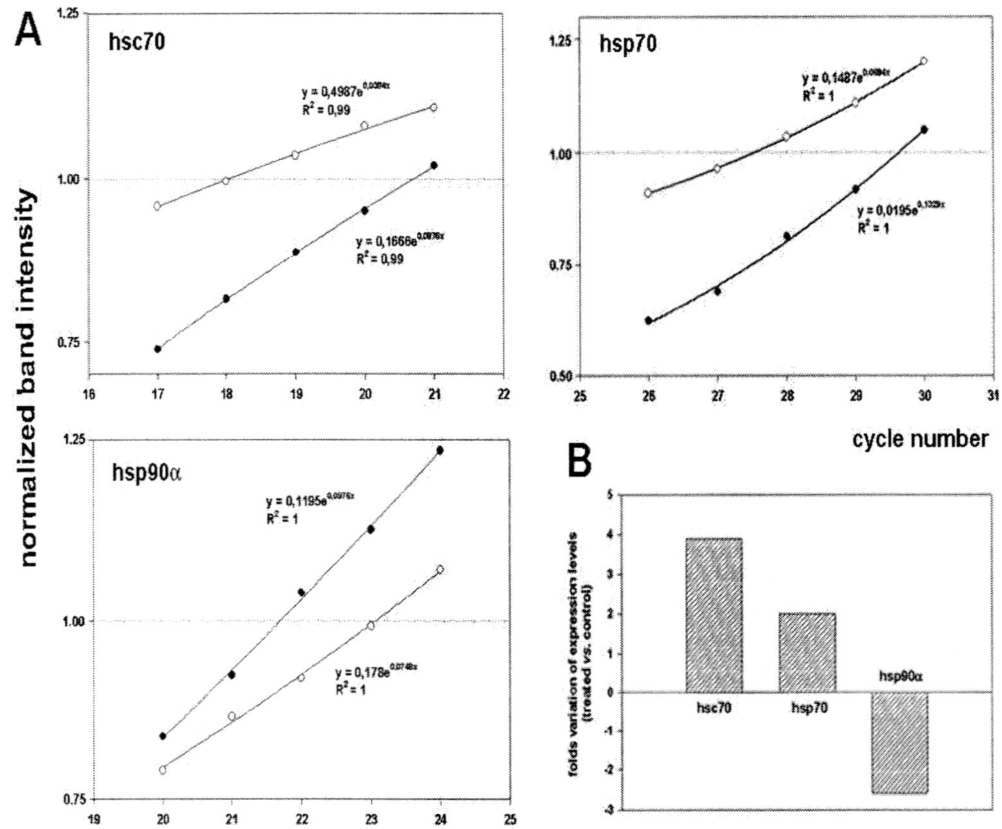

Figure 4. A) SM-PCR for stress response genes hsc70, hsp70 and hsp90α. Representative plots of normalized data vs. cycle number fit with an exponential curve for control (●) and midregion PTHrP-treated (○) MDA-MB231 cells. B) Histogram showing changes of gene expression levels in treated MDA-MB231 cells *versus* controls, as resulted from SM-PCR assays.

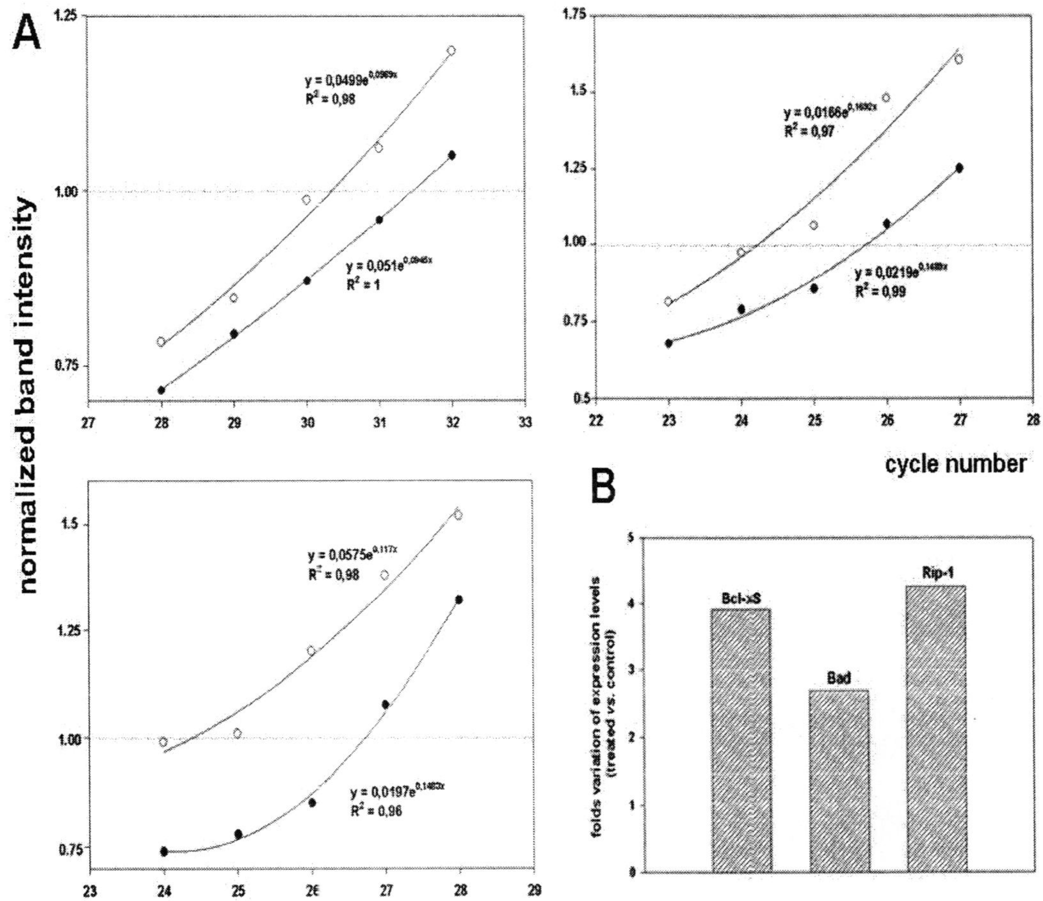

Figure 5. A) SM-PCR for apoptosis factors Bad, Bcl-xS and Rip-1. Representative plots of normalized data vs. cycle number fit with an exponential curve for control (●) and midregion PTHrP-treated (○) MDA-MB231 cells. B) Histogram showing changes of gene expression levels in treated MDA-MB231 cells *versus* controls, as resulted from SM-PCR assays.

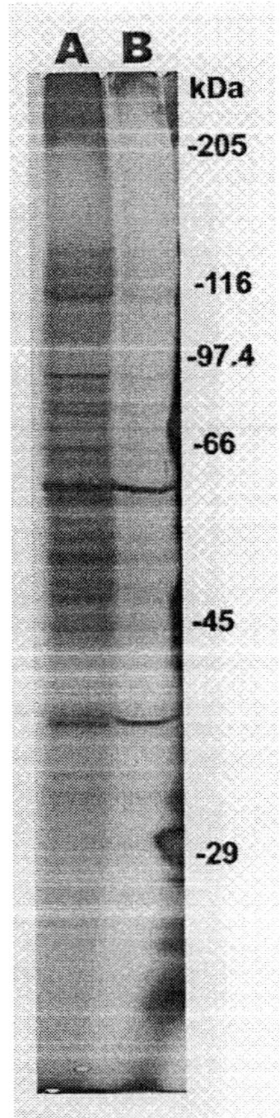

Figure 6. Electrophoretogram of protein lysates from control (A) and PTHrP-treated (B) MDA-MB231 cell preparations. 10% SDS-PAGE, silver stain.

PTHrP [38-94] Treatment Induces a Potential Massive Protein Degradation in MDA-MB231 Breast Tumor Cells

In a third set of experiments, still at the preliminary stage, we wanted to check the global electrophoretic protein pattern of preparations from control and PTHrP-treated MDA-MB231 cell cultures. To this purpose, cells were directly lysed in flasks and lysates submitted to protein extraction according to Wang et al. (1996); after colorimetric dosage, equivalent amounts of proteins from triplicate samples were submitted to SDS-PAGE in a sequencing gel apparatus and to silver stain, according to Luparello (2000), in order to reveal the expanded protein patterns in both experimental conditions of culture. Interestingly, as shown in figure 6, although starting with equivalent amounts of proteins, preparations from treated cells displayed a noticeable weakening of the staining of all electrophoretic bands with respect to control samples, except for two protein bands of apparent M_r of about 38 and 64 kDa, whose characterization remains to be determined. This result can be tentatively interpreted on the basis of the augmentation of protein degradative events in PTHrP-treated cells, leading to loss of small protein fragments during the electrophoretic run. It is worth-mentioning that full-length PTHrP, as well as various PTHrP domains such as [1-34], [1-40] and [67-86] were proven to promote up-regulation and activation of matrix metalloproteases and UBP41, an ubiquitin-specific protease, in different biological system (Hoekman et al., 1991; Kawashima-Ohya et al., 1999; Maioli et al., 2002; Miles et al., 2002; Luparello et al., 2003a). Whether additional experiments confirm that midregion PTHrP is also a stimulator of intracellular protease production and/or activity, such observation will provide further support to the postulate of massive intracellular damage following incubation of breast cancer cells with 1 nM midregion PTHrP.

Perspectives and Conclusion

In the present chapter we have summarized our more updated data on midregion PTHrP regulation of breast cancer cell phenotype, with the MDA-MB231 cell line as a model system. Although future work is needed to define the precise nature of molecular events underlying PTHrP cytotoxicity and to expand the list of neoplastic cytotypes tested, the data so far obtained allows the following considerations.

Clear indications have been produced that PTHrP [38-94]-amide gains access inside MDA-MB231 cells and is imported into the nucleus where it is likely to bind chromatin in accordance with the ability demonstrated "in vitro". Parallel data strongly suggests that the peptide actively controls gene expression, since cell treatment induces modifications in the expression level of selected genes encoding for stress response and apoptotic factors. Noteworthy, this hypothesis is supported by additional results we have recently obtained from differential display-PCR assays, revealing other mRNAs whose expression in MDA-MB231 cells is modulated by midregion PTHrP, including those from homeotic genes involved in complex intracellular networks such as *MSX-1* (Sirchia and Luparello, 2007). Thus, new sets of experiments will be designed with the aim to supplement even further the catalogue of mid-region PTHrP-responsive genes in MDA-MB231 cells, in order to better characterize the molecular basis of the putative "anti-breast cancer" effect of the peptide. On the other hand, to check its transcriptional factor-like role, it will be of interest to perform reporter gene studies to confirm "in vivo" the effect of midregion PTHrP on the modulation of gene expression.

From the preliminary data obtained, the lethal effect exerted by the peptide shows aspects amenable to both apoptosis and necrosis type of death. It is therefore conceivable that midregion PTHrP activates one of those alternative pathways of apoptosis, such as necrosis-like programmed cell death, which display mixed characteristics (e.g Leist and Jaattela, 2001, for a review). Within this context, a particular interest will be devoted to the observed up-regulation of *Rip-1* and its biological significance. In fact, its protein product, whose key role in life/death cellular decisions has been cited before, was also proven to have properties of both apoptosis and necrosis factor. In particular, Holler et al. (2000) reported that activation of Rip-1 kinase was responsible for the onset of cell necrosis due to accumulation of reactive oxygen species (ROS). Moreover, Lewis et al. (2000) and Vanden Berghe et al. (2003) have also demonstrated that hsp90, whose underexpression was observed in our model system for the α isotype, associates with Rip-1 thereby regulating its stability and activity. Future investigation will be designed to check whether i) mitochondrial respiration levels and the intracellular redox state may be involved in PTHrP-mediated lethal effect; ii) hsp90α may play a role in the Rip-1-controlled cellular events in our model system; iii) The activation of extensive intracellular proteolysis by incubation with the peptide will be evaluated more in detail, and the involved enzymes identified.

In conclusion, these studies provide evidence that PTHrP, in addition to its ability to activate endocrine, paracrine and autocrine receptor-mediated processes, also likely possesses intrinsic DNA binding and transcriptional modulation capability, which appears to account, at least in part, for the well-documented nuclear localization of PTHrP, and for the altered function of NTS-deleted forms of PTHrP. Moreover, these studies further support the concept that the physiology of PTHrP in normal breast development and function might include forms of PTHrP beyond those which have been studied most extensively to date, i.e. PTHrP [1-36] and full-length PTHrP (e.g. Falzon and Du, 2000; Guise et al., 2002). Based on the current observations, mid-region PTHrP may seemingly play physiologic roles in mammary ductular development, fat pad invasion, branching morphogenesis, and/or lactation. Characterization of these possibilities will require further analysis.

Acknowledgments

This work was supported by a grant from the University of Palermo (R.S. ex 60%). We thank Prof. A.F. Stewart (University of Pittsburgh, USA) for generous gift of purified PTHrP(38-94)-amide and for helpful suggestions.

References

Aarts, M. M., Rix, A., Guo, J., Bringhurst, R. & Henderson, J. E. (1999) The nucleolar targeting signal (NTS) of parathyroid hormone related protein mediates endocytosis and nucleolar translocation. *J. Bone Miner. Res.*, *14*, 1493-1503.

Agarraberes, F. A. & Dice, J. F. (2001) A molecular chaperone complex at the lysosomal membrane is required for protein translocation. *J. Cell Sci.*, *114*, 2491-2499.

Birch, M. A., Carron, J. A., Scott, M., Fraser, W. D. & Gallagher, J. A. (1995) Parathyroid hormone (PTH)/PTH-related protein (PTHrP) receptor expression and mitogenic responses in human breast cancer cell lines. *Br. J. Cancer.*, *72*, 90-95.

Budayr, A. A., Halloran, B. P., King, J. C., Diep, D., Nissenson, R. A. & Strewler, G. J. (1989) High levels of a parathyroid hormone-like protein in milk. *Proc. Natl. Acad. Sci. USA*, *86*, 7183-7185.

Byers, S., Park, M., Sommers, C. & Seslar, S. (1994) Breast carcinoma: a collective disorder. *Breast Cancer Res Treat.*, *31*, 203-215.

Ciocca, D. R., Fuqua, S. A., Lock-Lim, S., Toft, D. O., Welch, W. J. & McGuire, W. L. (1992) Response of human breast cancer cells to heat shock and chemotherapeutic drugs. *Cancer Res.*, *52*, 3648-3654.

Clemens, T. L., Cormier, S., Eichinger, A., Endlich, K., Fiaschi-Taesch, N., Fischer, E., Friedman, P. A., Karaplis, A. C., Massfelder, T., Rossert, J., Schluter, K. D., Silve, C., Stewart, A. F., Takane, K. & Helwig, J. J. (2001) Parathyroid hormone-related protein and its receptors: nuclear functions and roles in the renal and cardiovascular systems, the placental trophoblasts and the pancreatic islets. *Br. J. Pharmacol.*, *134*, 1113-1136.

Cros, M., Cataisson, C., Cho, Y. M., Berthois, Y., Bernard-Poenaru, O., Denne, M., Graulet, A. M., De Vernejoul, M. C., Foley, J. & Bouizar, Z. (2002) Constitutive production of parathyroid hormone-related protein (PTHrP) by fibroblasts derived from normal and pathological human breast tissue. *Oncol. Res.*, *13*, 137-146.

Dunbar, M. E., Young, P., Zhang, J. P., McCaughern-Carucci, J., Lanske, B., Orloff, J. J., Karaplis, A., Cunha, G. & Wysolmerski, J. J. (1998) Stromal cells are critical targets in the regulation of mammary ductal morphogenesis by parathyroid hormone-related protein. *Dev. Biol.*, *203*, 75-89.

Dunbar, M. E., Dann, P. R., Robinson, G. W., Hennighausen, L., Zhang, J. P & Wysolmerski, J. J. (1999) Parathyroid hormone-related protein signaling is necessary for sexual dimorphism during embryonic mammary development. *Development*, *126*, 3485-3493.

Ethier, S.P. (1995). Growth factor synthesis and human breast cancer progression. *J. Natl. Cancer Inst.*, *87*, 964-973.

Falzon, M. & Du, P. (2000) Enhanced growth of MCF-7 breast cancer cells overexpressing parathyroid hormone-related peptide. *Endocrinology*, *141*, 1882-1892.

Fiaschi-Taesch, N. M. & Stewart, A. F. (2003) Minireview: parathyroid hormone-related protein as an intracrine factor--trafficking mechanisms and functional consequences. *Endocrinology*, *144*, 407-411.

Fiaschi-Taesch, N., Takane, K. K., Masters, S., Lopez-Talavera, J. C. & Stewart, A. F. (2004) Parathyroid-hormone-related protein as a regulator of pRb and the cell cycle in arterial smooth muscle. *Circulation*, *110*, 177-185

Garrido, C., Gurbuxani, S., Ravagnan, L. & Kroemer, G. (2001) Heat shock proteins: endogenous modulators of apoptotic cell death. *Biochem. Biophys. Res. Commun.*, *286*, 433-442.

Grzesiak, J. J., Smith, K. C., Chalberg, C., Truong, C., Burton, D. W., Deftos, L. J. & Bouvet, M. (2005) Heat shock protein-70 expressed on the surface of cancer cells binds parathyroid hormone-related protein in vitro. *Endocrinology*, *146*, 3567-3576

Guise, T. A., Yin, J. J., Taylor, S. D., Kumagai, Y., Dallas, M., Boyce, B. F., Yoneda, T. & Mundy, G. R. (1996). Evidence for a causal role of parathyroid hormone-related protein in the pathogenesis of human breast cancer-mediated osteolysis. *J. Clin. Invest.*, *98*, 1544-1549.

Guise, T. A., Yin, J. J., Thomas, R. J., Dallas, M., Cui, Y. & Gillespie, M. T. (2002) Parathyroid hormone-related protein (PTHrP)-(1-139) isoform is efficiently secreted in vitro and enhances breast cancer metastasis to bone in vivo. *Bone*, *30*, 670-676.

Hastings, R. H., Asirvatham, A., Quintana, R., Sandoval, R., Dutta, R., Burton, D. W. & Deftos, L. J. (2002) Parathyroid hormone-related protein-(38-64) regulates lung cell proliferation after silica injury. *Am. J. Physiol. Lung Cell Mol. Physiol.*, *283*, L12-21.

Hastings, R. H., Quintana, R. A., Sandoval, R., Duey, D., Rascon, Y., Burton, D. W. & Deftos, L. J. (2003) Proapoptotic effects of parathyroid hormone-related protein in type II pneumocytes. *Am. J. Respir. Cell. Mol. Biol.*, *29*, 733-742.

Hens, J. R. & Wysolmerski, J. J. (2005) Key stages of mammary gland development: molecular mechanisms involved in the formation of the embryonic mammary gland. *Breast Cancer Res.*, *7*, 220-224.

Hoekman, K., Lowik, C. W., vd Ruit, M., Bijvoet, O. L., Verheijen, J. H. & Papapoulos, S. E. (1991) Regulation of the production of plasminogen activators by bone resorption enhancing and inhibiting factors in three types of osteoblast-like cells. *Bone Miner.*, *14*, 189-204.

Hoey, R. P., Sanderson, C., Iddon, J., Brady, G., Bundred, N. J. & Anderson, N. G. (2003) The parathyroid hormone-related protein receptor is expressed in breast cancer bone metastases and promotes autocrine proliferation in breast carcinoma cells. *Br. J. Cancer*, *88*, 567-573.

Holler, N., Zaru, R., Micheau, O., Thome, M., Attinger, A., Valitutti, S., Bodmer, J. L., Schneider, P., Seed, B. & Tschopp, J. (2000) Fas triggers an alternative, caspase-8-independent cell death pathway using the kinase RIP as effector molecule. *Nat. Immunol.*, *1*, 489-495.

Iezzoni, J. C., Bruns, M. E., Frierson, H. F., Scott, M. G., Pence, R. A., Deftos, L. J. & Bruns, D. E. (1998) Coexpression of parathyroid hormone-related protein and its receptor in breast carcinoma: a potential autocrine effector system. *Mod. Pathol.*, *11*, 265-270.

Ikeda ,K., Mangin, M., Dreyer, B. E., Webb, A. C., Posillico, J. T., Stewart, A. F., Bander, N. H., Weir, E. C., Insogna, K. L. & Broadus, A. E. (1998) Identification of transcripts encoding a parathyroid hormone-like peptide in messenger RNAs from a variety of human and animal tumors associated with humoral hypercalcemia of malignancy. *J Clin. Invest.*, *81*, 2010-2014.

Izzo, V., Asaro, M. R., Forte, G. I. & Barbieri, R. (2000) Use of voltage gradient gel electrophoresis in apoptotic DNA analysis. *J. Chromatogr. A*, *890*, 371-374.

Kawashima-Ohya, Y., Satakeda, H., Kuruta, Y., Kawamoto, T., Yan, W., Akagawa, Y., Hayakawa, T., Noshiro, M., Okada, Y., Nakamura, S.. &, Kato, Y. (1999) Effects of parathyroid hormone (PTH) and PTH-related peptide on expressions of matrix metalloproteinase-2, -3, and -9 in growth plate chondrocyte cultures. *Endocrinology*, *139*, 2120-2127.

Kumari, R., Robertson, J. F. & Watson, S. A. (2006) Nuclear targeting of a midregion PTHrP fragment is necessary for stimulating growth in breast cancer cells. *Int. J. Cancer*, *119*, 49-59.

Lam, M. H., Thomas, R. J., Martin, T. J., Gillespie, M. T. & Jans, D. A. (2000) Nuclear and nucleolar localization of parathyroid hormone-related protein. *Immunol. Cell Biol.*, *78*, 395-402.

Lam, M. H., Hu, W., Xiao, C. Y., Gillespie, M. T. & Jans, D. A. (2001) Molecular dissection of the importin beta1-recognized nuclear targeting signal of parathyroid hormone-related protein. *Biochem. Biophys. Res. Commun.*, *282*, 629-634.

Leist, M. & Jaattela, M. (2001) Four deaths and a funeral: from caspases to alternative mechanisms. *Nat. Rev. Mol. Cell. Biol.*, *2*, 589-598.

Lewis, J., Devin, A., Miller, A., Lin, Y., Rodriguez, Y., Neckers, L. & Liu, Z. G. (2000) Disruption of hsp90 function results in degradation of the death domain kinase, receptor-interacting protein (RIP), and blockage of tumor necrosis factor-induced nuclear factor-kappaB activation. *J. Biol. Chem.*, *275*, 10519-10526.

Li, G., Tolstonog, G. V., Sabasch, M. & Traub, P. (2003) Type III intermediate filament proteins interact with four-way junction DNA and facilitate its cleavage by the junction-resolving enzyme T7 endonuclease I. *DNA Cell Biol.*, *22*, 261-291.

Lim, K. B., Ng, C. Y., Ong, C. K., Ong, C. S., Tran, E., Nguyen, T. T., Chan, G. M. & Huynh, H. (2001) Induction of apoptosis in mammary gland by a pure anti-estrogen ICI 182780. *Breast Cancer Res. Treat.*, *68*, 127-138.

Luparello, C., Ginty A. F., Gallagher, J. A., Pucci-Minafra, I. & Minafra, S. (1993) Transforming growth factor-β1, β2, and β3, urokinase and parathyroid hormone-related peptide expression in 8701-BC breast cancer cells and clones. *Differentiation*, *55*, 73-80.

Luparello, C., Burtis, W. J., Raue, F., Birch, M. A. & Gallagher, J. A. (1995) Parathyroid hormone-related peptide and 8701-BC breast cancer cell growth and invasion in vitro. Evidence for growth-inhibiting and invasion-promoting effect. *Mol. Cell. Endocrinol.*, *111*, 225-232.

Luparello, C., Birch, M. A., Gallagher, J. A. & Burtis, W. J. (1997) Clonal heterogeneity of the growth and invasive response of a human breast carcinoma cell line to parathyroid hormone-related peptide fragments. *Carcinogenesis*, *18*, 23-29.

Luparello, C., Schilling, T., Cirincione, R. & Pucci-Minafra, I. (1999) Extracellular matrix regulation of PTHrP and PTH/PTHrP receptor in a human breast cancer cell line. *FEBS Lett.*, *463*, 265-269.

Luparello, C. (2000) Electrophoresis of unlabeled proteins in a sequencing gel apparatus. *Biotechniques*, *28*, 36-38

Luparello, C., Santamaria, F. & Schilling, T. (2000) Regulation of PTHrP and PTH/PTHrP receptor by extracellular (Ca^{++}) and hormones in the breast cancer cell line 8701-BC. *Biol. Chem.*, *381*, 303-308.

Luparello, C., Romanotto, R., Tipa, A., Sirchia, R., Olmo, N., Lopez de Silanes, I., Turnay, J., Lizarbe, M. A. & Stewart, A. F. (2001) Mid-region parathyroid hormone-related protein inhibits growth and invasion "in vitro" and tumorigenesis "in vivo" of human breast cancer cells, *J. Bone Miner. Res.*, *16*, 2173-2181.

Luparello, C., Sirchia, R. & Pupello, D. (2003a) PTHrP (67-86) regulates the expression of stress proteins in breast cancer cells inducing modifications in urokinase-plasminogen activator and MMP-1 expression. *J. Cell Sci.*, *116*, 2421-2430.

Luparello, C., David, F., Campisi, G. & Sirchia, R. (2003b) T47-D cells and type V collagen: a model for the study of apoptotic gene expression by breast cancer cells. *Biol. Chem.*, *384*, 965-975.

Luparello, C. & Sirchia, R. (2005) Type V collagen regulates the expression of apoptotic and stress response genes by breast cancer cells. *J. Cell. Physiol.*, *202*, 411-421.

Maioli, E,. Fortino, V., Torricelli, C., Arezzini, B.. &, Gardi, C. (2002) Effect of parathyroid hormone-related protein on fibroblast proliferation and collagen metabolism in human skin. *Exp. Dermatol.*, *11*, 302-310.

Majumder, B., Wahle, K. W., Moir, S., Schofield, A., Choe, S. N., Farquharson, A., Grant, I. & Heys, S. D. (2002) Conjugated linoleic acids (CLAs) regulate the expression of key apoptotic genes in human breast cancer cells. *FASEB J.*, *16*, 1447-1449.

Meylan, E. & Tschopp, J. (2005) The RIP kinases: crucial integrators of cellular stress. *Trends Biochem. Sci.*, *30*, 151-159.

Miles, R. R., Sluka, J. P., Halladay, D. L., Santerre, R. F., Hale, L. V., Bloem, L., Patanjali, S. R., Galvin, R. J., Ma, L., Hock, J. M. & Onyia, J. E. (2002) Parathyroid hormone (hPTH 1-38) stimulates the expression of UBP41, an ubiquitin-specific protease, in bone. *J. Cell. Biochem.*, *85*, 229-242.

Ogata, M., Naito, Z., Tanaka, S., Moriyama, Y. & Asano, G. (2000) Overexpression and localization of heat shock proteins mRNA in pancreatic carcinoma. *J. Nippon Med. Sch.*, *67*, 177-185.

Orloff, J. J., Ganz, M. B., Nathanson, M. H., Moyer, M. S., Kats, Y., Mitnick, M., Behal, A., Gasalla-Herraiz, J. & Isales, C. M. (1997) A midregion parathyroid hormone-related peptide mobilizes cytosolic calcium and stimulates formation of inositol trisphosphate in a squamous carcinoma cell line. *Endocrinology*, *137*, 5376-5385.

Powell, G. J., Southby, J., Danks, J. A., Stillwell, R. G., Hayman, J. A., Henderson, M. A., Bennett, R. C. & Martin, T. J. (1991) Localization of parathyroid hormone-related protein in breast cancer metastases: increased incidence in bone compared with other sites. *Cancer Res.*, *51*, 3059-3061.

Ratcliffe, W. A. (1992) Role of parathyroid hormone-related protein in lactation. *Clin. Endocrinol. (Oxf.)*, *37*, 402-404.

Shakoori, A. R., Oberdorf, A. M., Owen, T. A., Weber, L. A., Hickey, E., Stein, J. L., Lian, J. B. & Stein, G. S. (1992) Expression of heat shock genes during differentiation of mammalian osteoblasts and promyelocytic leukemia cells. *J. Cell. Biochem.*, *48*, 277-287.

Shekhar, M. P., Pauley, R. & Heppner, G. (2003) Host microenvironment in breast cancer development: extracellular matrix-stromal cell contribution to neoplastic phenotype of epithelial cells in the breast. *Breast Cancer Res.*, *5*, 130-135.

Shen, X. & Falzon, M. (2003) Parathyroid hormone-related protein upregulates integrin expression via an intracrine pathway in PC-3 prostate cancer cells. *Regul. Pept.*, *113*, 17-29.

Shen, X., Qian, L. & Falzon, M. (2004) PTH-related protein enhances MCF-7 breast cancer cell adhesion, migration, and invasion via an intracrine pathway. *Exp. Cell Res.*, *294*, 420-433.

Sirchia, R., Priulla, M., Sciandrello, G., Caradonna, F., Barbata, G. & Luparello, C. (in press) Mid-region parathyroid hormone-related protein (PTHrP) binds chromatin of MDA-MB231 breast cancer cells and isolated oligonucleotides "in vitro". *Breast Cancer Res. Treat.*, Nov 24; [Epub ahead of print].

Sirchia, R. & Luparello, C. (2007) Mid-region PTHrP and gene expression of MDA-MB231 breast cancer cells. *Biol. Chem*, *388*, 457-465.

Soifer, N. E., Dee, K. E., Insogna, K. L., Burtis, W. J., Matovcik, L. M., Wu, T. L., Milstone, L. M., Broadus, A. E., Philbrick, W. M. & Stewart, A. F. (1992) Parathyroid hormone-related protein. Evidence for secretion of a novel mid-region fragment by three different cell types. *J. Biol. Chem.*, *267*, 18236-18243.

Sopel, M. & Lis, A. (2000) Coexpression of PTHrP and PTH/PTHrP receptor in a myoepithelial cell line derived from normal human breast. *Folia Histochem. Cytobiol.*, *38*, 65-69.

Southby, J., Kissin, M. W., Danks, J. A., Hayman, J. A., Moseley, J. M., Henderson, M. A., Bennett, R. C. & Martin, T. J. (1990) Immunohistochemical localization of parathyroid hormone-related protein in human breast cancer. *Cancer Res.*, *50*, 7710-7716.

Spencer, W. E. & Christensen, M. J. (1999) Multiplex relative RT-PCR method for verification of differential gene expression. *Biotechniques*, *27*, 1044-1046.

Stewart, A. F., Wu, .T, Burtis, W. J., Weir, E. C., Broadus, A. E. & Insogna, K. L. (1987). The relative potency of a human tumor-derived PTH-like adenylate cyclase-stimulating preparation in three bioassays. *J. Bone Miner. Res.*, *2*, 37-43.

Strid, H., Care, A., Jansson, T. & Powell, T. (2002) Parathyroid hormone-related peptide (38-94) amide stimulates ATP-dependent calcium transport in the basal plasma membrane of the human syncytiotrophoblast. *J. Endocrinol.*, *175*, 517-524.

Sugimura, M., Sagae, S., Ishioka, S., Nishioka, Y., Tsukada, K. & Kudo, R. (2004) Mechanisms of paclitaxel-induced apoptosis in an ovarian cancer cell line and its paclitaxel-resistant clone. *Oncology*, *66*, 53-61.

Sumantran,V. N., Ealovega, M. W., Nunez, G., Clarke, M. F. & Wicha, M. S. (1995) Overexpression of Bcl-XS sensitizes MCF-7 cells to chemotherapy-induced apoptosis. *Cancer Res.*, *55*, 2507-2510.

Tolstonog G. V., Wang, X., Shoeman, R. & Traub, P. (2000) Intermediate filaments reconstituted from vimentin, desmin, and glial fibrillary acidic protein selectively bind repetitive and mobile DNA sequences from a mixture of mouse genomic DNA fragments. *DNA Cell Biol. 19*, 647-677.

Torricelli, C., Fortino, V., Capurro, E., Sacchi, G., Ponzo, P., Pacini, A., Muscettola, M. & Maioli, E. (2005) Role of PTHrP and PTHrP-engaged pathways in MCF-7 cells migration/invasion. *Matrix Biol.*, *25*, 104-111.

Tovar Sepulveda, V. A., Shen, X. & Falzon, M. (2002) Intracrine PTHrP protects against serum starvation-induced apoptosis and regulates the cell cycle in MCF-7 breast cancer cells. *Endocrinology*, *143*, 596-606.

Tudor, G., Aguilera, A., Halverson, D. O., Laing, N. D. & Sausville, E. A. (2000) Susceptibility to drug-induced apoptosis correlates with differential modulation of Bad, Bcl-2 and Bcl-xL protein levels. *Cell Death Differ.*, *7*, 574-586.

Vanden Berghe, T., Kalai, M., van Loo, G., Declercq, W. & Vandenabeele, P. (2003) Disruption of HSP90 function reverts tumor necrosis factor-induced necrosis to apoptosis. *J. Biol. Chem.*, *278*, 5622-5629

Van Steensel, B., Delrow, J. & Bussemaker, H. J. (2003) Genomewide analysis of Drosophila GAGA factor target genes reveals context-dependent DNA binding. *Proc. Natl. Acad. Sci. USA*, *100*, 2580-2585.

Vargas, S. J., Gillespie, M. T., Powell, G. J., Southby, J., Danks, J. A., Moseley, J. M. & Martin, T. J. (1992) Localization of parathyroid hormone-related protein mRNA expression in breast cancer and metastatic lesions by in situ hybridization. *J. Bone Miner. Res.*, *7*, 971-979.

Wang, K. K., Posner, A. & Hajimohammadreza, I. (1996) Total protein extraction from cultured cells for use in electrophoresis and western blotting. *Biotechniques*, *20*, 662-668.

Wang, E., Marcotte, R. & Petroulakis, E. (1999) Signaling pathway for apoptosis: a racetrack for life or death. *J. Cell. Biochem.*, *Suppl 32-33*, 95-102.

Wang, Q., Tolstonog, G. V., Shoeman, R. & Traub, P. (2001) Sites of nucleic acid binding in type I-IV intermediate filament subunit proteins. *Biochemistry*, *40*, 10342-10349.

Weaver, V. M., Fischer, A. H, Peterson, O. W. & Bissell, M. J. (1996) The importance of the microenvironment in breast cancer progression: recapitulation of mammary tumorigenesis using a unique human mammary epithelial cell model and a three-dimensional culture assay. *Biochem. Cell Biol.*, *74*, 833-851.

Wu, T. L., Vasavada, R. C., Yang, K., Massfelder, T., Ganz, M., Abbas, S. K., Care, A. D., Stewart, A. F. (1996) Structural and physiologic characterization of the mid-region secretory species of parathyroid hormone-related protein. *J. Biol. Chem.*, *271*, 24372-24381.

Wysolmerski, J. J., McCaughern-Carucci, J. F., Daifotis, A. G., Broadus, A. E. & Philbrick, W. M. (1995) Overexpression of parathyroid hormone-related protein or parathyroid hormone in transgenic mice impairs branching morphogenesis during mammary gland development. *Development*, *121*, 3539-3547.

Wysolmerski, J. J., Philbrick, W. M., Dunbar, M. E., Lanske, B., Kronenberg, H. & Broadus, A. E. (1998) Rescue of the parathyroid hormone-related protein knockout mouse demonstrates that parathyroid hormone-related protein is essential for mammary gland development. *Development*, *125*, 1285-1294.

Yang, K. H., de Papp, A. E., Soifer, N. E., Dreyer, B. E., Wu, T. L., Porter, S. E., Bellantoni, M., Burtis, W. J., Insogna, K. L. & Broadus, A.E. (1994) Parathyroid hormone-related protein : evidence for isoform- and tissue-specific posttranslational processing. *Biochemistry*, *33*, 7460-7469.

Zhang, M., Guo, R., Zhai, Y. & Yang, D. (2003) LIGHT sensitizes IFNgamma-mediated apoptosis of MDA-MB-231 breast cancer cells leading to down-regulation of anti-apoptosis Bcl-2 family members. *Cancer Lett.*, *195*, 201-210.

INDEX

A

B

D

E

F

G

H

I

J

K

L

M

N

O

R

S

U

V

W

Y